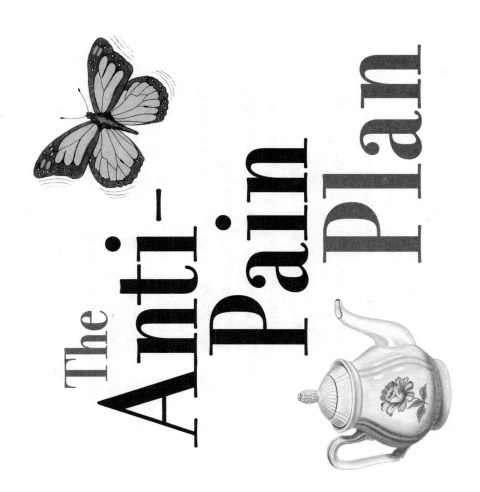

A Jerry Baker Health Book

The Anti-Pain Plan

www.jerrybaker.com

Other Jerry Baker Good Health Series books:

Jerry Baker's Homemade Health

Jerry Baker's Oddball Ointments, Powerful Potions & Fabulous Folk Remedies

Jerry Baker's Giant Book of Kitchen Counter Cures

Jerry Baker's Herbal Pharmacy

Jerry Baker's Good Gardening Series books:

Jerry Baker's Giant Book of Garden Solutions

Jerry Baker's Flower Garden Problem Solver

Jerry Baker's Perfect Perennials!

Jerry Baker's Backyard Problem Solver

Jerry Baker's Green Grass Magic

Jerry Baker's Terrific Tomatoes, Sensational Spuds, and Mouth-Watering Melons

Jerry Baker's Great Green Book of Garden Secrets

Jerry Baker's Old-Time Gardening Wisdom

Jerry Baker's Flower Power!

Jerry Baker's Good Home Series books:

Jerry Baker's Supermarket Super Products!

Jerry Baker's It Pays to Be Cheap!

Jerry Baker's Eureka! 1001 Old-Time Secrets and New-Fangled Solutions

To order any of the above, or for more information on Jerry Baker's amazing home, health, and garden tips, tricks, and tonics, please write to:

Jerry Baker, P.O. Box 1001, Wixom, MI 48393

Or visit Jerry Baker on the World Wide Web at www.jerrybaker.com

A Jerry Baker Health Book

The Anti-Pain Plan

467 No-Nonsense Ways to Avoid Arthritis, Heal a Headache, Beat a Backache, Trounce Carpal Tunnel, Relieve Sore Joints, and MORE!

Rick Chillot

Published by American Master Products, Inc./Jerry Baker
Kim Adam Gasior, Publisher

**A Jerry Baker Health Book and
a Blackberry Cottage Production**
Editorial: Ellen Michaud, Blackberry
   Cottage Productions
Design: Nest Publishing Resources
Editor: Mathew Hoffman

Book Composition: Wayne F. Michaud
Illustrator: Wayne F. Michaud
Researchers: Anita Small, Bernadette
   Sukley, Roe DeLuca Blumenthal
Copy Editor: Jane Sherman

Printed in the United States of America

Illustrations copyright © 2003 by Wayne F. Michaud

Publisher's Cataloging-in-Publication

Chillot, Rick.
  The anti-pain plan : 467 no-nonsense ways to avoid arthritis, heal a headache, beat a backache, trounce carpal tunnel, relieve sore joints, and more! / Rick Chillot.
    p. cm. — (A Jerry Baker health book)
  Includes index.
  ISBN: 0-922433-49-6
  1. Pain—Popular works.   I. Title.

RB127.C474 2003   616'.0472
                  03-200332

4 6 8 10 9 7 5 3 hardcover

Foreword

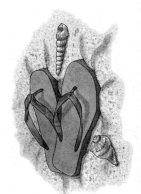

Simple pleasures are life's treasures; that's a fact. A cup of coffee with a friend, Sunday dinner with the family, or a quiet afternoon walk—those everyday, ordinary moments that we tend to take for granted in our wildly busy lives are really what's important. Unfortunately, often it isn't until something interferes with those moments that we realize how much we miss them.

That's one of the reasons why, come the first Saturday of every month, I get together with my old friend George for breakfast down at Martha's Diner here in town. We spend an easy hour or so enjoying a great meal and razzing each other about what's going on. It may not seem like much, but it's something I look forward to all month.

On our last visit, however, George just wasn't his usual self: His eyes were bloodshot and rimmed with dark circles, his skin was pale—why, he looked absolutely miserable! He looked so bad that I finally asked him what was going on. He tried to act like it was nothing, but as he sipped his cup of coffee, he finally admitted that his back was acting up again.

Like a lot of folks, George worked hard during his younger days and had suffered through his share of backaches. Over the years, he'd gotten used to them. He thought they'd go away when he eased up on his work schedule, but he was wrong. Instead, they had been getting worse, and no matter what his doctor prescribed, it just wasn't doing the trick.

Things had gotten so bad that George had had to cancel his Sunday morning fishing trip with his son. And forget about Wednesday night's bowling league—he couldn't even sleep at night, let alone lift a bowling ball! That Saturday, poor old George was in so much pain that he barely touched the food on his plate before he said goodbye and headed for home.

Well, needless to say, I left the diner with a heavy heart. I tried to forget about George by working in my garden (my favorite form of therapy), when, wouldn't you know it, my Aunt Betty dropped by. I helped her out of the car and onto the porch, then headed inside to get us some iced tea. When I handed Aunt Betty her tea, I watched in horror as she gulped down a couple of pain pills that were big enough to choke a horse! When I asked her what the heck she was taking them for, she told me that her hip just wasn't up to the trip. As a matter of fact, she added, these days her hip wasn't up to much of anything. Instead of taking her customary evening strolls, she sat for an hour on her porch. Her yard was a mess, and she couldn't even stand up in the kitchen long enough to cook dinner. On top of all that, the medication she was taking was wreaking havoc on her stomach!

Talking to George and Aunt Betty got me thinking about all of the miserable aches and pains that so many folks have to deal with, myself included. There's still nothing like a bright, sunny day to lure me outdoors, but these days, a few strenuous minutes in the spring are enough to send me and my aching knees right back inside. It seems that all those years of planting and weeding have finally caught up

Foreword

with me. What started out as a little morning stiffness every now and then has turned into a whole lot of throbbing pain. Now don't get me wrong—I wouldn't trade a minute of those thousands of happy hours I've spent working in the garden. But all this pain is ridiculous!

Finally, I said enough is enough. Between George's back, Aunt Betty's hip, and my old gardener's knees, I figured it was time to find out what could stop the pain. I asked my friend Rick Chillot to check out what pain experts have to offer besides surgery, medications, and a whole lot of misery.

Rick's a former editor at a major health magazine, and if he doesn't know what to do about something, well then, I guarantee that he knows a doctor who does! Rick spent more than a year talking to one doctor after another—more than 85 in all—finding out what works best for fast relief. What he discovered is that if you're in pain, you don't have to grin and bear it any more! There are hundreds of quick remedies and easy tricks to get rid of pain—whether it's from an aching back, a hurting hip, creaky knees, or a good, old-fashioned pain in the you-know-where!

Now, everyone knows that I can't keep a secret, and there's no way I could keep quiet about all the *amazing* remedies Rick uncovered. So we worked hard to put all those powerful pain pulverizers into this fantastic book.

When it comes to pain, we've covered just about everything—from the top of your head to the tips of your toes—in nine relief-packed sections that'll help stop the hurt in your head, arms, legs, chest, stomach, and places I don't care to discuss in front of my grandchildren. And to be complete, we didn't forget about those all-around aches such as flu, sore muscles, and tendinitis. Inside, you'll discover how to get rapid relief from more than 100 different painful ailments.

In addition to all the great remedies, we've added a bunch of terrific tips in some fabulous features. If you're looking for a tasty tea to heal your hurts, look for a "Cup of Comfort" that'll put the brakes on your aches. For the therapeutic power of massage, there's "Healing Hands" to relax you and ease your discomfort. Then there's a whole host of "Soothing Salves" to bring relief for everything from arthritis pain and headaches to muscle spasms and tender burns. Plus, there's my personal favorite—"Instant Ahhh…"— where you'll learn the quickest ways to relieve your most awful aches. You'll find all these and hundreds more no-nonsense pain busters right at your fingertips.

So, the next time you're in pain, don't just head for the medicine cabinet or decide that you simply have to grin and bear it. Instead, talk to a physician about the treasure trove of soothing solutions in this great book and let the doctor help you figure out which ones are just right for you. The hundreds of remarkable remedies inside will help you end your pain-filled misery and start enjoying life's simple pleasures again—just like George, Aunt Betty, and I did!

Contents

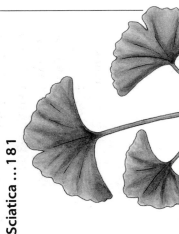

ix

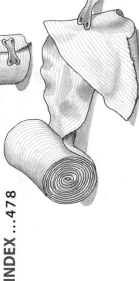

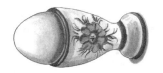

Pain in Your Head

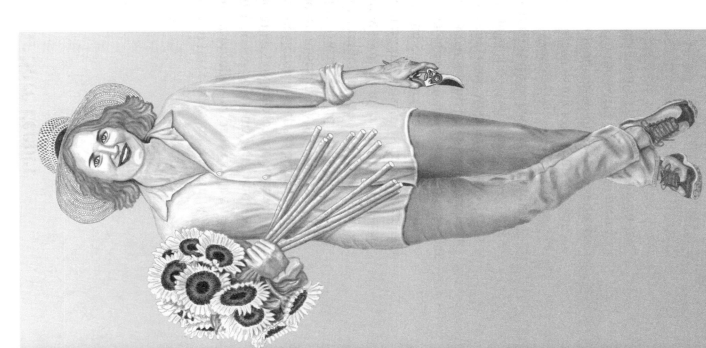

Black Eye
Burning Tongue or Mouth Syndrome
Canker Sores
Chapped Lips
Cluster Headaches
Cold Sores
Denture Pain
Earache
Eye Pain
Gum Pain
Hangover Headache
Migraine
"Moe Poke"
Neck Pain
Pierced-Ear Pain
Pizza Mouth
Sinus Headache
Sore Throat
Temporomandibular Disorder
Tension Headache
Toothache
Tooth Trauma
Trigeminal Neuralgia
Whiplash

Black Eye

Pamper Your Sore Peeper

As the youngest of three boys, my cousin Mike grew up with his fair share of bumps and bruises. One of his more notable escapades happened when my aunt and uncle were away for the day, and Mike's older brothers threw a party. At some point, a stray dog—a German shepherd the size of a mule—wandered onto the premises, and Mike was put in charge of the animal until its owners could be found.

All was going well until a rather fast car sped down their usually sleepy street. The dog took off after it, and my cousin, with the leash wrapped around his wrist, was dragged halfway down the front walk before he could let go. During his short trip, Mike clocked his head against a stone, giving him a shiner that threw his brothers into a panic. The boys knew their parents would be furious when they saw Mike's blackened eye. Worse, they would never believe a cockamamie story about a stray dog and would think the brothers had been fighting (again).

Mike's brothers had two things going for them, though. They both played high school football, so they knew how to treat hard knocks. And, thanks to the party, there was plenty of ice around. So they sat Mike in a comfy chair and kept an ice bag on his eye. By the time their folks came home, Mike was feeling a lot better, the swelling had gone down, and the injury looked a lot less traumatic. My aunt and uncle reached only about a 4 on the "angry parents' scale" instead of the 7 that had seemed imminent earlier. (There were no more parties at the house that summer, and the dog, as far as I know, was never seen again!)

SCHOOL OF HARD KNOCKS

The tissues surrounding your eyes are pretty tough, but they aren't impervious to hard knocks from balls, bats, and those everyday encounters with doors or low-hanging shelves. Bump into something hard enough, and there's a good chance that you'll be sporting a black eye for at least a week.

The term *black eye* isn't really accurate, because most shiners are more blue, purple, or even yellow. You can think of them as bad bruises. When blood vessels beneath the skin are broken, blood leaks into nearby tissues, causing swelling and a lot of tenderness. It takes a week or two for the damage to heal completely. In the meantime, chemical changes in the skin give black eyes their astonishing range of hues.

SHINER SOLUTIONS

A black eye almost always gets better on its own, but it's sometimes difficult to tell how serious the injury really is. Since shiners always look terrible, you can't go by appearance alone.

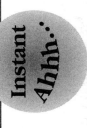

Instant Ahhh...

Terrific Tea Tannins

One of the quickest ways to soothe a black eye is with a tea bag. Black and green teas contain tannins, chemical compounds that help reduce swelling. After brewing a cup of tea, let the tea bag cool for a few minutes, then squeeze out the excess moisture. Lie back, close your eyes, and hold the tea bag against the injured area for 10 minutes or so.

So if you have vision changes—double vision, for example—after the injury, get to a doctor right away. The same goes for pain in your eyeball (as opposed to pain in the surrounding area) or bleeding in your eye. These are signs that your eye itself may be damaged, so you need to get medical help right away.

Fortunately, most black eyes involve nothing more than pain and swelling—and, of course, that ugly eggplant color. Here are a few ways to reduce those problems and help speed healing.

Ice it fast. As my cousins knew, nothing is better for a black eye than applying ice right away. Cold causes blood vessels to constrict, or narrow, which reduces internal bleeding, swelling, and those unsightly color changes, says Priscilla Natanson, N.D., a naturopathic physician in Plantation, Florida. Cold also numbs the area and helps ease the throbbing.

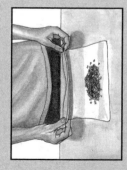

Make an ice pack by wrapping some ice cubes in a washcloth or small towel, then gently hold it against the area for 15 to 20 minutes every few hours during the 24 hours following the injury, Dr. Natanson advises.

Follow up with heat. You don't want to apply heat to a black eye right away because it may increase bleeding inside the skin. Within the 24- to 48-hour period after the injury, how-

Comfrey Compress

The herb comfrey is among the best treatments for minor wounds and bruises, and it's perfect for a black eye, says Priscilla Natanson, N.D. If you're using fresh leaves, mash them into a paste and apply it directly to the bruise. If you're using the dried form, crush the leaves between your fingers and add just enough water to moisten. Wrap the powder in a piece of cheesecloth, then hold it on the area. Apply either form of the herb for about 20 minutes twice a day. Comfrey is available at health food stores.

ever, a warm compress is just the thing. The heat promotes circulation and helps flush pain-causing substances from the area. Soak a washcloth in warm water, wring it out, and apply it for a few minutes as often as necessary to reduce discomfort.

Switch back and forth. You can also try a technique called contrast hydrotherapy, in which you alternate warm and cold compresses. It's a wonderful treatment for a black eye, says Dr. Natanson. The combination of heat and cold helps the body remove toxins from the tissues and will help your eye heal more quickly.

Start by applying a warm compress for about 3 minutes. Switch to cold for 30 seconds, then go back to heat. Repeat the process two or three times, always ending with the cold application. Use this technique three times a day until your eye is completely healed.

Load up on vitamin C. This mighty vitamin does more than relieve the sniffles. When you have a black eye, it helps strengthen and repair tiny blood vessels called capillaries. As long as you don't have stomach or kidney problems, think about trying 2,000 to 3,000 milligrams of vitamin C daily until the black eye is gone.

One problem with vitamin C, though, is that high doses can cause diarrhea or stomach upset. To avoid this, take divided doses at different times of the day. Taking it with food also helps.

Hold the aspirin. Even though it's a great remedy for pain, aspirin reduces the ability of blood to clot normally, which could result in even more bruising in the days following the injury. A better choice is acetaminophen, which has the same painkilling properties as aspirin but is less likely to cause additional bleeding or bruising.

Burning Tongue or Mouth Syndrome

Fight the Oral Flames

Imagine for a moment that your mouth, tongue, or lips feel as though they're on fire. The pain might be constant or come and go without warning. Naturally, you'd go straight to the doctor—only to be told that you're imagining everything.

What a terrible experience! Yet that's what frequently happens to people who have what's called burning tongue or mouth syndrome, or BTMS.

"We see people who've suffered for 10, 20, or even 30 years," says Joseph L. Konzelman Jr., D.D.S., a professor at the medical college of the Georgia School of Dentistry in Augusta.

If you're ever unlucky enough to develop this maddening condition, remember that you don't have to let it take over your life.

MOUTH OF FIRE

In rare cases, BTMS is caused by a readily identified problem, such as a fungal infection. Most of the time, however, its origin is a mystery. That's why doctors refer to it as a syndrome—a problem without a known cause.

What's more, pain isn't the only symptom you're likely to experience. People with BTMS sometimes complain of dry mouth; a strange, metallic taste; or even the total loss of all taste sensation.

BEAT THE HEAT

Because medical doctors are often unfamiliar with BTMS—many, in fact, have never seen a single case—you'll probably do better if you start by seeing your dentist. Dentists have more training in oral medicine than typical family doctors. The American Academy of Oral Medicine (www.aaom.com) can refer you to an expert in your area.

Do keep your doctor in the loop, though. There are several serious illnesses that can cause burning mouth symptoms, such as diabetes or diseases that affect the immune system.

The important thing is to be persistent, says Dr. Konzelman. It will take some time, but experts can nearly always solve the problem, often with a combination of home remedies and med-

---

Healing Hands

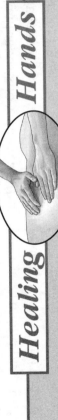

Stressed, tense, or injured muscles in your head or neck sometimes cause symptoms of burning tongue or mouth syndrome. Doctors call this curious phenomenon "referred pain," which means that a problem in one part of your body sends pain signals to a totally different part. Take the time to gently massage the muscles in your neck and scalp and apply moist heat several times a day. Once your muscles relax, you may find that the burning sensation disappears.

ications. Here are a few of the approaches you'll probably be advised to try.

Eliminate headaches. Don't be offended if your dentist says the pain is all in your head. Nearly 75 percent of people with BTMS also have headaches or facial pain, says Ira M. Klemons, D.D.S., director of the Center for Headaches and Facial Pain in South Amboy, New Jersey. "We can often solve the burning tongue syndrome by treating other symptoms," he says. So getting your headaches under control—with an over-the-counter painkiller, for example, or by practicing meditation or other stress-reduction techniques—could quench the fire in your mouth as well.

Boot the yeast beast. The common fungus known as yeast thrives in warm, humid places, and your mouth is nearly ideal. A yeast infection called oral candidiasis, or thrush, is often a side effect of antibiotics, which alter the natural balance of organisms in the body. If you notice whitish patches or sores in your mouth, see your doctor. Yeast infections are easily diagnosed by scraping a few cells from your mouth and examining them under a microscope. A few weeks of treatment with antifungal drugs will knock out the infection and return your mouth to normal.

Bone up on Bs. If you're not getting enough vitamin B_{12} in your diet, you could very well end up with BTMS, says Dr. Konzelman. Low levels of iron can cause it, too. It's easy to get more iron by eating more meat or shellfish, or your doctor may

Question the Experts

For a long time, doctors blamed burning tongue or mouth syndrome (BTMS) on psychological problems. Some doctors still believe this, but that doesn't mean that you should believe *them*. Research has clearly shown that people with BTMS are no more likely than anyone else to be depressed or have psychological problems, says Joseph L. Konzelman Jr., D.D.S.

advise you to take iron supplements.

If you're low on B$_{12}$, however, it may be time to roll up your sleeve. You may need an injection of this vitamin because oral forms are not well absorbed in your stomach, Dr. Konzelman explains.

This spice ain't nice. Cinnamon contains chemical compounds that can trigger allergic reactions in some people—reactions that may include a burning sensation, says Dr. Konzelman. Your doctor may advise you to avoid anything that contains cinnamon, from cookies and pumpkin pie to cinnamon-flavored gum or candy.

Check your medicine cabinet. It's worth making a list of all the drugs you're currently taking, prescription as well as over-the-counter, and asking your doctor if any of them may be causing your problems. Aspirin and other analgesics, along with some antibiotics and drugs used to treat diabetes or gout, may cause BTMS in some people.

Put the squeeze on toothpaste. Many popular brands contain a chemical compound called sodium laurel sulfate (SLS), a sudsing agent that can trigger a burning sensation. "Switch to products that don't contain SLS," Dr. Konzelman advises. Good choices include Biotene, Tom's of Maine, and Rembrandt SLS-Free.

Canker Sores

Purge the Pain

There's nothing like a canker to remind you just how often your mouth moves. When one of these pesky sores erupts, the slightest movement—chewing, talking, yawning, or merely shifting your tongue to the wrong place—can set off amazing amounts of pain. And should you accidentally touch the sore with a fork or a toothbrush—YEOW! You'll feel as if you'd just met the business end of an angry hornet.

ANNOYING BUT HARMLESS

Canker sores are sometimes confused with cold sores, but they're not the same. Cold sores (see page 22) usually crop up on the outside of your lips, while canker sores are tiny patches of damaged tissue that occur only inside your mouth—on your cheeks or gums or inside your lips.

No one's figured out what causes canker sores. Emotional stress seems to bring them on in some people. So can minor injuries, such as biting the inside of your cheek. There may be a food connection as well, because some people get canker sores only when they eat the "wrong" things.

SIMPLY COMPLEX

The most common type of canker is the "simple" variety. The sores may appear a few times a year, stick around for four days to a week, then disappear. Simple canker sores hurt like crazy, but they're nothing to get too worked up about. "Complex" canker sores are another story, because as soon as an old sore heals, a new one appears. Some people have to endure them for as much as 50 percent of their lives.

If you have a particularly nasty canker, or if sores keep coming back, see your doctor or dentist. You may need a prescription mouthwash to promote healing and possibly a topical anesthetic to numb the pain. Your doctor may also test for immune-system problems or nutritional deficiencies, which sometimes play a role in cankers.

Most of the time, however, you won't need special help to reduce the pain and help cankers heal more quickly. Here's what doctors advise.

Pull the triggers. "Foods that contain gluten, such as oats, wheat, rye, and barley, can trigger canker sores," says John Hibbs, N.D., a naturopathic physician and professor at Bastyr University near Seattle. Acidic foods, such as tomatoes and oranges, are also common culprits. When you get cankers, think back to what you were eating for a few days before they appeared, he advises. Giving up the

A Cup of Comfort

An herbal tea made with peppermint is a great way to calm cantankerous cankers. Put several tea bags in a saucepan, cover them with water, and simmer, covered, for about 30 minutes. Let the tea cool to room temperature, swish it around in your mouth for 30 to 60 seconds, then swallow the tea, suggests John Hibbs, N.D. Repeat the treatment several times a day until the sore is completely gone.

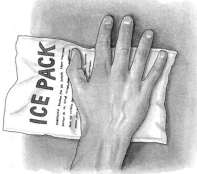

problem foods may be all it takes to eliminate the attacks.

Got milk? Swishing milk or an acid-neutralizing medicine such as Maalox liquid around in your mouth will coat the canker and protect it from acids and other irritating substances, says David A. Sirois, D.M.D., Ph.D., chair of the department of oral medicine at New York University College of Dentistry in New York City.

Ice is nice. As soon as you feel the first twinge of a canker sore, apply a small ice cube to the area. Cold temporarily numbs nerve endings and relieves pain. It also constricts, or narrows, blood vessels and reduces inflammation.

Try a dull diet. When you have cankers, the last thing you need is to scrape the insides of your lips or cheeks with hard, sharp foods. Avoid crunchy snacks such as pretzels and crackers.

Think hygiene. Brushing your teeth after every meal and flossing once or twice daily will keep your mouth clean and free of food particles that can trigger painful sores.

Don't go overboard. You don't want to use a lot of elbow grease when you brush your teeth. Scrubbing away with a hard-bristled brush is one of the quickest ways to irritate the delicate tissues inside your mouth. Dentists advise using gentle pressure when brushing your teeth

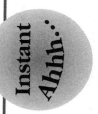

Instant Ahhh...

Mighty Mint Oil

Peppermint tea is renowned for its ability to combat canker pain, but it doesn't work right away. A faster approach is to dab a tiny amount of peppermint essential oil, which you can find at a health food store, right on the sore. The pain will disappear almost instantly—and peppermint is great for your breath, too!

and gums, especially if you already have a canker sore. Also, be sure to use a soft-bristled brush until the area heals, and be very careful not to poke the sore with the bristles.

Get some sleep. Eat well, too. Canker sores tend to erupt during times of stress, when your body's defenses are low. My fiancée, Susan, is a photographer. She used to get cankers like clockwork every winter, when clients were clamoring for their holiday portraits. She's since learned to control her stress during this busy time—and the sores have stopped making their annual visits.

Vitamins are vital. Folic acid and vitamin A, along with the mineral zinc, are especially important. Your body uses them to strengthen and maintain healthy membranes. You'll get plenty of protective nutrients just by eating a healthy diet, but a daily multivitamin is also a good idea.

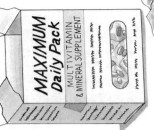

Don't forget your iron. Canker sores may be your body's way of telling you that you're low on this tissue-strengthening mineral. Iron is found in many foods, but your doctor may advise you to get a little extra to prevent iron-deficiency anemia, a condition that can lead to cankers. You may be told to take a daily iron supplement that contains 18 milligrams (the Daily Value).

Lick 'em with licorice. This sweet-tasting herbal remedy is prized for its ability to soothe inflamed tissues. As long as you don't have high blood pressure, drop by your local health food store and pick up licorice root extract, which has a molasses-like consistency. "Dab a little bit right on the sore," suggests Dr. Hibbs. Don't bother with licorice candy, however; it doesn't contain the same active ingredient.

Chapped Lips

Soothe Those Smackers

A while back, I used to wake up with chapped lips every morning during the late fall and winter. What I didn't realize was that inside air tends to be much drier in cold weather, especially in a house with oil heat. Since I'd always forget about the problem as the day went on, I never did anything about it, and I might have continued waking up dry as a mummy if I hadn't started taking guitar lessons. When I bought a new guitar, the salesperson told me that it would last much longer if I kept the wood from drying out during the cold months. So I bought a humidifier, and I found that it kept both my guitar and my lips well hydrated all winter long!

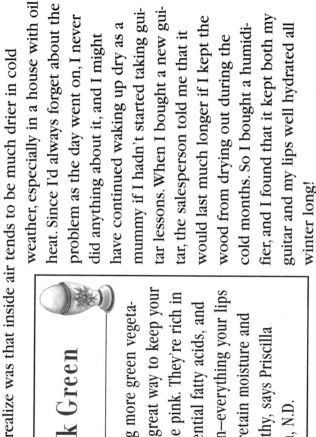

Think Green

Eating more green vegetables is a great way to keep your lips in the pink. They're rich in zinc, essential fatty acids, and riboflavin—everything your lips need to retain moisture and stay healthy, says Priscilla Natanson, N.D.

READ YOUR LIPS

Most of the time, of course, all your lips need is a good protective balm to keep them moist and shield them from sun and

Trouble from the Inside Out

Chapped lips usually indicate nothing more serious than too much exposure to sun or wind. In some cases, however, they may be signaling that something isn't right in your body. If your lips stay chapped for weeks at a time, or if they get better for a while, then get chapped again, you should probably see your doctor. "You may not be absorbing all the nutrients you need from your diet," says Priscilla Natanson, N.D.

Continually chapped lips can also be a sign of chronic stress. When you're stressed out for a long time, your adrenal glands can get out of whack and disrupt your body's sodium balance. This, in turn, can make your lips dry and chapped, no matter how much water you drink.

wind. It turns out, though, that your lips are more than just a mechanism for kissing or keeping soup from spilling out of your mouth. They're a barometer of what's going on elsewhere in your body. If you often get chapped lips, you may have to look beyond your mouth for the solutions.

MORE THAN LIP SERVICE

The skin on your lips sheds and is replaced more rapidly than other tissues, says Priscilla Natanson, N.D., a naturopathic physician in Plantation, Florida. If you aren't getting enough key nutrients in your diet, for example, the problem may start to show up on your lips before you notice other symptoms. Also, dry lips may be a signal that your body isn't retaining fluids as well as it should.

So don't think of chapped lips as just a nuisance. At the very least, a lack of proper TLC can result in deep, painful cracks that are agonizingly slow to heal. Lip balm should always be the first line of defense for parched lips, but if yours still seem rough enough to scour pots, consider these additional tips.

Bet on Bs. Chapped lips or cuts at the corners of the mouth are classic signs of a B vitamin deficiency, says John

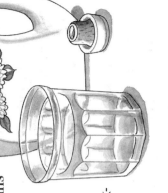

Hibbs, N.D., a naturopathic physician and professor at Bastyr University near Seattle. "B vitamins are required for cell division and reproduction," he explains. "When the tissues in the corner of the mouth are weak from lack of B vitamins, cracks or splits appear." A good multivitamin that contains all of the B vitamins should put your lips back in working order.

Refill the tank. Sometimes, chapped lips are simply a signal that your body's water tank is low. Try drinking several large glasses of water daily to give your lips the moisture they're craving.

Make your own rainforest. Okay, that's a bit of an exaggeration, but humidifying the air is a great way to keep your lips supple and healthy. It's especially important to use a humidifier during cold winter weather because indoor heat draws moisture out of the air.

Block the sun. Too much sun does more than just dry your lips; it can give them a ferocious burn, says Dr. Natanson. She recommends using a lip balm with the highest sun protection factor (SPF) that you can find. Be sure it's waterproof, and use it as often as the directions on the package recommend.

Bag the balm. "I'm not real keen on using petroleum-based products,"

Use Natural Balms

Herbal lip balms that contain marigold or calendula are better than synthetic goop from the cosmetics counter because they contain natural compounds that promote healing, says John Hibbs, N.D. Other lip-healing ingredients to look for in balms include lanolin, olive oil, and echinacea.

Instant Ahhh...

says Dr. Natanson. Rather than covering your lips with an oil slick, she recommends protective products that contain beeswax or other natural forms of oil.

Keep your tongue in cheek. If you find that your lips get severely chapped during stressful times—when visiting your in-laws at Thanksgiving, for example—you could be licking them more than usual, says Dr. Natanson. "Licking your lips actually dries them out," she says. Her advice: Chew gum or suck on lozenges when you're nervous.

Ditch the cigarettes. Need another reason to quit smoking? Smoking dries your lips and makes them more prone to chapping. And I hear it's bad for your lungs, too.

Inspect your foundation. Some people get chapped lips when they use foundation makeup or lipstick. In fact, almost any cosmetic ingredient that comes near the mouth can cause reactions in some people, says Dr. Natanson. If chapping is a frequent problem, try using different kinds of makeup until you find the brands that agree with you.

Change your mouthwash. Or try a new toothpaste. As with makeup, these products may contain ingredients that cause chapping. A simple thing like changing brands may make a big difference.

Cluster Headaches

Ease the Agony

If an ordinary headache feels like someone is whaling away at your skull with a sledgehammer, then a cluster headache is like being attacked by an entire road crew wielding picks, shovels, and jackhammers.

"Cluster headaches are terrible things," says David C. Haas, M.D., a headache specialist in the neurology department at the State University of New York Upstate Medical University in Syracuse. "People who get them are in agony."

The pain is so intense, in fact, that experts sometimes refer to clusters as suicide headaches. Some people get them throughout their lives, never knowing just when that bomb in their head is going to explode.

THE MOTHER OF ALL HEADACHES

As the name suggests, cluster headaches tend to occur in groups. You may have several headaches a day for several weeks, then none at all for months, or even years. Experts still aren't sure what causes clusters, but they suspect that the pain erupts when blood vessels in the head dilate, or expand, and press against nearby nerves.

The pain, which usually affects just one side of your head near or around your eye, peaks in 5 to 10 minutes. Most cluster headaches fade in about 45 minutes, but some have been known to last for hours. The affected eye will often droop and weep, and the nostril on that side of your face may run or be congested.

Fortunately, cluster headaches are the rarest type. Although they usually occur in men, women can get them, too.

ATTACK THE PAIN

Anyone who has cluster headaches needs to be under a doctor's care. There are a number of prescription drugs that can help prevent them, and some treatments can stop the pain, or at least ease it once it starts. But your greatest weapon against clusters is persistence: Not every drug works for every person, and you may need to try a variety of treatments before finding the one that's right for you. In the end, the odds are in your favor—but only if you get involved and manage the headaches yourself. Here's how.

Heed the 2-minute warning.
One reason that cluster headaches are difficult to control is that the pain comes on very quickly—too quickly to get to a

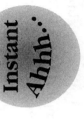

Instant
Ahhh...

Breathe Deeply

For years, doctors have treated cluster headaches by giving people pure oxygen. It causes blood vessels to constrict, or narrow, reducing painful nerve pressure. "It's a wonderful old-time cure for cluster headaches," says Seymour Diamond, M.D. Your physician may advise you to keep a portable oxygen tank at home and a smaller version in your car or in a backpack. Breathing pure oxygen will often reduce or eliminate symptoms in just a few minutes.

doctor before it starts. Once you know the warning signs, you can take medication at the earliest possible time, or at least find a quiet place to wait out the attack. Most people who get cluster headaches experience minor symptoms, such as pressure behind the eyes or a mild burning sensation on one side of the head, about 2 minutes before the attack.

Take a stab at it. Even if you hate shots, learning to use a syringe is the best strategy for halting clusters. A prescription drug called sumatriptan (Imitrex), taken at the first sign of pain, will often stop them in their tracks. "One of my patients, a policeman, always keeps a syringe with him while he's on patrol," says Dr. Haas. "If he feels a headache coming on, he gives himself an injection—and 7 minutes later, it's entirely gone."

If you're truly shot-phobic, sumatriptan is also available in tablets and as a spray, although neither works as quickly as injections.

Monitor your medications. Some of the drugs used to treat cluster headaches, such as steroids, can't be taken all the time because of side effects. But they're completely safe if you use them only when you're going through a cluster cycle, says Seymour Diamond, M.D., director of the Diamond Headache Clinic in Chicago. "You can use them for

When All Else Fails

If cluster headaches are taking over your life, and none of the usual treatments have helped, your doctor may recommend surgery. In one procedure, the trigeminal nerve—the source of most cluster pain—is cut. While surgery often works, it also has potentially serious side effects, including facial numbness. Your doctor will advise it only if you can't get relief in any other way.

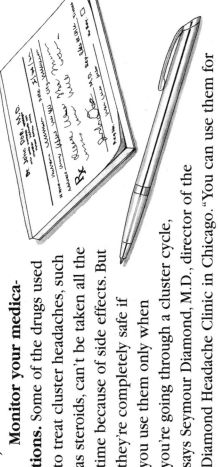

two or three months without worrying about long-term side effects," he explains.

Abandon headache triggers. If you're a dinosaur from the last century who still smokes, now's the time to quit—and ditch the alcohol as well. Both have been linked to cluster headaches, probably because they can cause blood vessels to temporarily dilate. Not only can alcohol and tobacco trigger attacks, they can also make existing headaches worse. Even if you don't give them up completely, you'll certainly want to avoid them when clusters are making their painful appearances.

Check your usual medicines. Any drug that causes blood vessels to dilate can trigger cluster attacks. Two common offenders are nitroglycerine, a drug commonly used by heart patients, and antihistamines, for allergies. If you're taking these or other drugs regularly, ask your doctor or pharmacist if they could be putting you at risk for cluster pain. If they are, ask your doctor to suggest some safe alternatives.

Prepare for "cluster season." Cluster headaches are often unpredictable, but some people have them like clockwork at certain times of the year, often in spring or fall. Try to anticipate problems by making sure that you have the medicines you need when cluster season approaches. You'll also want to adjust your schedule so the headaches don't catch you at the worst possible time—during a long-awaited trip to Hawaii, for example.

A Cup of Comfort

To make a pain-relieving tea, just buy some dried feverfew, lemon balm, and ginger at a health food store, then add 1 teaspoon of each to a cup of hot water. Steep for 10 minutes, strain out the herbs, and sip. Caution: Feverfew may cause mouth irritation in sensitive people, and since it's a uterine stimulant, pregnant women should not use it.

Cold Sores

Be a "Sore Loser"

I t's impossible to say anything good about cold sores. They're unsightly. They hurt. And, for many people, they keep coming back, year after year.

When I was in school, one of my classmates got cold sores almost like clockwork whenever midterms or finals rolled around. He used to say he was allergic to textbooks, but the real reason, I'm sure, was stress. When your life is in turmoil and your immune system is weaker than it should be, that's precisely when these painful sores are most likely to make an appearance.

THE VIRUS THAT WON'T VANISH

Despite the name, cold sores—also known as fever blisters—don't have anything to do with colds or fevers. They're caused by a virus called herpes simplex type 1. (A close relative, herpes simplex type 2, is responsible for genital sores.) Millions of Americans are infected with the virus but never get symptoms. Others aren't so lucky. The virus, which can survive in the body forever, spends most of its life in dormancy. Periodically, it "wakes up," travels up nerves to the skin, and erupts in a painful, fluid-filled blister on or near the lips. The blister goes away in about a week, but that doesn't mean the virus is gone. It's just gone back into hiding and will stay dormant until the next time conditions are right for it to reappear.

SAY SAYONARA TO SORES

Most people don't get cold sores often enough to worry much about them. If you're one of the exceptions—maybe you get sores every month, for example, or they're unusually large or painful—your doctor may write a prescription for acyclovir (Zovirax), which can shorten the duration of outbreaks if taken within a day or two after symptoms appear. There are also topical creams available, such as Abreva. Whether or not you decide to use medication, though, you'll certainly want to take steps to eliminate the sores as quickly as possible—and help keep them from coming back. Here's how.

Put licorice to work. Not licorice candy, but natural licorice root extract, sold in health food stores. It contains chemical compounds that inhibit the activity of the virus and can help cold sores heal more quickly, says John Hibbs, N.D., a naturopathic physician and professor at Bastyr University near Seattle. As soon as a cold sore appears, dab it with the molasses-like extract four to six times a day.

Apply a multiple "herpicide." You can buy cold creams that are specifically designed for people who get cold sores.

Soothing Salves

BABY THEM WITH BALM

The herb lemon balm, also known as melissa, is a traditional remedy for cold sores. In fact, anti-herpes creams sold in Europe often have lemon balm as the main ingredient. Here in the United States, you can buy lemon balm cream in health food stores. There's some evidence that when applied daily, it may help cold sores heal more quickly.

They usually contain a variety of virus-stopping ingredients, including licorice, lavender, lemon balm, marigold, vitamin E, vitamin A, or zinc.

Banish 'em with balm. The herbal balms sold in health food stores reduce cold sore pain and keep the skin moisturized as the blisters dry and crust. In addition, some balms help combat the virus directly. "Marigold and calendula balms are healing and have antiviral properties," says Dr. Hibbs.

Dab on some oil. Both lavender and St. John's wort oils, available in health food stores, inhibit the activity of herpes simplex, says Dr. Hibbs. Once or twice a day, use a cotton swab to dab a small amount of oil on the sore. Be careful not to get the oil in your mouth, though. Even in tiny amounts, these oils should not be taken internally.

V is for victory. The "V" stands for Vaseline petroleum jelly, and it's an easy way to soften the skin surrounding cold sores to prevent cracks or bleeding. Apply a generous layer of Vaseline to the area once or twice a day and

Instant Ahhh...

Ice It Early— And Often

It's often possible to stop cold sores in their tracks by applying ice at the earliest sign. Most people experience a slight tingling sensation days before cold sores erupt, and that's the time to apply an ice cube to the area. Keep it there for about 30 minutes and repeat the treatment throughout the day. "If you catch it early enough, it could abort the whole outbreak," says John Hibbs, N.D.

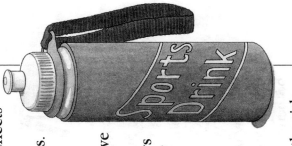

keep applying it until the cold sore is gone.

If you don't like the smell or consistency of petroleum jelly, vitamin E is a good alternative. Open a vitamin E capsule and spread the oil on the sore and the surrounding area. It's a good moisturizer, and it may also help cold sores heal more quickly.

Avoid arginine. The cold-sore virus can't thrive without an amino acid called arginine, so as soon as you feel a cold sore coming on, avoid arginine-rich foods such as chocolate.

Load up on lysine. Like arginine, lysine is a naturally occurring amino acid. Unlike arginine, it inhibits the effects of the herpes simplex virus. "Take 3,000 to 4,000 milligrams of lysine daily during outbreaks," says Dr. Hibbs.

Drown your sorrows. Even if you don't drink a lot of water most of the time, you really want to tank up when you have a cold sore. The more fluid you have in your body, the easier it is for immune cells to get where they're needed to start the healing process, says Dr. Hibbs. He recommends drinking 8 to 12 glasses of water a day until the sore is gone.

Take it easy. The virus tends to awaken during times of stress, probably because tension and anxiety make the immune system work less efficiently. It's impossible, of course, to eliminate all the stress from your life, but keeping it at manageable levels reduces the risk of getting cold sores. Even if you already have an outbreak, reducing stress can prevent one sore from triggering another.

Everyone controls stress in different ways. Daily exercise is a great stress reducer. Relaxation techniques, such as meditation and deep breathing, can help, as can setting aside time to do things you enjoy, such as going to the movies or spending time with friends.

Denture Pain

Get a Better Grip

My Uncle Frank was not someone who was embarrassed about wearing dentures: When I was a kid, he used to make us all laugh by taking them out after dinner and making funny faces. For some reason, this drove my Aunt Betty crazy. She'd yell at him to put them back in; he'd wink at us and yell back that he had to keep them out because his mouth was sore.

Now that I think about it, though, maybe Uncle Frank wasn't completely kidding when he claimed his dentures were bothering him. If that's the case, then he was smart to take them out and give his gums a chance to heal. I also hope he was smart enough to talk to his dentist and get a better fit.

Denture technology has come a long way since George Washington wore his famous artificial teeth. Today, it's almost impossible to distinguish dentures from natural teeth, at least by the way they look. Wearing them, on the other hand, does take some getting used to. If the fit isn't perfect, dentures can feel clumsy or uncomfortable. And even if they fit perfectly, they simply don't feel like real teeth. There's always an adjustment period—and the adjustment, in some cases, can be downright painful.

IT'S ALL ABOUT FIT

Your own teeth come properly fitted, and even the best dentist can't compete with Mother Nature. When you get dentures, your dentist will do everything possible to make sure that they fit properly and that the pressure on your gums is evenly distributed. For various reasons, however—changes during adjustments, for example, or even changes in your mouth—the way dentures fit can vary over time. You'll know there's a problem because you'll probably develop a sore spot somewhere along your gum line. It's similar to the blisters you get when your shoes don't fit right, and the pain increases every time the area is rubbed the wrong way.

NOTHING DENTURED, NOTHING GAINED

Denture pain is incredibly common, but that doesn't mean it's normal. Pain always means that something's wrong. If your dentures start hurting, you need to visit your dentist to have them adjusted. Otherwise, the problem will keep coming back. In the meantime, here are a few ways to reduce the pain and help the sore spots heal properly.

Stick with soft foods. New dentures are always uncomfortable at first. "In the first two months, most patients will probably need to have their den-

A Cup of Comfort

Here's a quick (and tasty) way to ease denture-related gum pain. Drop a teaspoon of dried chamomile (available at health food stores) into a cup of hot water, and steep for 10 to 20 minutes. When it's cool, take a mouthful of tea, swish it around for 30 seconds or so, and spit it out. Keep rinsing with the tea until it's all gone. You shouldn't use chamomile if you're allergic to ragweed.

tures adjusted two or three times," says David Austin, D.D.S., a dentist in Columbus, Ohio, and a member of the American Academy of Orofacial Pain. During that time, you can keep soreness to a minimum by sticking to foods that are soft and easy to chew, such as pasta or steamed vegetables.

Take 'em out. Once you get a sore spot on your gums, your best bet is to wear your dentures as little as possible until it heals. Otherwise, they will continue to irritate the area. Most sores heal completely within 10 to 14 days, although you'll probably be able to wear your dentures comfortably before then.

Gargle and spit. Antibacterial mouthwashes can help gum sores heal more quickly because they prevent bacteria from irritating the open wound. Be sure you choose a brand that's formulated to kill germs, not just freshen breath.

Load up on vitamin C. It's an essential nutrient for gum health. If your dentures have rubbed you the wrong way, take 2,000 to 3,000 milligrams of vitamin C daily to help the sore heal more quickly. Don't take this amount of C, however, if you have stomach or kidney problems. And since high doses can cause stomach upset or diarrhea in some people, take it in two or three smaller doses during the day. It also helps to take it with food.

Fix it with folic acid. This B vitamin is another nutrient that's good for the gums. Folic acid helps the body replace cells

---

It's an Emergency!

If you wear dentures, the last thing you would expect is to have a "toothache" in your lower jaw. Don't ignore it—you could be having a heart attack. "I've had two patients call me under those circumstances, and both times it turned out that they were having heart attacks," says David Austin, D.D.S. "If you wear dentures and are having what seems to be tooth pain in your lower jaw, call 911 just to be safe."

that were damaged by poorly fitting dentures. Until the sore heals, take at least 400 micrograms daily.

Increase O₂ with Q₁₀. Available in health food stores, drugstores, and supermarkets, coenzyme Q_{10} is a supplemental nutrient that promotes gum healing by increasing the amount of oxygen that's available to tissues in the mouth. Check with your doctor first, but it should be okay to take anywhere from 30 to 200 milligrams daily until the sore spots heal. Keep your mouth properly lubricated by drinking at least eight full glasses of water daily. You don't have to drink it all at once; just sip it throughout the day to keep your tissues moist.

Check the scale. Have you lost or gained weight recently? If so, you may have found the reason for your denture pain. "The gums can shrink with weight loss or swell if you gain weight," says Dr. Austin. Even small changes in the size and shape of your gums can throw your denture fit out of whack. If you aren't able to maintain a stable weight, stay in touch with your dentist, who will adjust your dentures to compensate for weight changes.

Keep them clean. Plaque and tartar, the same nasty substances that promote tooth and gum disease, can adhere to dentures just as easily as they cling to natural teeth. Once plaque and tartar build up, they can push your dentures out of alignment. "Brush your dentures at least twice a day, before you put them in and again after you take them out," Dr. Austin advises. It's a good idea to use a toothbrush that's specially made for dentures and designed to get into all the cracks and crevices.

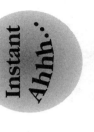

Cure It with Cloves

A traditional remedy for tooth pain is to dab on some clove oil, which you can buy at a health food store. This remedy works just as well for gum sores, and it takes effect almost instantly. Simply dip a cotton swab in the oil and apply it directly to the sore.

Instant Ahhh...

Earache

"Ear's" the Good News

I have a good friend, Luke, who has suffered from ear pain most of his life. It seems that every time he catches a cold, those pesky germs refuse to stay put in his nose. They travel into the area behind his eardrum, where they kick up a lot of irritation. Luke is normally very good-natured, but when his ears are hurting, he's not a happy camper—and he lets everyone know it, as loudly as he can! I can't say that I blame him, especially since he's only one year old.

PRESSURE AND PAIN

Adults get ear infections sometimes, but they're a lot more common in kids. And if you really want to get, well, an earful of complaints, talk to almost any parent. You'll hear a long litany of complaints about missed school days, last-minute visits to the doctor, and the difficulty of giving eardrops to pain-racked children who won't stop screaming.

I always thought that children get ear infections because their immune systems simply aren't up to the task of fighting off germs. When I talked to Emily A. Kane, N.D., a naturopathic physician in Juneau, Alaska, though, I heard a different story.

Most ear infections occur when cold germs take up residence in the eustachian tubes, the narrow passageways between the throat and eardrum. In children, the tubes are nearly horizontal, which means that it's hard for mucus to drain out. As more and more mucus accumulates, there's a rise in internal pressure, which is what makes ear infections so painful.

Ear infections gradually taper off as children get older because their heads and necks get longer, causing the eustachian tubes to assume a more vertical position. The more easily the mucus drains out, the less likely it is that infections will occur.

OPENING THE DRAIN

Ear infections are hardly ever serious, but that doesn't mean you should ignore them (as if you could!). If the infection isn't eliminated quickly (the usual treatment is antibiotic eardrops or pills), there could be scarring or other damage that can result in hearing loss. "Besides being painful, an infection in the ear can cause long-term damage to the ear's delicate mechanisms," says Dr. Kane.

As long as the pain is mild, it's okay to wait a day or two before seeing a doctor. But if the pain is severe or comes on very suddenly, go to an emergency room, Dr. Kane advises. You may be referred to an otolaryngologist, a doctor who specializes in ear problems.

In the majority of cases, ear pain is caused by simple infections, she adds. You'll almost certainly need medications, but there are also things you can do at home to reduce irritation

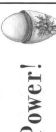

Potato Power!

The next time you have an earache, reach for a simple spud. Cut the potato in half, microwave it until it's soft, and let it cool to a comfortable temperature. Then hold the cut end against your ear for 10 to 15 minutes. The heat is very soothing, and the potato may help draw excess fluid from inside the ear. "I've tried it on kids with earaches, and though I'm not sure why, it really does work!" says Emily A. Kane, N.D.

and even eliminate the germs. Here's how to get started.

Heat things up. Gentle heat is probably the most soothing home treatment for aching ears, says John W. House, M.D., president of the House Ear Institute in Los Angeles. For adults, the easiest approach is to use a heating pad. Set it on low, cover it with a towel or pillowcase, and lie down for a while with your ear against the pad. As long as the pad doesn't get too hot, it's fine to lie there for 20 to 30 minutes, or until the pain subsides. Set a timer so you don't fall asleep.

If you don't have a heating pad, or if it's your child who's hurting, you can gently heat the ear with a hair dryer set on low. Hold the dryer at least 6 inches away from your ear, which should feel comfortably warm, but not hot, Dr. House advises. If your ear starts getting too warm, it's time to stop the treatment. To check the temperature for a child, put one hand over her ear when you turn on the dryer. Gradually move the dryer away until the airflow on the ear feels warm, but not hot.

▲ Cup of Comfort

Chicken soup is a traditional remedy for colds, and there's some evidence that it may relieve ear pain as well. Studies have shown that the soup stimulates immune cells and helps ease symptoms of infection. Try adding a few cloves of chopped garlic, which has powerful antimicrobial effects. After you cut the garlic, let it sit on your cutting board for 10 minutes before you toss it in the soup. This little "rest" allows its healing agents to form.

INSTANT HEAT microwaveable

Pop a pain reliever. Aspirin, ibuprofen, and acetaminophen aren't just for headaches. They quickly ease ear pain and also help control the fever that often accompanies infections, says Dr. House. These medications are very safe as long as you follow the directions on the label. There is one exception, however: Don't give aspirin or ibuprofen to children, because these drugs can increase the risk of Reye's syndrome, a serious neurological illness. Acetaminophen is safe for children of all ages.

Oil your ear. An oil made from mullein, a common weed, reduces inflammation and helps promote drainage from the ear canal. Available at health food stores, this oil also appears to help inhibit infection-causing cold germs. (Although mullein oil should be your first choice, you can substitute olive oil in a pinch.)

Warm the oil by putting the bottle in warm water. Test a

Healing Hands

A natural way to reduce pain-causing congestion is to massage the outer part of your ear. It helps the eustachian tubes drain normally, which reduces pressure on the eardrum, says Emily A. Kane, N.D. Simply put your index finger behind your ear and your middle finger right in front of the little triangular flap (the tragus) that covers the opening of your ear canal. Stroke with both fingers down toward the outer corner of your jaw, squeezing your fingers together as you pull. "This dislodges congestion and really promotes good drainage," says Dr. Kane.

The Swimmer's Bane

Most ear infections occur behind the eardrum, but it's also possible for the outer part of the ear canal to get infected. Doctors call this otitis externa. The more common name is swimmer's ear—and you don't have to be a swimmer to get it.

Here's what happens: Maybe you've spent an afternoon in the pool or merely lounged for a few minutes in a shower or bath. It's easy for water to flow in and out of the outer ear, but if some stays behind, it provides a warm, moist place for bacteria or fungi to set up camp. Once they start multiplying, you'll start scratching and rubbing your ear. The infections aren't serious, but they can be very uncomfortable, says John W. House, M.D.

Your doctor will probably recommend medicated eardrops to knock out the infection and relieve the itching and irritation. In the long run, a better approach is to make sure the infections never come back. Here's how.

Don't throw in the towel. Sure, you want to dry your ears drop on your skin; it should be comfortably warm, but not hot. Lie on your side with your sore ear facing up and use a dropper to let five or six drops of the oil slide into your ear canal. Hold still for 5 to 10 minutes, then roll over and let the oil drain out. Put a towel under your head to catch the oil.

Go for glycerin. Anhydrous glycerin, sold in drugstores, helps remove fluid from infected ears, says Dr. Kane, thus reducing painful pressure on the eardrum. To use it, put several drops in your ear, let it soak in for 5 to 10 minutes, then let it drain, she advises.

after swimming or bathing, but it's better to let the water evaporate naturally. Rubbing the corner of a towel or washcloth inside the ear will strip away some of the wax, the sticky substance that helps prevent infections from taking hold.

Swab no more. You may have heard a doctor say that you should never put anything smaller than your elbow in your ear. It's a humorous of way of saying that you should leave your ears alone—and that includes not scouring out the insides with cotton swabs. Using swabs to remove water or wax merely irritates your ears and makes them more vulnerable to infections. "You could wind up creating a rich area for bacteria to grow," says Dr. House.

Get the drop on moisture. One way to prevent swimmer's ear is to use eardrops that help water evaporate more quickly. You can buy them in drugstores, but it's easy to make your own by mixing equal amounts of rubbing alcohol and white vinegar.

Plug the holes. Hardly anyone wears a bathing cap any more, and earplugs are even less of a fashion accessory. You may want to ditch your style sensibilities, though, if you get frequent bouts of swimmer's ear. Wearing a cap or earplugs helps prevent water from getting inside and almost always guarantees that you won't have future problems.

Keep the channels open. Good mucus drainage is essential for preventing ear infections, especially when you have a cold or allergies. "You want to keep those passages open," says Dr. House. One solution, of course, is to take a decongestant, but the problem with these drugs is that they may cause drowsiness. A slightly messy but very effective alternative is to use a saline nasal spray, available at drugstores. Several times a day, spritz the spray into each nostril, then blow it out. It will help remove mucus before bacteria or other germs have a chance to take over.

Say sayonara to sweets. Sugary foods inhibit the body's ability to beat back infections, says Dr. Kane, so lay off the goodies until your ear is feeling better. This goes for honey and fruit juice, too.

Give the fork a rest. Going a little hungry is a great way to fight an infection, says Dr. Kane. "You want your body's resources to be oriented toward fighting the infection, not digesting food," she says. The idea isn't to go without food entirely, but just to eat a little less than you normally do until the infection is gone.

Make the dairy connection. Some people are sensitive to milk, cheese, and other dairy foods. Even a single serving may irritate mucous membranes inside the eustachian tubes, says Dr. Kane. "This creates more mucus and pressure and prevents the tubes from draining," she explains.

The next time you (or your child) get an ear infection, eliminate dairy products for a few days, she advises. There's a good chance that the pain will gradually get better.

Identify the culprits. Dairy foods are one earache trigger, but there are literally dozens of other foods, from nuts to wheat, that can stimulate pressure-causing mucus buildup. If you or others in your family get frequent infections, take the time to keep a complete diet record. You may have to do this for weeks or months, but eventually, you may find a pattern—a certain food or foods that always seem to precede the infections. Once you've made the connection, avoiding the food may be all that's needed for pain-free ears.

Eye Pain

Relief in a Blink

It was a classic case of wrong place, wrong time. One blustery day, my fiancée, Susan, stepped out of her house. About 10 seconds later, she felt a sudden, sharp pain in her right eye. Her eye turned red and filled with tears, and she could barely keep it open. Boy, were we scared!

I took her to the doctor right away. After a quick exam, he explained that she had scratched the cornea, the transparent membrane that covers the eye. A particle of dust or something else—we'll never know exactly what—had blown into her eye and scraped across the delicate membrane. It wasn't serious, but she had to wear an eye patch for a week to give the injury a chance to heal. I eventually ran out of pirate jokes, and her eye recovered just fine.

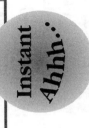

Instant Ahhh...

The Power of Positive Winking

The quickest way to ease aching eyes is to give them a few forceful blinks. Blinking spreads soothing tears over them and helps dislodge things that shouldn't be in there, says Donald Schwartz, M.D.

OPEN TO THE ELEMENTS

Eye pain is often like that. It hurts for a while, then disappears nicely. The darned thing is, though, that almost anything can cause it. That's not surprising, because your eyes are always open to the elements—and they're very sensitive. A tiny piece of dust can feel like a boulder. Even a day of staring at the computer screen can make you feel as if your eyes spent their summer vacation in the Sahara.

EASY EYE RELIEF

Dryness, overwork, and irritating particles are the main causes of eye pain. Because your eyes are so vulnerable to serious damage, though, you can never assume that everything's fine. Unless you're absolutely, positively sure that you know what's wrong, don't take any risks: Go to a doctor right away. There's a good chance that the treatment won't be any more complicated than using eyedrops to reduce irritation, although your doctor may need to do additional tests to figure out what's going on.

Most of the time, thank goodness, you can take care of eye pain easily at home. Here are a few simple tips to keep your peepers happy.

Bathe them from the inside out. Your eyes are always protected by a sheen of moisture, but if you're not drinking enough liquids, they may get dry and irritated. Drinking a few extra glasses of water a day will often solve the problem, says Donald Schwartz, M.D., associate clinical professor of ophthal-

It's an Emergency!

Never ignore sudden eye pain. It's especially important to call your doctor if you develop pain that doesn't go away within a few hours. You could have glaucoma, a group of diseases that increase pressure in the eye and can lead to blindness unless treated immediately. Glaucoma is usually painless, but one form, called angle-closure glaucoma, comes on very quickly and causes excruciating pain.

mology at the University of California, Irvine.

Soothe them from the outside in. Even if your eyes feel fine most of the year, you probably notice extra irritation in winter because the air is so dry. A humidifier can make all the difference. It's also helpful to stay out of the direct path of air blowing from heaters or fans, because it removes protective moisture.

Tear up. Tears aren't just a reaction to soap operas and IRS audits: They're designed to keep your eyes comfortably moist. Most of us produce fewer tears as we get older, and the hours we spend in front of the TV and computer screen can make our tears less effective. One easy solution is to use artificial tears. Available in drugstores, they closely resemble your eyes' natural fluids. Use the drops whenever your eyes feel itchy or irritated. "Pull open the lower lid to form a cup, then add the drop and close your eyes for a count of 10," advises Dr. Schwartz.

Flood it. When eye pain comes on suddenly, there's a good chance that something has gotten inside and is scratching the surface. "You want to flood the eye with water," says Dr.

Healing *Hands*

You instinctively rub your eyes when they're tired and overworked. It's worth doing, because a quick eye massage helps distribute the thin layer of fluid that keeps them moisturized, which tends to dry out in spots. But you don't have to rub hard; just close your eyes and apply a little pressure to your lids. You'll be *amazed* at how much better your eyes will feel!

Schwartz. Use a steady flow of water from a faucet or a pitcher and continue flushing until your eye feels better.

This is also a good technique for washing away irritating liquids, such as the jet of juice that shoots out when you're eating an orange or grapefruit.

Take the plunge. If flooding doesn't work, you'll need to use more water. Fill the sink or bathtub with body-temperature water, then submerge your head completely with your eyes open. The offending particle should float away.

Let there be dark. Irritated eyes can be intensely sensitive to sunlight. If you find yourself blinking and rubbing your eyes even in normal room light, you'll just have to spend some time in the dark—or at least dim the lights until your eye feels better.

Let there be light. Darkness helps when your eyes are hurting, but bright light will often prevent them from getting sore in the first place. Adequate illumination is especially important when you're reading, organizing your stamp collection, or doing anything else that requires close attention. Good light puts less strain on the muscles that move and focus your eyes.

Look into the distance. Do your eyes burn and itch when you've spent hours at the computer or the sewing machine? Join the crowd. Our eyes simply aren't

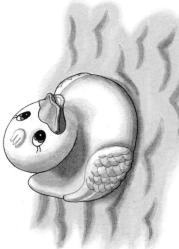

The 25¢ Solution

Eyebright is an old folk remedy for soothing achy eyes. Just add 1 teaspoon of eyebright, 1 teaspoon of fennel seeds (both available at health food stores), and a small, clean cloth to 1 cup of hot water. Steep for 10 minutes, then remove the cloth and wring it out. Drape it over your eyes as a warm compress for 20 minutes. You can repeat the treatment as often as necessary to get relief.

designed to stare at the same place for long periods of time. So at least once an hour—and preferably two or three times—take your eyes off what you're doing and look into the distance for about 5 minutes, suggests Dr. Schwartz. This reduces muscle strain and gives your eyes a chance to recover.

Monitor your monitor. If you spend a lot of time staring at a computer screen, sit at least 20 inches away, and be sure that the top of the screen is either right at or just below eye level. Improper monitor placement is a common cause of eye pain.

Relax with a compress. Covering your eyes with a warm, moist cloth is like giving them a relaxing bath. As soon as they start aching, soak a washcloth in warm water, wring it out, and drape it over your eyes. A compress works for dryness as well as for eyestrain and infections such as sties and conjunctivitis.

Don't patch up the problem. Eye patches provide valuable protection and can give an injured eye a chance to heal, but don't use one without checking with your doctor. Patches sometimes work loose and can scratch your cornea, Dr. Schwartz warns. Your doctor may recommend that you wear a special contact lens that protects your eye without blocking your vision.

Gum Pain

Get Rid of the Gunk!

I'm not one of those people who dread going to the dentist. When I was a kid, my grandmother was a receptionist at our family dentist's office, so I always thought of it as a friendly place. (The drawback, of course, was that everyone in my extended family knew about every cavity I ever had.)

I have to admit, though, that there's one aspect of dentist visits that always gives me the willies. It's the poster that shows, in full color, the horrible progression of gum disease. The first pictures show nice, healthy gums, and the last ones illustrate what happens when you don't take care of them—they look like something from *Night of the Living Dead*. Every time I see that poster, I wonder, How could anyone possibly let their gums get that bad?

GUM CONTROL

Unfortunately, gum disease can sneak up on you. The stuff that causes it, a toxin-filled, sticky film called plaque, is nearly invisible. It's produced by bacteria in your mouth, and every day, it clings to the surfaces of your teeth and underneath your gums. If you don't keep plaque under control with daily brushing and flossing, it proliferates like mold gone mad in a science experiment. Over time, chemicals and bacteria in plaque irritate your gums. If it's not stopped, your gums become red and swollen. They shrink and pull away from your teeth, and eventually, they can get so weak that your teeth loosen or fall out.

HOPE FOR GLUM GUMS

There's some good news and some bad news about gum pain. The bad news first: Once you have pain, you probably already have gum disease. If your gums bleed easily and are red and swollen, you're probably in the early stage, called gingivitis.

In a later stage, called periodontal disease or periodontitis, your gums are in really bad shape. It occurs when a long-time buildup of plaque causes chronic irritation and inflammation. Unless it's stopped, periodontitis weakens the gums and supporting bones so much that there's a risk of losing your teeth. Signs include gums that have pulled away from your teeth, discharge between your teeth and gums, or a change in the way your teeth come together when you bite. If you have any of these symptoms, go to a dentist immediately. Periodontitis allows bacteria that can inflame your heart to be dumped into your bloodstream. It can be stopped, but only if you act quickly.

Healing Hands

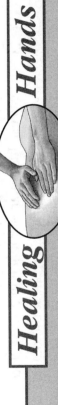

Massage is good for all sorts of aches and pains, including gum pain. It also speeds healing because it increases circulation and promotes better blood flow. Using the tip of your finger, rub your gum firmly where it hurts. Then massage all the way around your upper and lower gums. If you do this every day, your gums will feel better—and they'll heal more quickly, too!

Now, here's the good news. Gum pain caused by gingivitis is entirely reversible. All you have to do is be more diligent about flossing and brushing. Severe gum disease always requires a dentist's care, but there is no reason at all to let things go that far. If you follow these tips, you'll keep your gums in the pink—and totally free of pain.

Brush in circles. As I mentioned, regular brushing is the best way to reverse—and prevent—gum pain. But don't make the mistake of using too much elbow grease. You're not trying to sandblast the sides of a building, just break up the thin layers of plaque that may have formed. To be sure you get it all, move the brush in little circles rather than up and down, says Emily A. Kane, N.D., a naturopathic physician in Juneau, Alaska. If you've only recently started having problems, a week or two of gentle brushing is often enough to erase the pain.

Out with the old, in with the new. Don't forget to change your toothbrush a few times a year. Old brushes are often full of bacteria, which means you could actually be causing more problems. You can also clean your brush periodically. "From time to time, I soak my toothbrush in hydrogen peroxide overnight to kill bacteria," says Dr. Kane.

Make nice with ice. One of the most effective treatments for aching gums is also one of the easiest: Just wrap some ice in a washcloth or small towel and place it against the outside of your mouth for about 20 minutes. Cold acts as a local anesthetic, quickly numbing the pain.

Put water to work. Here's a nearly instant way to take away gum pain: Mix $1/2$ teaspoon of salt in a cup of warm water. Take a mouthful of the solution, swirl it around in your mouth, then spit it out. The soreness will disappear like magic, and it probably won't come back for at least an hour or two. You can repeat the saltwater rinse as often as necessary to get relief.

Pop a pill. Aspirin, ibuprofen, and other over-the-counter pain relievers work very quickly when you need relief from gum pain. Unless you're sensitive to these drugs, take one every 4 hours or as directed on the label.

The squeeze that pleases. Pressing the acupressure point for headaches, the web of skin between your index finger and thumb, is often effective for gum pain. Give the area a firm squeeze, hold it for a moment, then release. Do this several times in a row to see if it helps.

Eat some oranges. Or have a few servings of pineapple, grapefruit, or other fruits and vegetables that are rich in vitamin C. This all-purpose nutrient is essential for gum health. Eating vitamin C-rich foods will help keep your gums healthy, especially when they're recovering from gingivitis.

Fill up on folic acid. This B vitamin helps repair and replenish gum cells that have been damaged by gingivitis. The best way to get enough folic acid (the recommended amount is 400 micrograms a day) is to take a daily multivitamin. You can also get plenty of folate (the natural form of folic acid) by eating plenty of plant foods, along with folate-fortified breakfast cereals.

Say thank-Q. Talk to your doctor

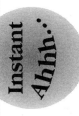

Instant Ahhh...

Clove-Oil Relief

Clove oil is a natural painkiller that works well for just about any kind of oral pain. Dip a cotton swab in the oil, which you can find at a health food store, and dab a little on the sore areas of your gums. Don't have clove oil? Open the spice rack, take out a whole clove, and tuck it between your teeth and gums. It's not as effective as the concentrated oil, but it will turn the throbbing down a notch.

about taking coenzyme Q_{10} (CoQ_{10}). This supplement increases the amount of oxygen that's available to cells inside your mouth. The extra oxygen helps gum cells grow and reproduce, and it kills gum-damaging bacteria. Until your gums are better, consider taking 30 to 200 milligrams of CoQ_{10} daily.

Try a tree tincture. Two herbal tinctures, prickly ash bark and Jamaican dogwood, are traditional favorites for reducing gum pain. Moisten a cotton ball or swab with the tincture and apply it where it hurts two or three times a day.

Use the right paste. Toothpaste with baking soda and peroxide kills the germs that cause gum disease and keep plaque from forming. It's a double whammy that prevents gum problems in the first place. So use it early, and use it often.

A Cup of Comfort

A swish of chamomile tea will bring soothing relief to sore gums. Steep a tea bag in hot water for 10 to 20 minutes, then let the tea cool. Take a mouthful, swirl it around for about 30 seconds, then swallow it or spit it out. Continue the process until you've used all the tea. Avoid using chamomile if you are allergic to ragweed.

Hangover Headache

12 Ways to Clear Your Head

I lived in a fraternity house when I was in college, and I'm embarrassed now to admit that hangovers arrived as regularly as the Sunday paper. Each guy, it seemed, had his own way of dealing with those miserable morning-after headaches. Some took a preventive approach and scarfed down an aspirin before drinking. A good friend of mine ate a handful of pistachios as soon as he woke up. One guy I knew drank his beer through a straw on the theory (wrong, I'm sure) that he'd suffer less if he took in less air while he was drinking. Me, I stayed in bed for as long as possible: I wanted to sleep through as much of the hangover as I could.

THE MORNING AFTER

Alcoholic beverages can certainly add some social lubrication to parties and nights on the town, but the cost can be a throbbing headache the next day. Alcohol causes blood vessels in the head and scalp to swell and press against nearby nerve fibers. It's also dehydrating, since it removes fluids from the membranes surrounding the brain, causing them to lose some of their "give." The result: Nerve fibers that are a little more sensitive than they should be.

HERE'S TO LESS PAIN

I'm not aware that anyone's ever had to see a doctor for relief from hangover headaches. The pain usually fades by the end of the day, even if you do nothing more than complain and look miserable. But why suffer any longer than you have to?

Sure, responsible drinking is the obvious solution, but it's easy to make mistakes from time to time. Here are a few ways to take the edge off those happy-hour headaches. Unlike the cockamamie schemes of my frat brothers, these methods actually work.

Pace yourself. "You should spread your drinks out over time," says Frederick Freitag, D.O., associate director of the Diamond Headache Clinic in Chicago. "The faster you drink, the worse your hangover will be."

For most people, one drink an hour is the upper limit. If you drink more than that, you're pushing your luck.

It's a clear choice. Clear alcoholic beverages, such as white wine, champagne, and vodka, tend to cause fewer hang-

A Cup of Comfort

One of the best ways to nurse a hangover headache is to sip some soup. Soups help soothe a queasy stomach, and they replace the fluids and minerals that you lost on your night on the town. If your stomach's feeling particularly uneasy, stick with thin soup, such as beef or chicken bouillon. If you're up to it, eating soup with vegetables or meat will give your body the energy it needs to make a more speedy recovery.

The Sweet Solution

Fructose, the kind of sugar that's found in all types of fruit, helps your body process alcohol and can reduce the likelihood of a hangover. It doesn't take much to do the trick, so after a night of drinking, you can munch on any fruit you like. You can also sip a glass of fruit juice, but choose a brand without added sugar. Tomato juice is also rich in fructose. And don't overlook honey, which is probably nature's richest source of fructose. Eat some on a cracker before bed, and you may wake up feeling fine.

over headaches than dark-colored drinks. This doesn't mean that you can down them with impunity, but your overall risk of waking up with a pounding head is lower if you stick to drinks you can see through. Even dark beers are more likely than light ones to provoke a hangover.

If you're a wine drinker, take note: Red wine contains tyramine, a chemical that appears to cause headaches in some people, so drinking in moderation is advisable.

Take B before bed. If you feel that you've overindulged, you can derail the next day's headache by taking vitamin B_6, or at least a B-complex supplement, either before going to bed or first thing in the morning. B vitamins appear to help your body cope with too much alcohol. You need about 50 milligrams of vitamin B_6, says Dr. Freitag.

Get moving. I used to try to sleep my way through hangovers, thinking that this would give my body more time to process the alcohol while I was oblivious to the symptoms. As it turns out, I was wrong. "It's better to get up and get moving," says Dr. Freitag. "You may exacerbate the headache by staying in bed too long."

Eat fatty foods. They aren't good for your cholesterol

level, but they can protect your head when you're drinking. Alcohol enters your system more slowly when you have food in your stomach. Fatty foods are particularly good at delaying the absorption of alcohol, so have some milk or indulge in those cheesy snacks.

Ice it. Applying an ice pack is a simple and effective way to numb the pain of a stubborn hangover headache. Cold blocks pain sensations and encourages swollen blood vessels to shrink. Keep the ice in place for 20 minutes or so, remove it for 20 minutes, then apply it again until you're feeling better.

Pop a pain reliever. Sometimes, all a hangover headache needs is an over-the-counter analgesic. As long as you're not sensitive to it, take two aspirins every 4 hours throughout the day. "Or take 600 milligrams of ibuprofen or naproxen (Aleve)," advises Dr. Freitag.

Get Gatorade. Quaffing a sports drink such as Gatorade can speed your recovery when your head is pounding. It will replace depleted levels of fluids and electrolytes and help bring your blood sugar back to normal.

Beware of the dog. I knew plenty of people in college who were convinced that the best treatment for a hangover was to drink some more. But taking a little "hair of the dog" is a terrible idea, says Dr. Freitag. "That's about the worst advice I can think of." Adding more alcohol to your system is likely to make you more dehydrated and exacerbate your headache.

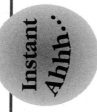

Instant Ahhh...

Quaff Caffeine

Ever wonder why coffee tastes so good when you're contending with a hangover headache? The caffeine in coffee is a vasoconstrictor: It shrinks the alcohol-swollen blood vessels that contribute to headache pain. You'll get all the caffeine you need from a cup of coffee or other caffeinated beverage, so don't drink more than one cup. Since caffeine is a diuretic, too much can make you dehydrated and increase your discomfort.

Pain in Your Head

Migraine

Ease the Anguish

At the company where I used to work, I shared an office with a woman named Peg, and you couldn't ask for a better friend. Lively and engaging, Peg could talk about anything, and her dry wit and clever observations always made me laugh. (She laughed at my jokes, too, which is just as important!) But there were times when Peg's smile just plain disappeared. I knew that those were days when she was struggling with migraines.

The sad thing is that Peg had to plan her entire life around her migraines. She loved getting together with family and friends, but for a long time, she had to limit her activities because she felt too lousy to leave the house. Her story has a happy ending, but before I tell you about it, let's take a look at what migraines are all about.

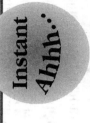

Instant Ahhh...

Ice Is Nice

One of the quickest ways to reduce throbbing migraine pain is to put a cold pack against the part of your head that hurts. Keep it in place for about 10 minutes. Cold shrinks blood vessels and helps reduce the pounding.

POUNDING PRESSURE

About 26 million Americans get migraines, and women are more prone than men to these miserable skull busters. As Peg could attest, it's almost impossible to exaggerate how awful migraines—which are to ordinary headaches what hurricanes are to gentle breezes—can make you feel.

Unlike garden-variety headaches, which are often caused by muscle tension, migraines occur when blood vessels in your scalp dilate, or expand, and press against nearby nerves. Intense, throbbing pain is just one part of the picture. Many people are so nauseated during migraine attacks that they can't leave the bathroom. They may experience "auras"—sparkling flashes of light or zigzag lines in their field of vision. They may also have weakness or tingling in their face or other parts of their body. It's common for migraines to persist for hours—and sometimes even days.

MANAGING MIGRAINES

It's generally fine to take ibuprofen at the first sign of a migraine. Over-the-counter treatments are surprisingly effective as long as you take them before the migraine really gets under way. But if the pain doesn't retreat fairly quickly, you'll want to see your doctor. This is especially true if you've had a recent head injury, if the pain occurs on both sides of your head, or if it's accompanied by difficulty speaking or mental confusion. Migraines can be a symptom of serious

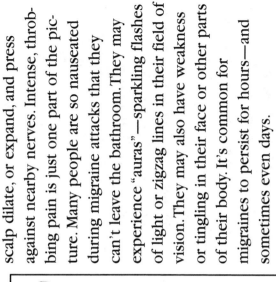

Ginger: It's a Snap

Here's a time-tested kitchen cure for coping with migraines: Spice up your diet with ginger. This pungent root appears to help keep blood vessels from dilating and pressing against sensitive nerves, says Terri Dallas-Prunskis, M.D., codirector of the Illinois Pain Treatment Institute in Chicago. Even small amounts of ginger seem to be effective, she adds. You can start by adding fresh or powdered ginger to stews, rice dishes, soups, and even fresh green salads.

underlying problems, such as brain tumors or blood vessel damage.

Even if you have only "simple" migraines, you should talk to your doctor at some point. There are a number of prescription drugs that can stop migraines within minutes, and there are other treatments that can help keep them from recurring. Most people with migraines, however, don't depend entirely on high-tech strategies. There are plenty of effective home-care approaches that can reduce your need for high-powered medications.

Try some herbal helpers. "Ginkgo, feverfew, and coleus are among my first approaches to treating migraines," says Chris Meletis, N.D., chief medical officer of the National College of Naturopathic Medicine in Portland, Oregon.

Ginkgo "thins" the blood and may inhibit the release of pain-causing chemicals. Take 60 milligrams in capsule form twice daily to relieve your pain. It's also good for preventing migraines, so you may want to take it daily to avert attacks.

Feverfew appears to inhibit the release of chemicals that cause blood vessels to dilate. It's used primarily to prevent migraines, but it can also help ease the pain once they're under way. The usual dose

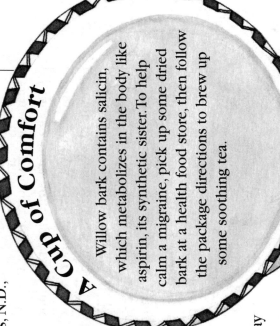

A Cup of Comfort

Willow bark contains salicin, which metabolizes in the body like aspirin, its synthetic sister. To help calm a migraine, pick up some dried bark at a health food store, then follow the package directions to brew up some soothing tea.

is 80 to 100 milligrams daily, usually in capsules.

The herb coleus lowers blood pressure and may help reduce blood vessel spasms that cause migraines. Talk to your doctor about taking 50 to 100 milligrams two or three times daily when migraine pain is flaring.

All three herbs are available at health food stores; you can find ginkgo and feverfew at drugstores and many supermarkets as well.

Don't fight the pain. Lie down immediately in a cool, dark place when you feel a migraine coming on. Moving around will only make the pain worse.

Pull the triggers. Most migraines are triggered by external factors. Everyone's different, so you'll have to be a bit of a detective to identify the things that tend to bring them on. "Many people have more than one trigger," adds Seymour Diamond, M.D., director of the Diamond Headache Clinic in Chicago. Common triggers include bright lights, changes in altitude, and even certain odors. Pay close attention to your environment when you feel a migraine beginning, suggests Dr. Diamond. Over time, you'll start to identify patterns, activities, or specific things that seem to bring them on.

Get plenty of exercise. Physical activity won't help once a migraine has started, but it's a very effective preventive strategy. Aerobic exercise—bicycling, jogging, or swimming, for example—seems to be the most effective, possibly because it helps maintain healthy circulation. Try to get at least 30 minutes of aerobic exercise most days of the week.

Pay attention to your diet. Foods are among the main migraine triggers. Chocolate, red wine, and aged cheeses, for example, contain a chemical called tyramine, which triggers

54   Pain in Your Head

blood vessel changes that can lead to migraines. All forms of alcohol may cause problems, as may smoked, cured, or fermented foods.

Keep to a schedule. Try to go to bed and get up at the same times every day. You may even want to eat and exercise at regular times. "Keeping a regular schedule is best for most people with migraines," says David C. Haas, M.D., a headache specialist in the department of neurology at the State University of New York Upstate Medical University in Syracuse.

"Being overtired can trigger migraines," he adds. "So can being hungry because you skipped a meal."

Dodge the rebound. A paradoxical thing about migraines is that the same treatments that make you feel better can also make things worse. If you take a lot of aspirin or other medication to control migraines, the pain may come back, or rebound, even more severely as soon as the medication wears off. The natural response is to take more medication, and the cycle continues.

That's exactly what happened with my friend Peg. When her doctor explained that she might be suffering from rebound headaches, she backed off from medication and started using nondrug approaches. Much to her surprise, her migraines became less and less frequent.

Obviously, you shouldn't stop taking a prescription drug without checking with your doctor first. But don't automatically reach for the aspirin or ibuprofen the next time you feel a migraine coming on. You may make things worse in the long run.

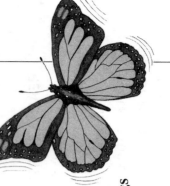

"Moe Poke"

Soothing Tips for a Sock in the Eye

When I was a kid, Saturday afternoons in front of the TV were special times because my friends and I were devoted to the antics of three classic performers. I'm talking, of course, about the Three Stooges. There was something about the spectacle of three grown men knocking each other around with slaps, shoves, and the occasional pipe wrench that we found uproariously funny. Best of all was the signature "Moe poke." Nothing stopped Larry and Curly (and later, Shemp) in their tracks like Moe's two-fingered jab to the eyes (punctuated by appropriate sound effects).

REALITY HURTS

The Three Stooges were practiced vaudevillians who knew how to pull off their stunts without injuring anyone. When real life hands you a Moe poke, though, it hurts. If you've ever taken a sock in the eye—from an accidental elbow shot during a soccer game, say, or from a toy hurled by your mischievous toddler—you probably still remember the sudden pain and dizziness that almost knocked you over.

THE EYES HAVE IT

Your eyes are delicate, and any sudden impact can do a lot of damage. Even if you think your eye is fine, there could be bleeding under the surface, so don't take any chances. Have it checked by a doctor right away. In the meantime, here are a few ways to take away the pain and help the injury heal more quickly.

Head for the shade. Any sharp blow to the eye will probably make it sensitive to light. Even normal indoor light can trigger torrents of tears, along with painful muscle spasms. One of the best things you can do is lie down in the dark for a while. If light still makes you uncomfortable when you get up, give your doctor a call. You could have iritis, a condition in which the iris (the colored part of the eye) becomes inflamed.

Pop the right pill. Aspirin and ibuprofen are great for all sorts of injuries, but not when you've been popped in the eye. Both of these drugs reduce the ability of blood to clot, which can be a real problem if there's bleeding inside your eye. A better choice for eye injuries is acetaminophen, the active ingredient in over-the-counter painkillers such as Tylenol, says Donald Schwartz, M.D., associate clinical professor of ophthalmology at the University of California, Irvine.

Put it on ice. As soon as possible after a Moe poke, wrap some ice cubes in a washcloth or small towel and hold them against your eye for a while. Cold causes blood ves-

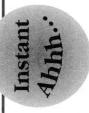

Instant Ahhh...

The Jolly Green Solution

Applying ice to an eye injury is probably the quickest way to stop the pain, but what if someone forgot to fill the ice cube trays again? Reach into the freezer and pull out a bag of frozen peas or corn. The bag will mold itself perfectly to the contour of your eye, putting the cold right where you need it.

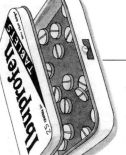

"Moe Poke"

sels to constrict, or narrow, which will help reduce swelling and irritation. Apply the ice for 15 to 20 minutes every 2 hours for the next 12 to 24 hours.

Start a warming trend. A day or two after using ice, switch to heat by applying a towel moistened with warm water, for example, or a heating pad swaddled in a soft towel. Heat will soothe the injured area and boost circulation, which will help your eye heal more quickly.

Run hot and cold. For particularly bad blows, a technique called contrast hydrotherapy can be extremely helpful. The idea is to alternate hot and cold compresses on your eye, which increases circulation, aids the removal of toxins, and decreases the swelling.

Here's how to do it. Apply a hot compress—a towel soaked in warm water works fine—for 3 minutes. Switch to a cold compress for 30 seconds, repeat the heat treatment, then switch back to cold. Repeat the cycle four or five times a day, always ending with the cold compress. "Keep doing it for 7 to 10 days," advises John Nowicki, N.D., a naturopathic physician in Issaquah, Washington. "That should be plenty of time for the injury to heal."

Incidentally, don't use the microwave to heat the towel. Microwaves often cause "hot spots," and you could end up with a nasty burn instead of a soothing cure.

Energize with enzymes. Available at health food stores and from physicians who practice complementary medicine,

It's an Emergency!

You can treat most minor eye injuries at home, but some pokes need immediate attention. If you see imaginary flashing lights or "floaters" or you've lost some of your side vision, go to an emergency room. The inner parts of your eye could be seriously damaged, and you may have a concussion, says Donald Schwartz, M.D. "These are big warning signs that there's a serious problem," he says. Don't ignore them!

HOT
COLD

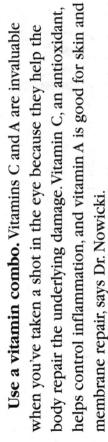

enzymes such as bromelain, papain, trypsin, and chymotrypsin can dramatically decrease swelling and speed healing, especially if you take them soon after the injury.

"Some studies show that they can cut healing time in half," explains Dr. Nowicki. It's fine to take a single enzyme or combine several different kinds. The usual dose is one to three capsules three times daily for 5 to 10 days. Don't take them with food, however, as the increase in digestive activity when you eat will make the enzymes less effective.

Use a vitamin combo. Vitamins C and A are invaluable when you've taken a shot in the eye because they help the body repair the underlying damage. Vitamin C, an antioxidant, helps control inflammation, and vitamin A is good for skin and membrane repair, says Dr. Nowicki.

As long as you don't have stomach or kidney problems, take 4,000 to 6,000 milligrams of vitamin C for a couple of days.

That's a lot more than the recommended daily amount, so it's a good idea to divide it into several doses throughout the day to help prevent diarrhea or stomach upset. It also helps to take your vitamin C with food.

There's nothing wrong with taking the small amounts of vitamin A found in a multivitamin, but you'll get better results with vitamin A eyedrops, which are available from most doctors.

Brighten up with eyebright. As the name suggests, this herbal remedy is believed to promote healthy eyes and vision. It reduces inflammation and has astringent properties, which means that it helps stabilize and support blood vessels in the eye, says Dr. Nowicki. Just follow the package directions.

Neck Pain

Be Nice to Your Neck

My friend Susan is really prone to neck problems, especially on long trips. She loves visiting her young nephew, Zach, but she doesn't like what the 2-hour car trip does to her neck. By the time she gets home, her muscles are so stiff and achy that she can barely hold her head up. I usually give her a quick massage, and I'm always amazed by how rigid her neck muscles are.

It's not a coincidence that we use the expression "a pain in the neck" for things that really bug us. Apart from the fact that neck pain really hurts, it also has a way of sticking around. Almost everything we do—driving, working on the computer, even rolling over in bed—affects the neck to some extent. And when the pain flares

Soothing Salves

THE CALENDULA CURE

When things get to be a pain in the neck, reach for a jar of calendula cream, available in health food stores and some drugstores. Just rub 1/2 teaspoon into the skin where it aches, then lie flat with a rolled-up towel under your neck. You'll be up and at 'em in 15 minutes.

up, it seems impossible to find a position that doesn't make it worse.

PAIN UNDER THE COLLAR

Most neck pain occurs when your muscles are overworked. This often happens when you've been holding your head in the same position for too long—while riding in the car, for example, or working on an overdue report. Neck pain can also be caused by sharp, sudden movements, such as your head lurching forward when you slam on the brakes. In either case, the pain means that the muscles are strained or inflamed. Sometimes, they lock up in agonizing spasms—and when that happens, you'll know it!

NO MO' NECK PAIN

When you think about how often you move your head, it's almost surprising that neck pain isn't more common. It's almost always caused by normal strains, and it's pretty easy to help the muscles relax and loosen up a bit.

The obvious exception is if you've had an accident of some kind—you've been in a car crash, for example, or taken a hard fall. Neck pain that flares up after a traumatic injury must be treated by a doctor, especially if you have symptoms such as weakness or tingling in one or both arms. These are signs of possible nerve damage, and you'll need professional help to make sure things don't get worse.

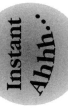

Instant Ahhh...

Unburden Your Shoulders

A lot of neck pain actually originates in the shoulders and upper back, says Dennis Dowling, D.O. One of the best ways to relieve it is to give your shoulders a relaxing workout. Here's a move you can do in a hurry: Put your right arm across your chest and grip your right elbow with your left hand. Slowly pull your elbow toward the left side of your body. Hold the stretch for a moment, relax, then repeat with your other arm.

Healing Hands

What's the best way to massage an aching neck? "If you just do what feels good, it will be helpful," says Sean Sapunar, N.D., a naturopathic physician and clinical faculty member at the Bastyr Center for Natural Health near Seattle. At the same time, good technique is important.

Press just hard enough. "You want to press hard enough so that the muscles relax, but not so hard that they hurt," says Dr. Sapunar. Close communication with your massage partner will help find the right touch.

Go easy at first. Be a little cautious if you've recently hurt your neck, because the injury is still vulnerable and prone to additional damage. Pressing a sore muscle too hard, for example, can delay healing time.

Move to the center. When giving a massage, always rub toward the center of the body. This helps push harmful muscle by-products, such as lactic acid, out of the sore area and back into circulation.

Rub across the muscle fibers. It's fine to massage muscles with the "grain," but going sideways across the fibers will help break up adhesions, or scar tissue, that may be forming between muscle groups.

Press and hold. When your neck's in spasm, apply firm pressure directly to the affected muscles. Keep up the pressure for a full minute, then relax. This will sometimes help stubborn muscles loosen up.

Practice strain/counterstrain. This is a massage technique in which you press against a tight muscle while at the same time flexing the muscle against the pressure.

STRETCHING

If your only symptom is sore muscles, though, you can easily take things into your own hands. Here's what the experts recommend.

Stretch that neck. A bit of a stretch can coax tense neck muscles into relaxing, says Dennis Dowling, D.O., chairman of the department of osteopathic and manipulative medicine at the New York College of Osteopathic Medicine in Old Westbury. "The stretching should be gentle enough that you can feel the muscles stretching, but it doesn't increase the pain," he says.

1. Start by slowly bending your neck forward and lowering your chin toward your chest.

2. Push gently on the back of your head with your hand to increase the stretch a bit.

3. Gently bend your neck backward while pushing lightly on your forehead.

4. Turn your head slowly to the right, then to the left.

5. Bend your neck sideways, lowering your right ear toward your right shoulder, then your left ear toward your left shoulder.

Do this series of stretches a few times a day until your neck is better, Dr. Dowling advises. Just be sure that you always move your head in a straight line, he adds. You don't want to twist your neck, which could make the pain worse.

Ice up. Applying a cold pack or ice cubes wrapped in a washcloth or small towel is a great way to numb neck pain. At the same time, it will reduce any inflammation, which makes the soreness worse. Apply cold for about 20 minutes every few hours until your neck feels better. Another good method is to hold a bag of frozen peas or corn against your neck. In some ways, this is actually the best approach because the bag will conform to the shape of your neck.

Do a pillow check. Does your neck hurt first thing in the morning? You may have a problem pillow that's not providing adequate support. Most people do better when they use a firm pillow that keeps their head and neck in proper alignment while they sleep. But you'll have to experiment: A pillow that provides good support for someone else may not necessarily be right for you.

Sleep on your side. People who sleep on their backs sometimes get neck pain because this position doesn't always provide enough neck support. You'll probably do better (and feel better) if you sleep on your side.

Rearrange your desk. If you spend a lot of time sitting at a desk, be sure you can reach everything you need without having to contort your neck and shoulders. Keep your computer monitor positioned so you can read it without bending your neck. If you're on the phone a lot, use a headset rather than holding the receiver in the crook of your shoulder.

Take a break. Or take several. "We have a tendency to work on things until they're done, no matter how long it takes, so we're doomed to hurt ourselves," says Dr. Dowling. As a general rule, you don't want to hold your neck in the same position for more than about 20 minutes at a time. When you're working, make it a point to take several breaks—by getting up and walking around, for example, or at least by swiveling your neck a few times each hour. (Set an egg timer so you don't forget.) On long car trips, pull over occasionally to stretch and enjoy the sights. You'll be glad you did.

Pierced-Ear Pain

Alleviate Sore Lobes

Just about every woman I know can remember when she got her ears pierced. It's almost like a rite of passage. A group of friends gathers in a dorm room. Someone sterilizes a needle, someone else grabs an ice cube, and a supportive pal holds the lucky girl's hands. And then—argh! The pain! The tears! The pretty earring!

You can think of pierced ears as proof of the body's wonderful ability to heal itself. Soon after your earlobe is pierced, it copes with the challenge of an embedded foreign object by forming scar tissue. This tough tissue envelops the earring post and prevents it from coming in contact with the soft tissue that surrounds it. As long as the soft tissue is protected, there's unlikely to be pain or infection.

When I talked to Avrim Eden, M.D., of the Ear Specialty Group of

Stick to the Lobe

It's been trendy in recent years to have piercings in the stiff cartilage of the ear. Here's some advice: Don't do it. "You can get very serious infections," says Avrim Eden, M.D. The only truly safe place to have your ears pierced is in the fleshy lobes.

Springfield, New Jersey, I was sure he'd have stern warnings about pierced ears. At the very least, I thought he'd warn about the risk of infection. To my surprise, he assured me that there's nothing particularly unhealthy about pierced ears. "It's just a cosmetic change," he says.

THE HOLE STORY

Millions, if not billions, of men and women have their ears pierced, and most never have any serious complications. But pierced ears are also like kids who have gone away to college: You only hear from them when there's some sort of problem. If you're experiencing any kind of pain, something is almost certainly wrong.

EARLY WARNING SIGNS

Ear piercings are most likely to cause pain when they're still fresh and vulnerable to infection. A little crusting is normal during the healing process, but if you've recently had your ears pierced and you notice pain, swelling, or yellowish discharge, you can be pretty sure that you're getting an infection.

Most infections start about three days after the piercing. It takes at least that long for infection-causing germs to get down to business. Although established piercings rarely become infected, it's not unheard of. Minor infections sometimes disappear on their own, but symptoms that persist for a week or more probably mean that you're going to need antibiotics.

Another potential problem is choosing the wrong types of

Dangerous Dangles

Those large, dangly earrings are beautiful, but they're notorious for catching on things and tearing loose. If that happens, remove the earring (assuming it didn't pull all the way out) and press your earlobe with gauze or tissue to stop the bleeding. Clean the area thoroughly, then get to a doctor. You may need antibiotics or even stitches to prevent infection and allow the lobe to heal properly.

earrings—and not only because they may clash with your nose ring. The body reacts in different ways to different types of metals, so you have to choose wisely. To ensure that piercings are problem-free, lend your ears to the following advice.

Keep it cold. Many ear-piercing services use a topical anesthetic to numb the pain during the procedure. You can get the same effect afterward by rubbing an ice cube on and near the piercing site.

Keep 'em clean. The best way to protect yourself while your piercings are healing—or to prevent a minor infection from getting worse—is to eliminate any bacteria that may be loitering nearby. "Clean your ear thoroughly with soap and water," Dr. Eden says. Be sure to dry it completely when you're done, since bacteria can't thrive in a dry environment.

It's also important to include your new earrings in your daily hygiene routine. "Use a little alcohol to clean the earrings that came with the piercing," says Dr. Eden.

Scrub your hands. Doctors always advise people not to touch the area of a recent piercing, and everyone routinely ignores this advice. The least you can do is thoroughly wash your hands before touching your earlobes.

Cream those germs. Over-the-counter antibiotic creams

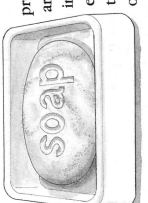

A Cup of Comfort

As soon as you notice signs of infection, start drinking echinacea tea. Studies show that it strengthens your immune system and makes it better able to fend off infection. Health food stores sell herbal tea bags, or you can use the dried herb. Add about a teaspoon of the herb to a cup of freshly boiled water, steep for about 10 minutes, then strain and drink.

and ointment are very effective at killing bacteria on your earlobes. If you have any kind of pain after a piercing, apply some at least two or three times a day. Many ear-piercing services will send you home with a small tube of antibiotic cream.

Go the herbal route. Tincture of St. John's wort, available in health food stores, is great for healing damaged skin because it quickly kills surface bacteria. Tinctures are alcohol-based, so you may feel a little stinging when you use this remedy. It doesn't last long, however, and the tincture will help keep the area problem-free.

Leave 'em in. Do you find that it hurts to put your earrings in when you haven't worn them for a while? Chances are the piercings have partially closed, and you're forcing the earrings through new skin. Apart from being painful, this can create all sorts of problems. "Forcing an earring may tear the skin and cause an infection," warns Dr. Eden. While your piercings are still healing, it's important to keep the holes open all the time. If you aren't in the mood to wear earrings, use small studs or "sleepers."

Lighten up. If you find that your earlobes ache at the end of the day, you may be wearing earrings that are too heavy. Here's an easy test: In the morning, put your usual earring in one ear. At the end of the day, compare how your ears feel. If the ear with the earring hurts or you notice that the earring has stretched the opening into an elongated or oval shape, you can bet that it's too heavy. Switching to lighter earrings may be all it takes to ease the pain.

Buyer beware. Inexpensive earrings often contain nickel, a lightweight metal that's a common cause of allergic reactions. If you notice that your piercings are persistently itchy or painful, or the surrounding skin is scaly and red, there's a good chance that you have a nickel allergy. Switch to earrings with posts made of gold (18 karat or higher) or surgical stainless steel, suggests Dr. Eden.

Pizza Mouth

Soothe a "Slice Attack"

There was a fantastic pizzeria just a few blocks from the house where I grew up, and my family did their best to keep it in business. Someone forgot to buy chicken for supper? "Let's have pizza!" The meat loaf will take an hour to cook? "Let's have pizza!" It looks like it might rain? "Let's have pizza!"

Since the restaurant was almost within shouting distance, we could count on the pizza being nice and hot when we got it home. One of my favorite memories is opening the box, leaning over, and bathing my face in that hot pizza steam. The pizza was so hot, in fact, that it posed something of a dilemma. I could barely restrain myself from diving right in, but I also knew the painful consequences of burning the roof of my mouth with all that hot, melted cheese. Sometimes, I did the smart thing and waited until the pizza cooled. More often than not, though, hunger won out—and my poor mouth paid the price for days!

PURE PIZZA PAIN

A burned mouth is no laughing matter—although my parents always thought it was pretty funny when I yowled and jumped around after taking a mouthful of scorching toppings. It happens so fast! It takes only a second for hot foods to burn the delicate tissues in your mouth. The area will usually heal within a few days, but it can be hard to eat in the meantime. I really advise my fellow pizza lovers to let the pie cool down a bit before diving in. I only hope you take this advice more seriously than I used to.

COOL TIPS FOR A HOT PROBLEM

If the pain of pizza mouth is really intense, it's probably worth checking with your doctor or dentist. The burn itself will heal easily enough, but until it does, you're vulnerable to infection because you've lost a protective layer of tissue. Your doctor may apply medications and a skinlike bandage to protect the area while it heals.

While it's unlikely that you'll burn yourself this badly with a mouthful of hot pizza, you'll still want to reduce the pain and help the burn heal more quickly. Here are some tips to try.

Bet on bicarbonate. Rinsing with a baking soda solution will reduce acidity in your mouth. That's important, because mouth acids cause additional pain, and their levels rise quickly after burns or other injuries. "Add a level teaspoon of

---

Best Bets for Mouth Bites

If there's anything more painful than pizza mouth, it's accidentally biting your tongue or cheek when you're eating. Here's how to reduce the pain in a hurry.

1. Press the area with a gauze pad or a clean washcloth to stop any bleeding. Don't use a paper towel or tissue because it will dissolve too quickly to be effective.

2. Put an ice cube in your mouth and let it rest against the painful area. It will numb the pain almost instantly and help stop bleeding.

3. Take acetaminophen or ibuprofen to reduce discomfort.

4. Dab on some Orabase or other adhesive mouth gel to protect the area and help it heal.

baking soda to an 8-ounce glass of water," advises Joseph L. Konzelman Jr., D.D.S., professor at the medical college of the Georgia School of Dentistry in Augusta. Swish the solution around in your mouth a couple of times a day until the discomfort is gone.

Be cool. The last thing your mouth needs after a close encounter with scorching pizza is even more heat. Remember, you've already burned off a protective layer of skin. Eating anything hot at that point will be doubly painful. "Stick to cool foods for a day or two when you've got a bad burn," says John Hibbs, N.D., a naturopathic physician and professor at Bastyr University near Seattle. Cool soups are good choices, as are salads and sandwiches.

Suck on ice. As with any burn, applying ice to the area will strip away residual heat, numb the pain, and constrict, or narrow, tiny blood vessels, which will inhibit inflammation or bleeding under the surface. The best way to use ice is to simply suck on an ice cube for a while. You can also swish ice water around in your mouth for about 20 seconds several times a day.

Ax the acids. Forget oranges, pineapple, tomatoes, or other acidic foods when you're recovering from pizza mouth. Apart from causing pain, they'll increase the time it takes the injury to heal.

Swear off salsa. The chemical compounds that put the heat in salsa, chili, and other spicy foods will really irritate the burn.

A Cup of Comfort

Slippery elm is one of the best herbal remedies for pizza mouth. "It's soothing, it reduces irritation and inflammation, and it shortens the healing time for burns," says John Hibbs, N.D. Buy the powdered form at a health food store and mix it with water. Several times a day, swish the solution around in your mouth, then swallow it or spit it out.

Salad, Anyone?

The next time you burn your mouth with hot pizza, make the second course a fresh green salad. Spinach, arugula, broccoli, and other leafy greens are loaded with folate (the natural form of folic acid), a B vitamin that helps damaged cells grow and reproduce to repair painful damage. While you're recovering, it's also a good idea to take a supplement that contains 400 micrograms of folic acid.

Eat soft foods. There's a good reason that people with pizza mouth often find themselves eating a lot of cottage cheese and similar foods. Anything with hard edges, such as pretzels or carrot pieces, can jab against the roof of your mouth and make the pain worse.

Apply St. John's wort oil. Available in health food stores, this oil soothes the pain of burns and helps them heal more quickly, says Dr. Hibbs. Put a tiny amount of oil on your finger and gently dab it on the sore area once or twice a day.

Put on a protective coating. You can't stick a bandage on your tongue or the roof of your mouth, but you can cover the area with an over-the-counter adhesive gel such as Orabase. It will protect the area from acids and other pain-causing substances, says Dr. Konzelman.

Forget the saltwater cure. A traditional remedy for mouth burns is to gargle with saltwater, but take this advice with a grain of salt, says Dr. Konzelman. Saltwater can actually increase discomfort and slow healing time. "Rubbing salt on any wound is not a good thing," he says. So don't do it!

Sinus Headache

Unclog the Caverns

It would probably be more accurate to call sinus headaches sinus "face aches." One of my best friends, who has had more than her share of these skull busters, says that head pain is only part of the problem. There's also the pain in the forehead, behind the eyes and nose, and even in the jaw. If that weren't bad enough, the discomfort tends to stick around for days. "You feel like you can't escape it," she says. "And it's not just pain, but also intense pressure. It feels kind of like someone stuck a bicycle pump in your ear and tried to inflate your head."

FIRE IN THE HOLES

Don't be offended if someone says that you have holes in your head. We all do. They're called sinuses—bony cavities above and below your eyes and on each side of your nose. Each sinus is lined with a spongy membrane. If you have allergies or an

---

soothing salves

SINUS SAVER

Applying eucalyptus nose cream, available at health food stores and some drugstores, to the insides of your nostrils daily can prevent sinus headaches.

upper respiratory infection, the membranes can become intensely irritated and inflamed, a condition called sinusitis. The main symptom, of course, is a sinus headache.

What's the connection between colds, allergies, and sinusitis? Colds and allergies cause congestion, which makes it difficult for mucus—and the bacteria and viruses that call it home—to drain away. The more germs you have in your sinuses, the more likely you are to get a sinus headache.

CONGESTION PROTECTION

Sinus headaches usually go away as soon as your sinuses begin draining again. At least, that's how it's supposed to work. If you're really unlucky, you could have a sinus headache that drags on for weeks, months, or even years. Chronic sinus headaches require serious treatment, sometimes with antibiotics or other drugs, and possibly even surgery. If you have a sinus headache for more than a day or so, see your doctor. You could have an infection that could spread to the brain.

If you're like most people, however, you probably get no more than a few sinus headaches a year. Here are a few ways to stop them fast.

Steam away congestion. The next time your sinuses start pounding, melt away congestion with an herbal steam. Put a few cups of water in a saucepan and bring it to a boil. Add 2 to 3 teaspoons of aromatic

Instant Ahhh...

Miraculous Menthol for Instant Relief

Here's a fast way to stop the pain of sinus headaches: Add a few drops of menthol or eucalyptus oil to hot water (just about as hot as you can stand it). Soak a small towel, wring it out, and drape it over your eyes, nose, or wherever else you hurt. The heat breaks up congestion and provides nearly instant relief. The oils are sold at health food stores.

Spice Away Sinus Pain

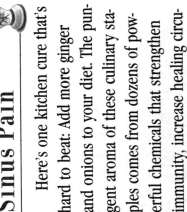

Here's one kitchen cure that's hard to beat: Add more ginger and onions to your diet. The pungent aroma of these culinary staples comes from dozens of powerful chemicals that strengthen immunity, increase healing circulation, and kill germs that can cause sinus headaches, says John Nowicki, N.D.

And don't forget the garlic. It's loaded with antibacterial, antiviral, and anti-inflammatory compounds. Raw garlic provides the biggest health punch, but cooked garlic retains many of the healing benefits.

herbs, such as thyme, rosemary, oregano, or basil. It's also good to add a few drops of eucalyptus oil, available in health food stores. Then carefully put the pot on a table or counter, drape a towel over your head to trap the steam, lean over the pot, and breathe deeply. Inhale the steam though your nose and exhale through your mouth. Do this for 10 to 15 minutes two or three times a day.

Keep your nose clean. Forget the old rule about not putting things in your nose. When you have a sinus headache, a nasal wash can make a real difference. It's not pretty, but it works. Mix 1 teaspoon of salt in 3 ounces of warm water and fill a dropper with the solution. Tilt your head back, put 10 drops in each nostril, and wait for 5 to 10 seconds. Then lean forward and let the fluid drain from your nose. You can repeat the nasal wash three times a day to treat an existing headache or prevent a new one.

Drink like a camel. Relief from sinus headaches may be as close as the kitchen faucet. "Drink 8 to 10 glasses of water a day," advises John Nowicki, N.D., a naturopathic physician in Issaquah, Washington. Water thins mucus in the sinuses and nasal passages so they drain more easily.

Clear the air. Okay, you already know

that inhaling cigarette smoke is a bad idea. If your sinuses are always in an uproar, however, you'll have to do whatever it takes to avoid smoke as well as other airborne irritants, such as pollen, dust, and even perfume.

Pop a multi. If you keep getting sinus headaches, it could be a sign that your body's defenses aren't up to par. Taking a multivitamin every day will shore them up, says Dr. Nowicki.

ACE it. Vitamins A, C, and E are among the best weapons against sinus headaches during the high-risk cold and allergy seasons, says Dr. Nowicki. Unless you're pregnant or planning to become pregnant, take 5,000 IU of vitamin A daily to strengthen your mucous membranes. As long as you don't have kidney problems, 4,000 to 6,000 milligrams of vitamin C daily will strengthen immunity, reduce congestion, and help protect against cold- and flu-causing germs. (Since that much vitamin C may cause diarrhea or upset your stomach, it's better to take it in two or three doses throughout the day. Taking it with food also helps.) Finally, 400 IU of vitamin E daily will also boost immunity.

Zinc about it. The mineral zinc is among the most potent immune boosters, and it also helps prevent headache-causing sinus infections. Take 30 milligrams of zinc daily during sinusitis season, suggests Dr. Nowicki. To maintain your mineral

---

Is It Really Sinusitis?

It's not always easy to tell if you have a sinus headache, a tension headache, or simply a painful head cold. Here's how to figure it out.

• If you have pain in the front of your head or your face, especially around your eyes, it's probably a sinus headache.

• Headaches that flare up at the end of long, stressful days and cause pain mainly in your scalp or the back of your head are usually tension headaches.

• Head colds are often accompanied by headaches, but if the pain in your head comes later, after the cold is gone, it's probably caused by something else.

balance, you should also take 2 to 4 milligrams of copper a day.

Battle back with bioflavonoids. Ever wonder what makes fruits and vegetables every color of the rainbow? It's the presence, among other things, of bioflavonoids, a large chemical family of plant pigments that fight off viruses and reduce allergic reactions that can trigger headaches. Produce is loaded with them, but if you get frequent sinus headaches, you'll probably need to take supplements. You can buy them at health food stores and drugstores. Make sure you follow the directions on the package.

Feast on fish. Two to four weekly servings of salmon, tuna, or other cold-water fish will load your system with inflammation-fighting fatty acids. If that's too much fish for your taste, you can try fish-oil or flaxseed-oil capsules, both of which are rich in fatty acids. Take 1 to 5 grams daily to combat sinus headaches, Dr. Nowicki suggests.

Herbs help. Humans have been getting sinus headaches for eons, and they've been easing them with herbal medicines for almost as long. One of the best of these is echinacea, which enhances the body's ability to fight infection. Eyebright, goldenseal, and elderberry are helpful for reducing congestion and inflammation. You can use dried herbs to make tea, but it's easier to take supplements, available at health food stores. Follow the directions on the label.

Move it and lose it. Walking and other forms of exercise are key for keeping your body strong enough to repel sinus infections and headaches. Exercise is also effective if you already have a sinus headache, because it promotes drainage of excess mucus.

Sore Throat

Super Soothing Solutions

Some time back, after years without so much as a sniffle, I woke up with a throat so raw that I felt as if I'd swallowed thumbtacks. It had been so long since I'd had a cold that I didn't have anything helpful in the medicine cabinet—not even one lozenge!

In desperation, I started scouring the kitchen cabinets. I found a few forgotten tea bags—green tea, my favorite kind. The tea, with a little honey thrown in, felt so good going down that I kept drinking it until my throat was back to normal. It wasn't until much later that I learned I'd stumbled onto a traditional remedy—just one of many, it turns out, that can coax a sore throat back to health.

HARD TO SWALLOW

The main causes of sore throats are bacteria and viruses, the same germs that cause colds and other upper respiratory infections. Seasonal allergies can also make your throat cry uncle because they often trigger inflammation in the tender tissues. Then there's plain old nasal congestion. The pesky dripping of mucus into the back of your throat can irritate it, and congestion forces you to breathe through your mouth, making your throat desert dry. And if you've been talking or yelling a lot recently, a sore throat may be your body's way of telling you that all that vocal action is taking its toll.

GO FOR THE THROAT

You'll want to see a doctor if your sore throat lasts longer than about a week; you could have a bacterial infection that won't go away unless you take antibiotics. While most sore throats get better on their own, they can make you mighty miserable in the meantime. Here are some time-tested remedies that really work wonders.

Wrap it up. Here's a throat soother that doesn't require a trip to the drugstore. Soak a washcloth or small towel in warm water. Wring it out, wrap it around your throat, and leave it on for about 5 minutes. Replace it with a cloth moistened with cool water, wrap a warm scarf around your neck, and keep both in place for about 30 minutes. The combination of heat and cold is wonderfully soothing, says Jane Hopson, N.D., a naturopathic physician in Hillsboro, Oregon.

"It helps clear congestion in your head and throat," she explains.

Load up on vitamins A and C. Both strengthen immunity and increase the activity of specialized cells that

---

Instant Ahhh...

The Ocean Potion

Your grandmother was right: The quickest way to soothe a sore throat is to gargle with saltwater. Mix 1 teaspoon of salt in a cup of warm water and gargle with the solution for about 30 seconds. Spit it out, then gargle again. The relief usually lasts anywhere from 15 minutes to an hour, and you can repeat the gargle as often as necessary.

fight infection. Take a multivitamin that contains both—plus (if you don't have stomach or kidney problems) 500 milligrams of vitamin C twice a day.

Eat plenty of garlic. This herb is one of the best remedies for sore throats as well as for colds and flu. It has anti-inflammatory, antiviral, and antibacterial properties, says Dr. Hopson. The problem with garlic, of course, is that you'd have to eat a few cloves a day to take advantage of its healing power—and that much garlic can give you a powerful aroma. To get the benefits without the pungency, Dr. Hopson recommends taking garlic capsules that have had the "stink" removed. Look for a supplement that provides about 10 milligrams of allicin, the active ingredient.

If you're a real garlic fan, though, go ahead and enjoy the real McCoy. Plan on eating one or two cloves a day. Raw or lightly steamed garlic provides more allicin than garlic that has been thoroughly cooked, Dr. Hopson adds. Just don't decide to visit with the neighbors until you've showered and brushed your teeth.

Soothe your throat with licorice. Licorice root is loaded with natural chemical compounds that soothe inflammation anywhere in your digestive tract, including your throat. Don't bother with licorice candy, though; it has only licorice flavor, not real licorice. What you want is licorice capsules, so visit your local health food store, then take 100 milligrams three

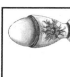

Juice It!

If you own a juicer, now's the time to rev it up. Juices are a great way to give your body the extra fluids and natural healing substances it needs to help a sore throat. All fruit juices are beneficial, but papaya, orange, and pineapple are good choices because they're loaded with vitamin C. Other throat-comforting produce includes carrots, spinach, blueberries, and dark cherries. The juice will be especially soothing if you warm it slightly before drinking it. If the flavor is too intense, just add a bit of water.

times a day. Since a substance in licorice called glycyrrhizic acid can cause high blood pressure in some people, look for deglycyrrhizinated licorice (DGL) products.

Enlist echinacea. The herb echinacea is like an inspirational general who rallies the troops: It stimulates immune cells that fight off throat-burning infections. You can brew echinacea tea, but it's easier to take capsules. The recommended dose is 350 milligrams three times a day.

Zinc it over. It may be at the end of the mineralogical alphabet, but zinc comes first when you need to soothe a sore throat. "It makes your throat feel better, and it boosts the immune system," says Dr. Hopson. She recommends sucking on zinc gluconate lozenges, available at most drugstores.

Add some color to your diet. The natural pigments that give fruits and vegetables their brilliant hues are called bioflavonoids—and they're loaded with anti-inflammatory agents. If your poor throat screams every time you eat, it may be easier to take bioflavonoid supplements. Two of the best for sore throats are quercetin and rutin. You'll want to take between 1,000 and 3,000 milligrams a day.

A Cup of Comfort

Green tea is among the best sore throat remedies because it's loaded with chemical compounds called bioflavonoids, which help quell irritation and inflammation, says Jane Hopson, N.D. If green's not your cup of tea, try chamomile—it's a traditional remedy for sore throat pain. And don't forget to add honey. It coats your throat and helps numb the pain.

Get allergies under control. If you tend to get sore throats during ragweed season (ragweed is one of the most common allergy triggers), you may want to take herbal supplements that contain nettle. The herb blocks the action of histamines, natural chemicals that fire up allergic reactions. Take 200 milligrams three times daily until your allergies—and your sore throat—are better.

Tap some liquid assets. Your throat will heal faster if you don't overuse it swallowing food. And if you happen to have a cold, you'll bounce back faster if your body doesn't expend a lot of energy in digestion. In other words, this is the best time to eat a bland diet—plenty of liquids and easy-to-digest foods. "Broths are a great choice," says Dr. Hopson. "No heavy, fatty meals; keep them light and liquid."

An important bonus of a diet that's heavy on liquids is that it will help make mucus thinner and more watery, so it will drain more easily and cause less throat irritation.

Suck down some slippery elm. This sweet-tasting herb coats your throat with a soothing film and reduces inflammation and irritation, says John Hibbs, N.D., a naturopathic physician and professor at Bastyr University near Seattle. Slippery elm lozenges work well, or you can buy slippery elm root powder at a health food store. Add about a tablespoon to a cup of hot water and stir it well. The tea has a gelatinous texture, which is what makes it such a good throat soother.

Temporomandibular Disorder

Calm That Jumpin' Joint!

When my friend Christine was a teenager, she woke up one morning and found that she couldn't open her mouth—not even enough to yawn. Her jaw was literally locked in place.

"I ran into my mom's bedroom to tell her what was happening, but I couldn't talk," she remembers. Her mom got the message, though, and together they were finally able to ease her jaw open. "It made a popping sound, kind of like when you crack your knuckles," Christine says with a laugh.

Apparently, they fixed the problem, because her jaw never locked up again. I'm glad, because there's nothing I enjoy more than hearing Christine laugh!

COMING UNHINGED

Christine's problem, TMD (short for temporomandibular disorder), is a common one. The temporomandibular joint is the hinge that allows your jaw to move up and down. Like any other joint in the body, it's vulnerable to things such as arthritis and sprains. The joint can also be looser than it should be, which can make it jump out of place on occasion. That's probably what happened to Christine, and the popping sound she heard was the joint slipping back into position. TMD isn't always painful, but it is always annoying, especially when you go through life hearing clicking and popping sounds every time you move your mouth.

TLC FOR TMD

Because TMD can be caused by so many different things, it's always worth checking with your doctor if the joint is sometimes painful or seems to be grinding instead of moving smoothly. Even if you don't have jaw-related problems, you should suspect TMD if you have frequent headaches, neck pain, or earaches, all of which are sometimes linked to problems with the jaw joint.

If TMD is causing you a lot of pain or your jaw is locking up with some regularity, you may need surgery to repair the joint. In the vast majority of cases, however, you can ease or even eliminate TMD with some simple home care. Here's how to do it.

Unlock That Jaw!

Most people with TMD don't experience jaw lock, but it can happen, and when it does, there are usually some warning signs. If you notice that your jaw is getting increasingly stiff or sore, or it seems to be getting harder to move, see your doctor right away. If you're lucky, the doctor will be able to correct the problem before your jaw takes itself totally out of action.

What do you do if you are caught by surprise? For starters, don't panic! Your jaw won't stay closed permanently, believe me. What you want to do is move it carefully as much as you can—a little bit from side to side or a little bit up and down. Flex and relax the muscles. The more you do this, the more your jaw will relax. Sooner or later, it should start moving normally again. If it doesn't get better within an hour or two, though, you may be out of luck, and you'll want to get to a doctor right away.

Supplement your jaw. Two over-the-counter dietary supplements, glucosamine and chondroitin, encourage the growth and repair of cartilage and other protective tissues in the joints. They may also help prevent age-related joint damage that can lead to TMD. The recommended dose is 500 milligrams of either (or both) three times daily. You can buy supplements that combine these helpful compounds in one caplet, capsule, or powder.

Load up on vitamin C. This helpful vitamin is an antioxidant nutrient that helps prevent harmful molecules called free radicals from damaging your joints. It also promotes the growth of collagen, a tissue that helps keep joints healthy, says Gerald J. Murphy, D.D.S., director of publications for the American Academy of Craniofacial Pain. He tells people to take 3,000 milligrams of vitamin C daily. Doses this large may cause diarrhea or other side effects, and they may be harmful for people with stomach or kidney problems, so check with your doctor before you start. You can minimize digestive side effects by

Healing Hands

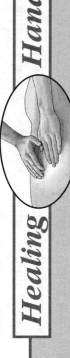

You can't always rub out TMD, but you can almost always rub it the right way. When you first notice pain, put your fingers on the side of your jaw, then open and close your mouth. The thick muscle that you feel is the one that controls your jaw. Put one finger on either side of the muscle and knead it gently, working all the way from your ear to your jaw. Rubbing and relaxing the muscle is one of the best ways to prevent—or ease—painful spasms.

dividing the amount into two or three doses and taking them at different times during the day. Taking vitamin C with food also helps alleviate side effects.

Do the Dixie chill-out. Flare-ups of TMD are usually accompanied by inflammation, which is what causes pain and swelling. Probably the quickest way to reduce inflammation is to immediately apply cold to your jaw. Cold causes blood vessels to constrict, or narrow, which reduces swelling. "Fill some Dixie cups with water and keep them in the freezer," Dr. Murphy advises. When TMD strikes, tear off part of the cup or push out an inch or two of ice, then apply it right where it hurts. Apply the ice for about 20 minutes every few hours throughout the day.

Heat the area. You don't want to apply heat to your jaw joint right away because it can increase swelling. After a day or two of cold treatments, though, heat will increase circulation and help remove any buildup of fluids and painful toxins. Soak a washcloth in hot water, wring it out, and hold it to your jaw until the cloth cools. Then dip it again and repeat the treatment as often as necessary for relief.

Stop the Nightly Grind

Millions of Americans grind their teeth at night, a condition called bruxism. Hour after hour of nighttime jaw action is a common cause of TMD, says Gerald J. Murphy, D.D.S. Most people who grind their teeth don't know it, so you may need to ask the person who shares your bed to watch (and listen) while you sleep. A minute or two of grinding isn't a big deal, but if you do it a lot, you'll have to work with your doctor to find ways to keep your jaw still.

People who grind their teeth are often under a lot of stress, so your doctor will probably recommend a relaxation strategy such as biofeedback, meditation, or yoga. You also may need to wear a bite guard while you sleep. Available from dentists, these devices reduce the frequency of grinding and help protect your teeth from long-term damage.

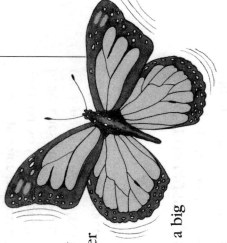

Splint your jaw. Don't worry, it sounds worse than it really is. One of the most successful strategies for easing TMD is to use an oral splint that guides the jaw back into its proper position, says Dr. Murphy. The splints are custom-made by doctors and dentists, and they're usually worn only at night—although if your TMD is serious, you may have to wear a splint night and day for a while.

It takes time to get used to a splint, but it works very quickly. "In a week, most people don't want to do without them because their jaws are feeling so much better," says Dr. Murphy.

Don't bite off more than you can chew. When TMD is acting up, it's important to give your jaw a rest, just as you'd stay off your feet after spraining your ankle. Stick to foods that are easy on your chops and avoid those that require a lot of jaw action, such as apples and corn on the cob. And by all means, let the silverware do the work. Cut food into small pieces, so you don't have to chew as much.

Stand up straight. And no slumping while you work! "Postures that create the least stress on your upper body will also produce the least stress on your jaw," says Dr. Murphy. This means standing and sitting up straight and always making an effort to keep your head and neck in line with the rest of your body. It really does help!

Reduce your stress. Any kind of emotional stress makes TMD worse, because it makes muscles tense and tighten. It also increases levels of body chemicals that aggravate pain. Whatever it is that you do when you relax, do it even more often when TMD is acting up. "Things like meditation, yoga, or just getting away for a while can make a big difference," says Dr. Murphy.

Tension Headache

Muscle In on Tightness

I've known Wendy for years, and she's one of the most productive people anywhere. She runs her own design firm—a full-time job if ever there was one. Yet she also works part-time at a small publishing company, and in what little free time she has, is a volunteer at the local animal shelter. Just thinking about her daily schedule makes me want to take a nap!

Despite her packed calendar, Wendy never seems tired or stressed, so I was surprised when she said that she often gets headaches. "It usually happens when a meeting's been going on too long," she says. "My whole head starts throbbing."

Her solution, characteristically, involves even more activity. "I go for a short walk. I'll take an aspirin, too, but I think it's the walk that really helps."

BLAME IT ON MUSCLES

Tension headaches are the most common type of head pain, and they're aptly named. Whenever you're tense, muscles in your scalp, neck, and shoulders contract and tighten up. Tight muscles have to pull against something, and it's often your head that feels the squeeze.

Most tension headaches cause achy pain and pressure in your neck, forehead, or scalp—sometimes all three places at once. Some headache remedies work from the inside out, but most are designed to get all those muscles to loosen up. Once your muscles relax, the pain usually goes away.

TAKE THE TENSION OUT

Nearly everyone gets headaches sometimes. It's worth checking with your doctor if you get them all the time or if the pain interferes with your daily activities, but you'll probably be able to manage most headaches on your own. The vast majority of headaches (about 95 percent) are "primary" headaches, which means that they aren't caused by some dangerous underlying illness.

It's fine to take aspirin, ibuprofen, acetaminophen, or other over-the-counter headache medications as long as you're not sensitive to them. Keep in mind, however, that these drugs don't eliminate the underlying problems, and they may cause side effects that are more uncomfortable than the headaches themselves. Doctors usually advise starting with gentler

Healing *Hands*

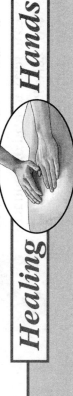

Don't feel like taking aspirin for tension headaches? Here's an acupressure technique from Traditional Chinese Medicine that can literally help in a pinch: Grip the skin between your thumb and index finger and give it a firm pinch. "Pressing that area often takes the pain away," says Terri Dallas-Prunskis, M.D.

approaches. Here's what they mean.

Think on your feet. It's hard to imagine that foot problems could cause head pain, but that's exactly what happens, especially in women. "Wearing high heels or shoes without good support can cause muscle strain that causes headaches," says Chris Meletis, N.D., chief medical officer of the National College of Naturopathic Medicine in Portland, Oregon. Always buy shoes with plenty of padding, he advises. If you wear high heels, slip out of them now and then to give the muscles in your legs and feet—as well as in your scalp—a chance to relax.

Heat your head. You've probably seen movies or television shows that portray headache sufferers holding comically large ice bags on their heads. Ice can certainly help in some cases, but heat is usually better for tension headaches because it causes muscles to relax instead of contract, says Terri Dallas-Prunskis, M.D., codirector of the Illinois Pain Treatment Institute in Chicago. She recommends putting a heating pad or a washcloth soaked in warm water on the areas that hurt. You can also hang out in a bath or shower for 10 to 15 minutes.

Push and flex. A quick way to ease tension headaches is to press your fingers firmly where it hurts while flexing those

Instant Ahhh...

Take a Swipe at Stress

You don't want a heavy-duty workout when your head is hurting, but gentle exercise, such as walking or yoga, will relieve tension headaches fast. Exercise helps eliminate muscle-tensing stress hormones from your body and stimulates the release of painkilling chemicals called endorphins.

INSTANT HEAT
microwaveable

muscles against the pressure. Doing this a few times helps tense muscles relax, says Dr. Meletis.

Suppose that your shoulder muscles are unusually tight, and you're feeling the pain in your scalp. Press your fingers into the muscles and shrug your shoulders at the same time to increase the pressure. Next, while maintaining the finger pressure, relax your shoulders for a few seconds, then shrug them again. The combination of pressure and relaxation knocks out tension in a hurry, Dr. Meletis explains.

Work magic with magnesium. This common mineral appears to promote muscle relaxation, says Dr. Meletis. The next time you have a tension headache, take anywhere from 250 to 750 milligrams of magnesium and see if it helps. Start by taking the lower amount and increase the dose only if you don't get relief, he advises. Taking more than 400 to 500 milligrams of magnesium a day can cause diarrhea in some people. If this occurs, reduce the dose.

Vitamin C pain relief. This all-purpose nutrient has powerful anti-inflammatory properties, which is important because inflammation plays a role in some tension headaches. You can try taking 1,000 to 2,000 milligrams of vitamin C at the first sign of a tension headache. If it's going to work, you should feel the benefits within an hour or two. (If you have stomach or kidney problems, though, you shouldn't take high amounts of vitamin C. Also, to avoid diarrhea or stomach upset, take it in two or three smaller doses throughout the day.)

Correct your posture. If you spend a lot of time slumped in a chair or hunched over a keyboard, your head will pay the price. Poor posture is among the most common causes of tension headaches. "When you're sitting, you want your legs to be at a 90-degree angle to your hips," says Dr. Dallas-Prunskis. "Keep your shoulders back and don't let your head hang backward or forward; keep it in line with your spine."

Eat less salt. A lot of women get tension headaches during the week to 10 days before their menstrual periods. Eating salt during this time can make things worse because it promotes fluid retention and sometimes raises blood pressure. You may find that cutting back on salt—not only when you're premenstrual, but throughout the month—will prevent a lot of headaches, says Dr. Dallas-Prunskis.

Don't focus only on the saltshaker, she adds. Only a small percentage of the salt we eat is added at the table. Most is found in processed foods—canned soups, for example, or those hurry-up lunches at fast-food restaurants. If you eat plenty of natural foods, such as fruits, vegetables, and whole grains, you'll almost automatically reduce your salt intake to healthier levels.

Make the caffeine connection. Coffee is the most popular pick-me-up in America, but that pleasant morning jolt comes with a price. Your body literally gets addicted to caffeine, and you may start experiencing headaches or other withdrawal symptoms as soon as 2 hours after having a cup. Switching to decaf is one solution, but if you can't bring

A Cup of Comfort

Herbal teas not only taste good and give you the chance to relax for a few moments, they also reduce muscle tension and painful pressure in your head and neck, says Chris Meletis, N.D. The best teas for tension headaches include chamomile, passionflower, cramp bark, cinnamon, and ginkgo. When using dried herbs, add about 1 tablespoon to a cup of freshly boiled water and steep for 5 to 10 minutes. You should avoid chamomile if you're allergic to ragweed.

yourself to give up caffeine entirely, at least cut back to a cup or two a day. You'll still get the pleasant lift, but without the headaches later on.

Sleep on your back. It's the best position for supporting your head and neck muscles. Sleeping on your stomach, on the other hand, means that your head is turned to the side for hours at a time. This can be a real strain on the neck—and a pain in the head. "Imagine how you'd feel if you had to stand for hours with your head turned to the right or left," says Dr. Dallas-Prunskis. "You'd end up with quite a headache."

Check out different pillows. Some pillows do an excellent job of supporting your head and neck, while others are so soft that you might as well be sleeping on air. Firm pillows are usually best for preventing tension headaches, but you'll have to experiment to find the pillow that works best for you.

Stretch pain away. A good way to prevent tension headaches is with stretching exercises. Focus on your neck, because that's where tension headaches often originate. Several times a day, gently turn your head from left to right. Turn it as far as you comfortably can in each direction. Then lower your chin toward your chest, hold for a moment, and tilt your head all the way back until you're looking at the ceiling. This exercise is especially helpful on those days when you've been chained to the computer or stuck in rush-hour traffic, and your muscles are tighter than usual.

STRETCHING

Toothache

Take a Bite Out of Pain

In college, there was a guy who was renowned for his toughness. He just didn't seem to feel pain the way we lesser mortals did. I once watched him head-butt the soda machine to get it to release the cola he'd paid for. The machine was left with a dent, but he didn't even get a headache. One day during lunch, he developed a toothache that made it too painful to finish his chickenburger. All of us sitting at the table told him to go to the campus health center. But he was anxious to get to his afternoon classes (believe it or not, he was even more brainy than he was brawny), so he decided to live with the pain and have it checked the next day.

Since I happened to be going to the same class, I walked to cam-

---

Soothing Salves

SPICY SOLUTIONS

Relief from a raging toothache may be as close as your spice rack. Folk healers often advise people to spread a little ground ginger or red pepper around the tooth. Add a little water to the spice to make a paste, then spread it liberally around the point of pain. You may notice relief in as little as 5 minutes.

pus with him that afternoon. He made it all of two blocks before the pain made him change his plans, and he made a beeline to the dentist. Later, we found out that this six-foot-five tank of a man had been brought to his knees by a single sesame seed that had slipped beneath his gum.

FROM THE OUTSIDE IN

It's a wonder we all don't get toothaches more often, since the tiny nerves inside our teeth are just a fraction of an inch from the outside world. They don't cause any pain as long as they're well shielded. If there's a breach in the protective tooth enamel, however, or if your gum line recedes even a tiny bit, these nerves are exposed to air—or, in some cases, assaulted by inflammation or infection. They let you know what's happening immediately by causing excruciating pain.

TAMING TOOTH PAIN

It's not unusual for toothaches to disappear on their own, but you can bet that the pain's going to come back—probably sooner rather than later. You may as well bite the bullet and make an appointment to see your dentist. Toothaches are often caused by decay, explains Richard Price, D.M.D., a dentist in the

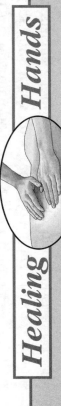

Healing Hands

According to Traditional Chinese Medicine, you can often relieve pain in one part of the body by applying pressure to another part. The next time you get a toothache, grip the web of skin between your index finger and thumb on the hand opposite the ache and give it a firm squeeze, suggests Flora Stay, D.D.S. "Sometimes it works, and sometimes it doesn't," she adds.

Soothing Sensitive Teeth

People keep their teeth a lot longer than they used to. That's a good thing, but there's also a downside: Natural wear and tear can rub away the protective enamel and make your teeth unusually sensitive to hot or cold temperatures. To reduce sensitivity, try these tips.

Brush with a light touch. Brushing too vigorously tends to make the teeth more sensitive. So does using a hard toothbrush.

Avoid the same old grind. Millions of Americans grind their teeth at night, which wears teeth down and often makes them more sensitive. Tooth grinding, called bruxism, is usually caused by stress, explains Flora Stay, D.D.S. Practicing relaxation techniques such as meditation and yoga can help keep your jaws still while you sleep. If that doesn't work, your dentist may need to make a bite guard that will protect your teeth from all that nighttime action.

Use a special paste. Toothpastes made for sensitive teeth often work, but not right away. "It may take a tube or two before you notice results," says Richard Price, D.M.D. "Pastes for sensitive teeth have different ingredients, so you may have to experiment until you find the one that works for you."

Get your teeth checked. Old fillings or caps can loosen over time, making a tooth sensitive. Ask your dentist to take a look. Simply replacing the old dental work may be all it takes to stop the pain.

Boston area and consumer advisor for the American Dental Association. There's a good chance you'll need a filling or even a root canal. Once the damage is repaired, the toothache will be gone for good.

There's a curious thing about toothaches, though. It seems that they never happen on weekdays or during business hours, when it's easy to see your dentist. They have an unfortunate way of cropping up late at night or at the beginning of three-day weekends. When that happens, you have to find ways to ease the agony until you can get some help. Here are a few terrific tips to try.

Fix it with floss. Sometimes, as with my burly classmate, a toothache is caused by a particle of food lodged between your teeth or between your teeth and gums. It's worth it to take a few minutes to gently floss the area to see if anything pops out.

Keep on brushing. Even if it hurts a little when you brush, it's essential to keep your teeth clean until you can see a dentist. "Food and debris can collect on your tooth and make the pain worse," says Dr. Price.

Swish and spit. Thoroughly rinsing your mouth with a saltwater solution—made by mixing about 1/2 teaspoon of salt in a cup of warm water—will often reduce the pain of a toothache, says Dr. Price. The relief doesn't last very long, but you can repeat the swishing as often as necessary.

Numb it with ice. You wouldn't think that placing a cold pack—or a washcloth wrapped around some ice cubes—on the outside of your mouth would have much effect on a toothache, but it does seem to help. Hold it against

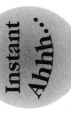

Instant *Ahhh...*

Rinse with Chamomile

Brew some chamomile tea by steeping 1 teaspoon of dried herb (available at health food stores) in a cup of hot water for 10 to 20 minutes. Strain the tea and let it cool, swish some around in your mouth for about 30 seconds, then swallow it or spit it out. Keep rinsing your mouth until you've used up all the tea. Avoid chamomile if you're allergic to ragweed.

the tender area for 15 to 20 minutes every few hours until you can see your dentist.

Take a pain reliever. The analgesics in your medicine cabinet are more effective than you might think. Acetaminophen can sometimes ease a toothache as effectively as mild prescription drugs. And as long as you're not sensitive to them, aspirin and ibuprofen may be even better. "They reduce inflammation and also stop the body's production of prostaglandins, chemicals that cause pain," says Dr. Price.

Keep things fluid. Toothaches can get a lot worse when your mouth is dry. Until the pain is gone, it's important to drink a lot of water to keep it lubricated. Have a glass of water handy at all times and keep taking small sips, Dr. Price advises.

If your mouth is always a little dry, it's probably time to make a list of all the medications you're taking and review them with your dentist. Anywhere from 200 to 400 common drugs, such as antihistamines, heart drugs, and anti-anxiety medications, cause dryness, says Dr. Price. A dry mouth not only aggravates a toothache, it also promotes tooth decay by making it easier for bacteria to thrive.

Cool it with cloves. This remedy has been used for generations for easing toothaches, and there's good evidence that it works, says Flora Stay, D.D.S., author of *The Complete Book of Dental Remedies*. You can buy clove oil in health food stores and some drugstores. Dip a cotton swab in the oil and rub it on the sore tooth. In many cases, the pain will disappear almost instantly.

Tooth Trauma

Tips to Save Your Smile

Forget the stress of crunching carrots. Your teeth have to withstand such things as olive pits hidden in green salads and those surprising bits of grit that sometimes turn up in three-bean salads. They also have to deal with the impact of other teeth—when you nervously clench your jaw, for example, or grind your teeth in the middle of the night.

Although they're strong, teeth, and their tough enamel coating, can stand only so much. At one time or another, nearly everyone develops small cracks or chips in their teeth. Apart from marring the beauty of your smile, even the smallest amount of damage can eventually weaken an entire tooth. Then it's denture city—and who wants that?

TOOTH AND CONSEQUENCES

You would think that the fear of going through life with a gap-toothed smile would get most people to the dentist if they even suspected that they'd damaged a tooth. In fact, the problem is easy to miss. The pain probably comes and goes—maybe only when you bite in a certain way, for example. Even if you discuss the problem with your dentist, it may be hard to identify. Chips are easy enough to spot, but hairline cracks in a tooth may be painful or visible only when the tooth is under pressure in a particular way. "It's often difficult to reproduce the pain when you're in the dentist's office," explains Richard Price, D.M.D., a dentist in the Boston area and consumer advisor for the American Dental Association.

RELIEF FROM TOOTH PAIN

A tiny chip or crack may not seem like a big deal, but think about it: There's now an opening in the hard, protective outer layer of your tooth. The sensitive nerves underneath are vulnerable to the harsh outside environment. Cracks and chips can also admit germs that may cause permanent damage.

This kind of damage is usually easy to repair, but only if you catch it early. Just like a chip in a car's windshield, damage to the surface of a tooth invariably begins to spread outward, weakening the entire structure.

Seeing your dentist right away could help you keep a tooth instead of losing it. You may need a cap, a hard covering that makes the whole thing stronger.

If you can't get to dentist right away, here are a few ways to minimize the pain and prevent long-term problems.

A Cup of Comfort

Chamomile tea, a traditional remedy for tooth pain, helps in two ways: It reduces inflammation and has a mild tranquilizing effect. Make a cup of tea, using one tea bag per cup of hot water. Steep the tea for 10 to 20 minutes, let it cool, then swish some around in your mouth for about 30 seconds. Swallow the tea (or spit it out), then repeat until the entire cup is gone. Avoid chamomile if you're allergic to ragweed.

Don't crack corn, Jimmy. "Our teeth are not designed for chewing on popcorn kernels," says Dr. Price. The same goes for ice cubes, the ends of pens, and other hard objects. Biting anything harder than a raw carrot is sure to make even the tiniest crack a whole lot worse.

All you need is clove. Clove oil has been used for generations for easing tooth pain, and dentists have found that it really works. "Clove oil is nature's tooth-pain remedy," says Dr. Price. When a tooth starts hurting, dip a cotton swab in the oil and apply it directly to the painful spot. The pain will disappear in just a few seconds. You can buy clove oil at health food stores and some drugstores.

Swallow that aspirin. Or take

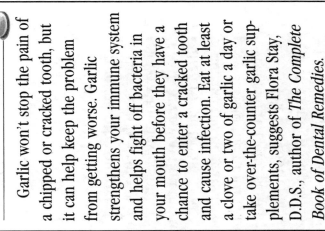

ibuprofen at the first painful twinge. Each of these pain relievers blocks the action of prostaglandins, chemicals in the body that cause pain. Since acetaminophen has no effect on prosta-

glandins, it won't work as well. Avoid aspirin if it bothers your stomach, however.

But don't apply it. Aspirin is for internal use only, so forget the old folk remedy about applying a tablet directly to a sore tooth. You'll get only small amounts of the pain-relieving ingredient, and the high acid content of aspirin could damage the tender tissues in your mouth.

Add water. If you've recently damaged a tooth, the worst

Grab Some Garlic

Garlic won't stop the pain of a chipped or cracked tooth, but it can help keep the problem from getting worse. Garlic strengthens your immune system and helps fight off bacteria in your mouth before they have a chance to enter a cracked tooth and cause infection. Eat at least a clove or two of garlic a day or take over-the-counter garlic supplements, suggests Flora Stay, D.D.S., author of *The Complete Book of Dental Remedies*.

thing to do is let the inside of your mouth dry out. Your tooth needs to stay lubricated to reduce potential damage as well as pain. Keep a glass of water nearby and take frequent sips until you see your dentist.

It's an Emergency!

Don't panic if a sudden accident temporarily separates you from a tooth you love. If you act quickly, there's a good chance that it can be happily reunited with its 30-odd companions. Just follow the advice of Richard Price, D.M.D.

1. After you find the tooth, pick it up by the top part, called the crown. Don't handle the root end, or you may permanently damage the delicate tissues.

2. Hold the tooth under gently running water to remove any visible dirt. Don't scrub; just give it a quick rinse.

3. Put the tooth back in its socket. You may think that only a doctor or dentist can do this, but it's really pretty easy. Be sure the tooth is facing in the right direction, then slip it in. You'll know right away if it's in the proper position.

4. If you aren't able to slip the tooth back into its socket, at least keep it moist by holding it between your cheek and gum. Another option is to put it in a glass of water—or better yet, milk. "Proteins in the milk will help keep the tooth alive," says Dr. Price. Even wrapping the tooth in a moist washcloth is better than nothing. A dry tooth won't reattach inside the mouth, he explains.

5. Get to a dentist immediately. You have only about 30 minutes to an hour to have a chance at saving the tooth. Teeth that have been out of your mouth for longer than that sometimes survive, but you can't count on it.

Trigeminal Neuralgia

Face the Pain

My friend Fayne Daniels was singing at a funeral when a jolt of intense pain flashed across her face. "It was like a sudden electric shock," she says. "I was barely able to finish, the song."

Fayne had never experienced anything like it before, but a week later, it happened again—and it kept happening off and on for more than 30 years. Her doctors told her she had trigeminal neuralgia (TN), sometimes called tic doloreaux. What they couldn't tell her (and still can't) is what exactly causes the pain in most people—and, more important, how to make it go away.

WHEN LIGHTNING STRIKES

Only a few thousand Americans have trigeminal neuralgia, so there are still a lot of doctors who don't know about it. The pain, which has been compared to being zapped by thousands of volts of electricity, tends to occur more often on the right side of your face than on the left. It may occur spontaneously, or it may be triggered by facial stimulation, such as brushing your teeth, for example, or putting on makeup.

The pain is clearly linked to a disturbance in the trigeminal nerve, which controls sensation in the face, but what causes the disturbance isn't always clear. It may be due to abnormal kinks in the nerve or, less often, inflammation of the tissue that covers it. Attacks can last seconds, minutes, or hours, and there's no predicting when the pain will strike. You may have daily pain, or there may be months or even years between episodes.

PULLING THE PLUG

Most people who have frequent TN episodes rely on muscle relaxants or other medications to control the pain. The problem with drug therapy is that the medicines often quit working, and they may also cause side effects such as dizziness and fatigue. As a result, people sometimes resort to surgery, which may be used to destroy the nerve that causes the pain.

It doesn't, however, have to go this far. Most people with TN can relieve, if not eliminate, the symptoms with some self-care strategies. Here are some things that can help.

Clear your schedule. "When people have more stress in their lives, that's when I get more phone calls," says Jeffrey Cohen, M.D., Ph.D., board member of the Trigeminal Neuralgia

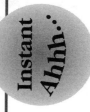

Instant Ahhh...

The Popsicle Prescription

It doesn't work for everyone, but sucking on a Popsicle or an ice cube will often take the edge off trigeminal neuralgia that affects the area around your mouth. As soon as you feel the pain coming on, get something cold in your mouth. Another option is to apply a cold pack to the outside of your face, but be gentle, because too much pressure can make the pain worse.

Association and director of the clinical neurophysiology laboratory at Beth Israel Hospital in New York City.

Do whatever it takes to make your life less hectic, he advises. Get a sitter to watch the kids occasionally. Take regular walks through the park. Do your holiday shopping throughout the year instead of during the busy season. The more you're able to relax, the fewer episodes you're likely to have.

Guard your face. For some people with TN, facial pressure is almost sure to set off attacks. Be sure to use a gentle touch when washing your face, brushing your teeth, or applying makeup. Also, take the time to write down whatever you're doing or feeling when you have the pain. You may be able to identify specific triggers.

Work your body. Regular exercise is a great stress buster, plus it's good for your overall health—and for reducing TN attacks. "Yoga helped me quite a bit," Fayne says.

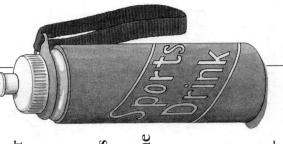

Prepare for dental visits. People with TN are understandably nervous about having dental work done, but don't let fear cause you to miss important dental appointments. Talk to your doctor, who may advise you to temporarily take higher doses of medication before dental appointments. This is often enough to keep the pain from flaring up.

Grab the knitting needles. Or get in the habit of doing crosswords, reading a good thriller or biography, or whatever else you normally do when you need distraction. Keeping your mind busy won't prevent attacks, but it can make the pain a lot less severe.

Bundle up. Cold air is a common trigger of TN. During the winter months, get in the habit of bundling up well and wrapping a scarf around your face. The one problem with this approach is that movement of the scarf may bring on attacks. An alternative is to wear a cold-weather face mask that fits snugly.

Laugh...a lot! It's hard to do when you're in pain, but one of the best ways to fight back is to take the time to feed your funny bone. "Believe it or not," says Fayne, "it really helps."

Go out to dinner. Take in a movie. Get together with friends. The last thing you want to do when you have TN is let the condition take over your social life. People who withdraw and get discouraged invariably experience more pain than those who stay active and involved in life.

Make some new friends. One of the most frustrating things about TN is that so little is known about it. People often feel that their friends, relatives, and even their doctors don't really understand what they're going through. This is what led Fayne to start a trigeminal neuralgia support group in the mid-Hudson area of New York State.

"It's so wonderful to be with people who have the problem and understand what it's about," she says.

If you want to find a support group in your area, or you'd like to start your own, contact the Trigeminal Neuralgia Association at 904-779-0333 or check out their Web site at www.tna-support.org. The group will even send you a handbook filled with practical advice from patients as well as doctors. (If you end up joining Fayne's group, be sure to tell her I said Hi!)

Soothing Salves

HOT CREAM GIVES RELIEF

An over-the-counter cream that contains capsaicin can sometimes reduce the frequency or severity of trigeminal neuralgia. The active ingredient is the same one that puts the "hot" in red pepper, and it appears to block the transmission of pain signals from your face to your brain. Just be sure to keep the cream well away from your eyes and mouth, and wash your hands thoroughly after using it.

Whiplash
Nix the Neck Pain

One night at a dinner party, a woman seated across from me told me that she'd been in a car accident and was recovering from whiplash. If it hadn't been for the airbag and seatbelt, she certainly would have been more seriously injured, but she could have walked away without a scratch except for one thing: The car's headrests were set too low. At the moment of impact, her head was thrown backward, causing the injury that necessitated the uncomfortable-looking brace wrapped around her neck.

When I got into my car after the party, you'd better believe that I checked the headrests to be sure they were positioned right at the back of my head. I now do the same each time I get into any car, just before buckling up the seatbelt.

SNAP TO IT

Whiplash is one of those words that sounds exactly like what it is

Pillow Talk

Is your neck so sore that you can't sleep? Try a cervical pillow. Available at most drugstores, these pillows are designed to give your neck extra support while you sleep.

(and it's easier to say than the medical name, hyperextension flexion injury). It happens when your head is suddenly thrown backward or forward, making your neck essentially snap like a whip. The sudden motion can damage soft tissues, producing pain that lingers for days or weeks. In more serious cases, whiplash can damage your spine. While car accidents are the most common way to get whiplash, any abrupt movement can cause it.

WIPE OUT WHIPLASH

One of the strange things about whiplash is that you don't always feel it right away. It's common for people to feel just fine after an accident, only to have an unbearably stiff neck a day or two later.

Whiplash injuries aren't always serious. Most people, in fact, don't experience anything worse than pain and stiffness. But whiplash can damage the bony vertebrae in the neck as well as the essential nerves in the spine. Even if you think the injury is minor, see a doctor. You may need x-rays or other tests to ensure that your spine is intact and the nerves aren't damaged. There's a good chance you'll need prescription drugs or physical therapy if the pain is intense. If the injury is minor, here are a few ways to heal a little faster.

Wear an ice collar. Use an ice pack as soon as possible after you've been hurt—even while you're on the way to the

---

Instant Ahhh...

The Paper-Cup Cure

An ice massage is an inexpensive, effective way to give whiplash the cold shoulder—and to relieve pain and help you sleep, says John Nowicki, N.D. Here's an easy way to do it: Fill a paper cup three-quarters full of water and put it in the freezer. When it's frozen, peel away the cup so that about half of the ice is exposed. Rub it vigorously over the painful part of your neck for 10 to 15 minutes.

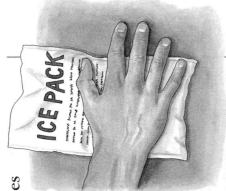

emergency room or the doctor's office. Ice does more than numb pain; it constricts blood vessels and curtails swelling and inflammation. For the first 24 hours after the injury, apply ice every few hours, holding it in place for about 20 minutes each time.

Keep it swivelin'. You obviously don't want to overuse your neck muscles after you've been hurt (as if the pain would let you!), but you don't want to totally immobilize them, either. Even a few days of zero activity can cause the muscles to weaken and contract, which will make the pain worse.

Your doctor may advise you to wear a neck brace or collar, but don't do it just because you think you're supposed to. Except in cases where your doctor wants to keep your neck completely still, allowing it to move more or less through its normal range of motion will help it heal more quickly, says John Nowicki, N.D., a naturopathic physician in Issaquah, Washington.

Pepper the pain. Capsaicin cream, available over the counter, contains the "hot" chemical found in red pepper. It reduces pain by making your body deplete its normal supply of pain-causing chemicals. Use it only as directed on the package—and be sure to keep it away from any area of open skin and wash your hands thoroughly after using it. It stings!

Roll with it. Gentle stretches will encourage healing in your neck and keep your muscles from getting stiff. An easy stretch to do is the neck roll. First, turn your head to the left, tuck your chin to your shoulder, and hold for a moment. Then gently turn your head to the right, keeping your chin down. Finally, repeat the same movement in the opposite direction. Never roll your head backward; it puts too much strain on your neck.

Get your doctor's okay before doing this or any other stretch, and be sure to stop if you feel more than very minor pain. That's your body's way of telling you that you need a little more recovery time.

Sit up straight. Your mother was right: Good posture is very important, especially while your body is repairing the damaged tissue in your neck. "Good posture helps your body align new tissue in the proper direction," says Dr. Nowicki.

When sitting, keep your shoulders back and your head in line with your neck, not bent forward or backward. If you can, sit in a chair that provides good neck and head support. Also, change positions frequently; you don't want your beleaguered neck muscles to stay in the same position for too long.

Try a passionate solution. The herb passionflower is a traditional remedy for easing muscle spasms after injuries, says Dr. Nowicki. It's a sedative that will help you relax, so never use it if you're taking antidepressants, anti-anxiety drugs, sedatives, or even a single glass of alcohol. Look for a tincture at a health food store and take one dropper twice a day.

Use the magic of magnesium. Many people don't get enough of this important mineral. Even though many foods are

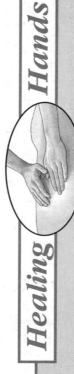

Healing Hands

People instinctively rub their necks to ease the pain of whiplash, but it doesn't do much good, because rubbing your own neck activates the same muscles that you're trying to relax. Having someone else do the massage, however, is a great way to relieve muscle tension, reduce spasms, and help injured tissues heal more quickly.

high in magnesium, you need extra-large amounts after injuries because it relaxes muscles and promotes healing. Take a supplement that supplies 400 to 600 milligrams daily. This amount of magnesium may cause diarrhea in some people. If this occurs, reduce the dose.

Supplement your joints. A few years ago, doctors scoffed at glucosamine and chondroitin, supplements that were purported to be good for injured joints. They've now changed their tune, since studies have shown conclusively that the supplements repair damaged cartilage and other tissues. When you're recovering from whiplash, take 500 milligrams of glucosamine or chondroitin (or a supplement that contains both) three times daily, then keep on taking it for at least a few more months.

Fish for oil. The essential fatty acids found in salmon, tuna, and other cold-water fish help reduce the inflammation caused by whiplash. Or you can take a teaspoon of fish oil once a day.

Be painfully careful. Modern drugs are remarkably effective at quelling neck pain. Keep in mind, however, that all drugs—from aspirin and ibuprofen to high-powered prescription products—only ease symptoms; they don't heal the injury. Don't let a few pain-free days lull you into resuming all of your usual activities. Your body still needs time to heal, so ease back into your regular routine slowly.

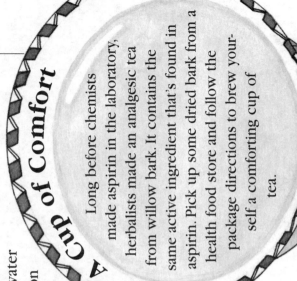

A Cup of Comfort

Long before chemists made aspirin in the laboratory, herbalists made an analgesic tea from willow bark. It contains the same active ingredient that's found in aspirin. Pick up some dried bark from a health food store and follow the package directions to brew yourself a comforting cup of tea.

Pain in Your Shoulders, Arms, and Hands

Carpal Tunnel Syndrome

Frozen Shoulder

Rotator Cuff Tear

Smashed Fingers and
Hammered Thumbs

Tennis Elbow

Wrist Sprain or Strain

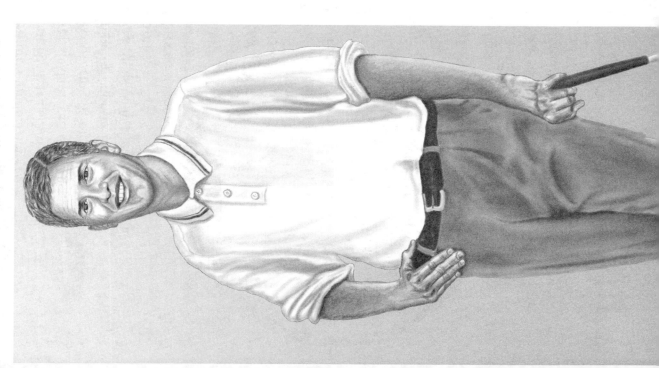

Carpal Tunnel Syndrome

Wipe Out Wrist Pain

Years ago, carpal tunnel syndrome wasn't as well known as it is today. I remember when a writer friend of mine first noticed that his hands and wrists started aching after a few hours at the keyboard. He chalked it up to weak muscles. He figured that his wrists ached for the same reason that his back hurt after he rearranged furniture—the muscles weren't as strong as they should be. His solution was to type even more. He reasoned that once the muscles were built up enough, the symptoms would go away, so he worked through the pain. As any doctor could tell him, that was about the dumbest thing he could have done.

PAINFUL PRESSURE

Carpal tunnel syndrome has nothing at all to do with muscle soreness and everything to do with nerves. There's a nerve in the wrist that passes through a narrow channel called the carpal tunnel. Even under normal circumstances, there's barely enough room in there for the nerve to move freely. If anything happens to make the tunnel smaller—swelling caused by too much typing, for example—the nerve gets a little mashed. That's what causes the tingling, numbness, and/or pain that are the telltale signs of carpal tunnel syndrome. The symptoms usually crop up in the thumb and first two fingers, which are connected to the affected nerve.

LIGHT AT THE END OF THE TUNNEL

Carpal tunnel syndrome can cause permanent disability in some cases, but my friend was lucky. He finally saw a doctor, who told him to give his hands a vacation. Afterward, he made sure that he didn't work for more than an hour or two without taking a break. The swelling went down, the nerve returned to normal, and his symptoms went away.

Unfortunately, carpal tunnel syndrome isn't always that easy to treat, especially if you've had symptoms for a long time. Even if the nerve isn't permanently damaged, scar tissue can form inside the carpal tunnel and permanently narrow the opening. When that happens, about the only long-term solution is to have surgery to remove tissue and relieve pressure on the nerve.

For most people, however, it never goes that far. There are a number of easier ways to reduce painful nerve pressure and keep the problem from getting worse.

Heed the pain. Don't make the mistake of ignoring tingling or other symptoms in your hands or wrists. Stop what

---

Instant Ahhh…

Sink the Pain

A fast way to ease carpal tunnel flare-ups is to flood your wrists with cold water, says Kevin Conner, N.D. Go to the kitchen or bathroom sink, turn on the cold water tap, and let the water flow over your wrists for 5 to 10 minutes. "It's the quickest, easiest way I know to reduce pain and inflammation," says Dr. Conner.

---

you're doing immediately. It may be that a few days' rest will reduce the internal swelling, though it's more likely that you'll have to give your hands a few weeks off—perhaps longer. It's worth doing because inflammation and swelling in the wrist can cause permanent nerve damage if it isn't stopped early enough. If the tingling continues, check with your doctor.

Make a splint decision. One of the best remedies for carpal tunnel pain is to wear a splint that holds your wrist straight while you work. A splint prevents your wrist from flexing and putting unnecessary pressure on the nerve, explains Kevin Conner, N.D., a naturopathic physician and faculty member at Bastyr University near Seattle. "Have it fitted by a doctor or physical therapist," he adds. Over-the-counter splints rarely fit correctly. A splint that's too loose won't work very well, and one that's too tight could cause circulation problems.

Sleep on it. Don't use your splint only when you're working. It's also important to wear it while you sleep. Most people sleep with their wrists bent at an angle at least some of the time, and this can aggravate carpal tunnel problems even while they're snoozing.

Take pineapple in a pill. An enzyme called bromelain, which is extracted from pineapples, works

A Berry Good Cure

Birds sit for hours with their talons wrapped around small branches, but as far as we know, they don't get "carpal claw syndrome." What are they doing that we aren't?

It may be that they fill up on berries. Blueberries, blackberries, strawberries, and boysenberries all contain natural compounds called bioflavonoids, which are nature's remedies for pain and inflammation. "Eating your fill of berries every day will help the healing process," says Kevin Conner, N.D.

as a natural anti-inflammatory, and it's unlikely to cause the stomach upset that people sometimes get when they take aspirin or ibuprofen, says Dr. Conner. You'd have to eat a luau's worth of pineapples to get enough bromelain, so it makes more sense to use a supplement. Take 375 milligrams three times daily on an empty stomach, he advises. If you take bromelain with meals, your digestive juices will make the enzyme ineffective.

Bet on B$_6$. It doesn't work for everyone, but there's some evidence that vitamin B$_6$ improves nerve function and can help reduce carpal tunnel pain. The usual advice is to take 50 milligrams twice daily, but ask your doctor if it's safe to take this large a dose. High amounts of B$_6$ may cause serious, nerve-damaging side effects.

Heat it up, cool it down. You don't want to depend on hot packs when you have carpal tunnel syndrome, because heat can increase swelling. What you can do, however, is combine heat and cold. This approach, called contrast hydrotherapy, helps reduce swelling and flushes pain-causing toxins from the area.

Start by applying a hot, moist washcloth to your wrist. Hold it there for 3 minutes, then replace it with a cold pack or a washcloth soaked in cold water. Leave it in place for 30 seconds, then switch back to heat. You can repeat this cycle three or four times, always ending with the cold treatment. Use it several times a day until the discomfort is gone.

Stretch, but don't strain. It's hard to reverse carpal tunnel syndrome once you have it. That's why doctors stress the preventive approach. Before working with your hands—typing, operating a cash register, or working in the yard, for example—take a few minutes to warm up with some gentle stretching. Here's one of the best wrist-protecting stretches. Extend

HOT

COLD

your arm in front of you with your palm facing down. Slowly raise your hand so your wrist flexes upward. Keep going until you feel a good stretch, then bend your hand down for another stretch. Do this at least a dozen times, up and down, and repeat it several times a day.

Hold your wrist like a lady. This isn't meant to sound sexist. The Asian body-movement discipline known as tai chi includes a wrist position called beautiful lady's wrist. "It means always keeping your wrist in a neutral position, in line with your arm," says Dr. Conner. In practical terms, it requires holding your wrist in positions that don't require upward or downward flexing. When you're typing, for example, keep your wrists as straight as possible. It's a lot easier to do this if you use an ergonomically designed keyboard to keep your wrists in the proper position.

Beat the bloat. Carpal tunnel syndrome tends to get a lot worse if you're retaining more water than you should, says Dr. Conner. It makes sense, because all that water has to go somewhere, and some of it winds up in tissues in your wrist. The more the tissues swell, the more likely you are to experience carpal tunnel pain. This is why women often develop symptoms during pregnancy or even at the bloating stage of their menstrual cycles.

There are a number of herbal treatments for easing water retention—dandelion and parsley are two of the main ones—but don't use them without checking with a doctor. Water retention is a sign that something's wrong with your body's natural balance, and you'll want to correct the underlying problem rather than merely treating the symptom.

Frozen Shoulder

Loosen Up Your Swing

Your shoulder isn't just something to shrug with or to let people cry on. It lets you reach out and touch the world. Think about it. Even if your arm's in fine shape, there's no way you can grab a bottle of aspirin from the cabinet, raise a spoon to your mouth, or throw a stick for your dog if your shoulder won't move.

It doesn't happen often, but sometimes your shoulder can almost completely lock in place. Doctors call this adhesive capsulitis, but people who have experienced it usually call it frozen shoulder.

COLD SHOULDER

A frozen shoulder isn't literally frozen, of course, but it may as well be. The problem usually starts with an injury—from throwing a softball too hard, for example, or pulling too many weeds in the garden. As happens with most injuries, you'll probably have pain, inflammation, and tissue damage within your shoulder. During the healing process, scar tissue may form in the wrong places. As a result, you'll lose some of the natural free movement of your muscles and tendons. The more extensive the "freeze," the more limited your range of motion—and the more painful your shoulder is likely to be.

A GRADUAL THAW

It's always a good idea to see your doctor if your shoulder stays frozen for more than a few days. You may need steroid injections or even surgery to eliminate the pain and restore the full range of movement. In most cases, however, a frozen shoulder will return to normal on its own.

The bad news is that the recovery can take anywhere from a month to a year. Can you imagine going an entire year without being able to move your shoulder normally? I certainly can't. When I asked doctors if there was any way to reduce pain and help hasten the healing process, I was surprised to discover how many options there are. The next time your shoulder freezes—or if you want to make sure it never does again—here are some expert tips that will help.

Cool it quickly. You already know that cold is among the best treatments for easing pain and stiffness. What you may not know is that it's essential to apply it immediately—preferably within minutes of the time you first notice discomfort. The quick application of cold

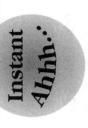

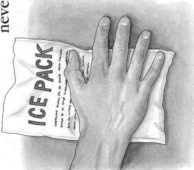

Instant Ahhh...

Ease the Pain with Arnica

If you've had a shoulder injury, you may be able to keep your shoulder from freezing just by using arnica, a traditional herbal remedy, at the first hint of pain. Go to the health food store and buy arnica gel. Apply it liberally to the sore area several times a day. It helps shoulder damage—or any other kind of skin or muscle injury—heal much more quickly.

can dramatically reduce swelling and tissue damage, which in turn can keep your shoulder from locking down entirely.

When you first notice shoulder pain, put a cold pack or a washcloth filled with ice cubes right where it hurts. Apply cold for 20 to 30 minutes every few hours for the first day or two. It acts as a local anesthetic, reduces blood flow, and helps prevent tissue-damaging inflammation.

Get the joint swinging. You may not have your full range of motion, but make the most of whatever you do have. Immobilizing an injured shoulder or wearing a sling makes the problem even worse. It also weakens your shoulder muscles. Don't do anything that aggravates the pain, but do use your shoulder to the degree that the injury permits during recovery.

"You want to get an injured shoulder moving, even just a little. Moving it is what increases your range of motion," says Sean Sapunar, N.D., a naturopathic physician and clinical faculty member at the Bastyr Center for Natural Health near Seattle. Even if your shoulder is so bad that you can't raise your arm, you can

---

Soothing Salves

FOR PEAT'S SAKE

Even if your gardening expertise is limited to raising houseplants, you probably have some peat around the house. It's a soil additive that grabs and holds onto moisture. In a slightly different form, it's also a good remedy for a frozen shoulder because it contains dozens of substances with anti-inflammatory properties. "I've seen peat therapy do incredible things for people in pain," says Sean Sapunar, N.D.

You can buy peat cream at health food stores. Apply it to the injured area and cover it with a warm, moist washcloth. Leave it on for 20 to 30 minutes and repeat the treatment several times a day. Keep in mind that peat cream can feel very warm on the skin, so be prepared to wash it off if the area gets too hot.

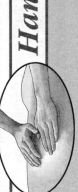

STRETCHING

still stretch and exercise it by letting it hang down and moving it in a figure-eight pattern, for example.

Stretch it out. Here's a simple stretching exercise that will help unlock your shoulder and get it moving normally again. Stand with your arms at your sides with your palms facing in. Raise your arms slowly to the sides and rotate them so your thumbs are pointing down and your palms are facing back. Repeat the exercise until your arms feel tired.

Don't try to raise your arms more than halfway; stop as soon as you notice pain. As the days (or weeks) go by, you'll find that you can gradually move your arms farther.

Let your fingers do the crawling. Here's another stretch that can increase your shoulder's range of motion. Stand a little less than arm's length away from a wall, with your fingers barely touching it. Slowly move your hand up the wall, letting your fingers do most of the work.

Swallow a pain pill. Over-the-counter analgesics help con-

Healing Hands

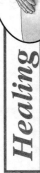

A massage is a good way to ease a frozen shoulder, but only if it's the right kind of massage. A technique called cross-fiber friction, in which the muscles are rubbed against the "grain" instead of lengthwise, can help break up scar tissue attachments, or adhesions, between muscle groups. It's these adhe-sions that often contribute to pain and stiffness.

"Just apply a little pressure with the side of your hand as you slide it across the muscle," says Sean Sapunar, N.D. You may find that it's easier, as well as a lot more pleasant, to have someone else to do the honors.

trol pain, but that's not all they do. Aspirin, ibuprofen, and similar drugs (but not acetaminophen) reduce the inflammation that can cause a frozen shoulder.

Slap on some oil. A castor-oil pack is a traditional remedy to soothe and heal injured muscles, and it's easy to use.

Just apply some castor oil to the injured area and cover it with plastic wrap. Then apply a warm compress or a heating pad set on low. The heat will help the oil penetrate the skin, where it will ease pain as well as stiffness. Leave the pack on for 20 to 30 minutes, then wash away the oil. Repeat the treatment several times a day.

Strengthen damaged cartilage. Two over-the-counter supplements, glucosamine and chondroitin, stimulate the production of cartilage, the connective tissue that's often damaged when you have a frozen shoulder. You can buy combination supplements that contain both of these compounds. Many experts recommend 500 milligrams three times a day.

Sip a fish. Fish is loaded with essential fatty acids that reduce inflammation and help repair cells that have been damaged by injuries. Since it's not always easy to eat enough fish to get healing amounts of these oils, an easy alternative is to take 1 to 3 teaspoons of fish oil daily.

Rotator Cuff Tear

Soothe That Shoulder!

I avoided most high school sports because I was nervous about anything that required me to interact with fast-moving objects. I stuck with track and cross-country running because I was reasonably sure that even with my poor coordination skills, I could still put one foot in front of the other.

My friend Matt, though, was a natural athlete. No one was surprised when he joined the baseball team and eventually became a pitcher. What did surprise me was the toll that pitching took on his throwing arm. It wasn't uncommon for him to ice his aching arm for hours after a tough game, and he always seemed to have shoulder pain, even when baseball season was over. I don't know for sure if he had a rotator cuff tear, but now that I think back, it sure sounds like he did.

TOO MUCH MOTION

The term *rotator cuff* refers to the group of tendons that surround your shoulder joint. Injuries are usually caused by the long-term wear and tear of repetitive motions, such as throwing a baseball for hours a day or painting houses year after year. Rotator cuff problems can also occur in an instant, such as when you lift a heavy suitcase from the ground into the trunk of a car.

Persistent shoulder pain or stiffness isn't always caused by a rotator cuff injury, but that should be your first suspect. Here's a quick test: If the pain gets worse when you raise your arm over your head or continues even when you're not using your shoulder, a rotator cuff injury is probably to blame.

SHRUG IT OFF

Your shoulder is a complicated piece of real estate, and all sorts of things can go wrong. If you have pain that lasts more than a week or two, you should see a doctor. You could have arthritis or another painful condition that could get worse without proper treatment. If it turns out that you've injured your rotator cuff, rest easy. It sounds like a serious diagnosis, but in nearly all cases, it will heal on its own without medical or surgical treatment. The pain won't go away overnight, however. Plan on giving your shoulder plenty of TLC for at least three to six weeks. Here's what doctors advise.

Ice it fast. Ice is the best treatment for joint and muscle injuries, but it has to be applied quickly, within the first 24 to 48 hours, to be effective. Icing the sore area right away will

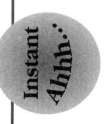

Instant Ahhh...

Chinese Heat

A quick way to ease shoulder pain and restore muscle flexibility is to apply Chinese balm several times a day. "Tiger Balm and White Flower Analgesic Balm are two of my favorites," says John Nowicki, N.D. The balms, available in health food stores, contain ingredients that give a sensation of heat, which penetrates deeply into the injured area.

Soothing Salves

TURMERIC TAMES PAIN

Turmeric does more than add a beautiful golden tint to stews and rice dishes; it's also a great remedy for shoulder pain. It contains a chemical compound that warms the joint and interrupts pain signals on their journey from the shoulder to the brain. Make a paste by adding a little water to dried turmeric. Mix well, then smear it on the injured area, cover with a moist cloth, and leave it on for about 20 minutes.

reduce swelling and inflammation. That's important because if inflammation isn't stopped, it can cause additional tissue damage.

As soon as you notice any shoulder pain, apply an ice pack—or ice cubes wrapped in a washcloth or small towel—to the area for about 30 minutes. Repeat the treatment every few hours for at least 24 hours.

Switch to heat. Applying heat to an injured area right away can increase swelling or internal bleeding. Using it a day or two after the pain starts, however, will relax the muscle, loosen the joint, and help prevent painful spasms. Hold a heating pad (set on low) or a warm compress against your shoulder for 15 to 20 minutes at a time whenever it starts feeling stiff. Just this short period of heat treatment can leave your shoulder feeling loose and relaxed for hours.

Take a painkiller. If you have any over-the-counter analgesics in the house, now's a good time to break them out.

Ibuprofen and aspirin are good choices because they inhibit the activity of prostaglandins, chemicals that cause pain and swelling after injuries. Acetaminophen is also good, although it has less effect than aspirin or ibuprofen on swelling.

Engage some enzymes. If taken within 24 hours after the pain starts, supplements that contain natural proteolytic enzymes can cut the healing time in half. "The sooner you take them after the injury, the more benefit they'll bring," says John Nowicki, N.D., a naturopathic physician in Issaquah, Washington.

Health food stores stock a variety of these enzymes. If you read the labels, you'll see ingredients such as bromelain, papain, trypsin, chymotrypsin, amylase, lipase, and cellulase. They all work equally well to ease shoulder pain. The usual dose is one to three capsules three times daily for 5 to 10 days. Don't take them with food, though; the increase in digestive juices after eating will deactivate the enzymes.

Pass the pepper. Creams or gels made with capsaicin, the hot chemical in red pepper, are good for rotator cuff injuries, says Dr. Nowicki. Capsaicin is a counterirritant, which means that it helps deplete the area of a body chemical called substance P, which transmits pain signals.

Capsaicin products are available at drugstores. Be careful not to get the cream near your eyes or any areas of broken skin, and wash your hands thoroughly after using it.

Make like the Three Wise Men. Gold and myrrh weren't the only precious gifts the kings carried to the infant Jesus. They also brought frankincense, an herb that can go a long way toward easing shoulder pain. Taken internally, it blocks a body enzyme that contributes to pain and tenderness. If you'd like to consider it, look for frankincense capsules, available at health food stores, that contain 60 percent boswellic acid, the active ingredient. Follow the package directions.

Stock up on supplements. Your body will need extra nutrients to rebuild damaged shoulder tissues and promote healing. Consider the following supplements.

- Vitamin C: 3,000 to 6,000 milligrams daily (unless you have stomach or kidney problems), divided into several doses. It helps the body rebuild tendons and other connective tissues.

- Glucosamine: 500 milligrams three times daily. It stimulates the production of cartilage.

- Fish oil: 1 to 3 teaspoons daily. It decreases inflammation and stabilizes cell membranes that may have been damaged by the injury.

Exercise the pain away. Exercise isn't appealing when you have a damaged rotator cuff, but it's essential for strengthening the muscles and helping the healing process. Here's a good one to start with: Lie facedown on a table with your sore arm and shoulder hanging over the edge. Rotate your shoulder and slowly raise your arm until it's even with your shoulder, with the palm of your hand facing down. Lower your arm slowly, then repeat the exercise until the muscle has had a good workout.

Take up arms. Stand straight with your arms at your sides, palms facing in. Slowly raise your arms to the sides, rotating them so your thumbs point down and your palms face back. Continue until you've had enough.

Use it, don't abuse it. Once the initial pain is gone, keeping your shoulder active will help it heal faster, but you need to be careful not to reinjure the damaged tendons. You should avoid any activity that causes pain, but anything else is okay. Just to be safe, though, don't lift anything over your head until your doctor says that your shoulder is fully recovered.

Smashed Fingers and Hammered Thumbs

Take the Ouch Out of Accidents

We put our precious fingers in harm's way all the time. Closing a car door, forcing open a stuck window, and moving furniture are just a few of the everyday tasks in which even the slightest miscalculation can result in a painful accident.

Not too long ago, for instance, two of my friends tried to move a heavy bookcase across the room—with the books still on the shelves. They bent down, slipped their fingers underneath, and hoisted with all their might. They managed to raise the monster about an inch off the floor before they realized they were overmatched. The bookcase slammed down—and one of the fingers involved didn't get out of the way fast enough. OUCH!

A SMASH HIT

When something clobbers one of your fingers—a poorly aimed hammer, for example—the impact crushes small blood

Pain in Your Shoulders, Arms, and Hands

vessels under the skin. It's the under-the-surface bleeding that causes those blue-black bruises that can last for weeks. The swelling usually goes away in a few days, but the area can stay tender for a long time. Plus, you may have a torn nail to deal with. It's no laughing matter.

FINGER TIPS

Unless the nail is torn or pulled loose, or the injury has left an open wound, you don't have to get too worked up over a smashed finger or hammered thumb. It will hurt like the dickens, but it will heal quite nicely on its own. The one exception is if you can't move the finger or thumb a day or two after the accident, or if the digit is locked into an abnormal position. It's possible that you fractured a bone, and you'll need x-rays to find out how serious the damage is. Otherwise, a few simple home remedies will reduce the pain and help the injury heal more quickly. Here are some suggestions.

Grab a cold one. The sooner you're able to get ice on that bruised finger or thumb, the sooner the swelling will go down—and the less pain you'll have in the long run. Put some ice cubes in a washcloth and wrap your fingers around it, or hold the ice on the injured area for 15 to 20 minutes. Repeat the treatment every 2 hours for the first 12 to 24 hours. Cold slows bleeding inside the skin, which will help reduce bruising and may also keep the finger from

---

Soothing Salves

PARSLEY POWER

Parsley is among the best herbs for banishing bruises because it helps remove excess moisture from the body. If you've smashed your finger or thumb, chop some fresh parsley as finely as possible, add a little water, and let stand for about 20 minutes. Then apply the paste to the injured area and cover it with a bandage, says Priscilla Natanson, N.D. If you don't have fresh parsley, it's fine to use the dried form, although it probably isn't as effective, she adds.

swelling to twice its normal size.

Follow up with heat. Once the swelling has gone down—it usually takes about 24 to 48 hours—apply heat. You can rest your hand on a heating pad set on low or wrap the finger or thumb in a washcloth moistened with warm water. Heat increases circulation, speeds the flow of healing nutrients to the area, and helps flush away pain-causing toxins.

Reach for the right bottle. A lot of people automatically take aspirin when they're hurting, but that's the worst thing to do when you've smashed a finger. Aspirin "thins" the blood and increases bleeding and bruising. Ibuprofen or acetaminophen is better. Both work just as well as aspirin to ease pain, but they're less likely to cause bleeding under the skin.

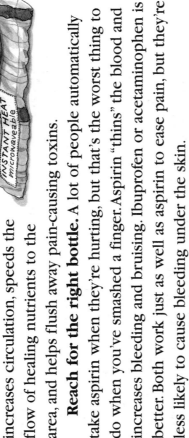

Wrap and raise. That's the advice of Priscilla Natanson, N.D., a naturopathic physician in Plantation, Florida. Wrapping the area snugly with a bandage prevents injured blood vessels from bleeding too much. Elevating it as much as possible puts gravity on your side. "There will be less pain and bruising when the blood has to run uphill. "Pressure and gravity keep the damaged tissue from swelling with fluid," explains Dr. Natanson.

Just don't get carried away when wrapping the injury, she adds. You want the bandage to be tight enough to slow bleeding, but not so tight that it cuts off circulation. It should be

It's an Emergency!

It doesn't happen often, but bashing a finger or thumb can sometimes push it out of joint. If the digit is stuck at an odd angle, don't try to reposition it. The pain will drive you crazy, and you could push it into the wrong position. Go to an emergency room right away. The sooner the digit is readjusted to its normal position, the more quickly the injury will heal.

just loose enough to allow you to wiggle one of your fingers underneath it.

Clean the scene. Infection is the main risk when an injury has broken the skin. Before wrapping the digit, clean the wound thoroughly with soap and water. Splash on some hydrogen peroxide if you have any in your medicine cabinet. The bubbling action will help float dirt or other debris out of the wound, and it has a mild disinfectant action.

Splash on St. John's wort.

Herbalists often recommend it for depression, but it's also helpful when a finger or thumb has been on the receiving end of something painful. "Tincture of St. John's wort is wonderful for wounds," says Dr. Natanson. Tinctures are alcohol-based solutions, which will kill any germs that happen to be lurking inside the wound, she adds. You can buy St. John's wort tincture at a health food store.

Protect the nail. Nothing is more painful than a torn nail. Nothing is riskier, either, because loose nails tend to snag on just about everything, which can make the original injury a lot worse. There's also a high risk of infection. So wrap the area carefully in a bandage and keep it protected until the nail grows back.

If the Skin Is Broken...

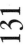

The herbs comfrey and calendula help broken skin heal more quickly. Get a cream containing one or both of these herbs at a health food store and slather it generously on the injured area, advises Priscilla Natanson, N.D. You can also use dried herbs by crumbling them into a powder and adding just enough water to make a paste. Spread it on and wrap the area with a moist cloth. Keep the injury covered for a day or two, changing the poultice every few hours.

Tennis Elbow

Take a Swing at Pain

One summer, my sister and I, along with some other kids from the neighborhood, took tennis lessons. A few mornings a week, the bunch of us would head over to the local park, where a college kid named Greg tried to teach us to knock the ball back and forth without hitting ourselves in the head.

I realize now that the whole thing was probably a scheme by our parents to get us out of the house for a few hours. At the time, though, I learned two things about tennis: First, hitting the ball over the net was a key strategy I had little hope of mastering, and second, if you swung the racket the wrong way, you could end up with a horrible affliction called tennis elbow.

The way Greg described it, tennis elbow was nastier and more painful than having your arm gnawed off by Bobby Riggs.

Soothing Salves

CALENDULA CREAM

Want fast, natural relief from an ouchy elbow? Grab a jar of calendula cream, available at health food stores, and rub $1/2$ teaspoon into the muscles surrounding your elbow. It can reduce the ache and help you heal more quickly.

TROUBLE AROUND THE BEND

It's true that playing tennis can give you tennis elbow, but there are plenty of other ways to get it, too. Hammering nails, carrying heavy suitcases, lifting a crying child several times a day—anything that requires repeated use of your elbow joint can overtax one of the many muscles attached there. Here's what happens: The muscles or tendons become inflamed, causing pain that can range from a dull throb at your elbow to an ache that radiates down your arm. Often, the pain starts off as a minor twinge, and it may or may not flare into major agony. It all depends on what you do next.

STRAIGHT ADVICE

In extreme cases, tennis elbow will go away only if you take powerful drugs to reduce the inflammation. Occasionally, it's necessary to have steroid injections or physical therapy to get things working properly again. Unless your symptoms persist for a few weeks or more or steadily get worse, you can almost always treat tennis elbow at home simply by putting down the tennis racket (or whatever it was that caused the pain). In the meantime, here are a few quick ways to reduce the discomfort and help the muscles and tendons heal more quickly.

Ice it right away. As soon as the pain starts, reach for an ice pack (with the other arm). You can't beat ice for reducing inflammation and numbing pain. For the first few days after the injury, apply it for 20 minutes at a time every few hours.

Brace yourself. Since moving your elbow too much is what causes tennis elbow, it makes sense that keeping it still will help it get better. You may want to pick up an arm brace at a drugstore or medical supply store. It will protect the injured

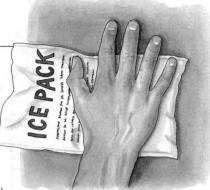

joint and prevent it from moving in an inappropriate (and painful) direction.

Play a waiting game. You shouldn't rush back into action as soon as your pain is gone. Wait a few days or a week to be sure you're really better, advises Kevin Conner, N.D., a naturopathic physician and faculty member at Bastyr University near Seattle. "The tissue's still healing," he says. "You don't want to aggravate it."

Eat like a bear. Essential fatty acids, especially the omega-3 fatty acids in cold-water fish (salmon, tuna, and mackerel, for example), help suppress the inflammation that causes the pain. You can also get plenty of omega-3's by eating a few tablespoons of ground flaxseed or taking a few capsules of fish oil or flaxseed oil.

Try the tropical cure. Pineapple does more than add delicious sweetness to fresh fruit platters. It's also rich in bromelain, a substance that acts as a natural painkiller, says Dr. Conner. In fact, bromelain has been shown to reduce the swelling around muscles and tendons that causes the pain of tennis elbow. You can't get healing amounts of bromelain by eating fresh pineapple, however. A better approach is to take

Healing Hands

A massage always feels good, but a special technique called cross-fiber friction is the best thing for tennis elbow, says Kevin Conner, N.D. When you rub the muscles across the fibers, rather than lengthwise, it helps relax muscle spasms and breaks up scar tissue that may have formed between muscle groups. Focus on the muscles above and below the joint. For extra relief, follow each massage session by applying cold to the area, Dr. Conner advises.

supplements; the usual dose is 375 milligrams three times a day on an empty stomach. Don't take them with meals, because your digestive juices destroy the active ingredient.

Feel berry better. Dark berries, such as blueberries, blackberries, and boysenberries, contain natural chemicals called bioflavonoids that relieve pain and inflammation. It's also a good idea to eat plenty of other fruits and vegetables while you're healing. They'll pump even more bioflavonoids into your system.

Listen to your body. You probably remember this old joke: A patient says to his doctor, "It hurts when I do this," and the doctor says, "Well, don't do that." Okay, it's a groaner, but there's a lot of truth behind it. "The single best thing you can do is find the movements that cause or aggravate the injury and then quit doing them," says Dr. Conner. Pain from tennis elbow tends to be very specific: It hurts when you move your arm one way, and it doesn't hurt when you move it a different way. Limit your movements to the non-painful ones, and let the healing begin.

Get bent. Some slow, gentle stretching will help your aggrieved elbow heal and strengthen. First, extend your arm straight in front of you, palm down, and slowly bend

Rebuild with Protein

When you're recovering from tennis elbow, you need a lot of protein, the nutrient that your body uses to repair muscle damage. The usual rule is to get 0.8 gram of protein for each kilogram of body weight. Here's an easy way to figure out how much you need: Divide your body weight by 2.2 (there are 2.2 pounds per kilogram), then multiply that number by 0.8 to get your daily target for protein. Thus, if you weigh 150 pounds, you'll need 54 grams of protein. That's roughly the amount you'd get in a cup of tuna salad, a cup of long-grain white rice, and a cup of milk.

Tennis Anyone?

Although any kind of repetitive elbow movements can trigger tennis elbow, quite often the culprit is (no surprise) tennis. I asked a few tennis pros what players should do to prevent it. Here's their advice.

Examine your backhand. It's the stroke that usually triggers tennis elbow. It may be worth having a tennis pro watch while you swing in order to refine your stroke. You could also switch to a two-handed backhand, which puts less stress on your elbow.

Change rackets. If your racket is too big, you have to grip harder to hold it, and the extra tension can lead to tennis elbow. Strings that are too tight are also a notorious elbow threat, because they transmit harder jolts into your arm.

Call it quits for a while. This could be the best way to save your game. If you push past the pain, the injury will only get worse, so give yourself a few weeks or even a few months away from the court. A long recovery period may be all you need to keep your elbow healthy.

your wrist so the back of your hand moves toward you. Then lower your hand and flex your wrist so that your fingers point down.

You can do a similar exercise with your elbow. Hold your arm out, palm up, and slowly bend your elbow so your palm moves toward you. Repeat both stretches a few times a day, but quit if they cause real pain. It's okay for stretches to be slightly uncomfortable, but they shouldn't hurt. If they do, you're overdoing it.

STRETCHING

Wrist Sprain or Strain

Take Away the Pain

I'm not a big fan of winter. It's not so much the cold I dislike, or the perpetual darkness, or the lack of baseball. What I really hate is the ice. As early as October, I haul out a huge bag of rock salt and keep it right next to the front door, so it will be handy at the first sign of freezing temperatures.

I don't believe for a minute that Old Man Winter is out to get me personally, but there's a reason for my caution. A few years ago, I slipped on the ice-coated concrete in front of my garage. I didn't break any bones, but when I fell, one of my wrists bent farther than I ever thought it could. The result was a nasty sprain—one that kept hurting long after the ice melted and baseball season was under way again.

MORE THAN A SLAP ON THE WRIST

We tend to use the words *strain* and *sprain* interchangeably, but there is a difference. A sprain is an injury to the ligaments, the tough tissues that connect bones to bones. You tend to get sprains when a joint is pushed beyond its usual range of motion. A strain, on the other hand, is a muscle injury. More specifically, it means that some of the tiny fibers that make up muscles have been stretched or even torn.

The reason it's so hard to differentiate strains from sprains is that the symptoms—mainly swelling and pain—are nearly identical. Even your doctor would be hard-pressed to tell the difference—not that it matters all that much. The treatments for sprains and strains, like the symptoms, are pretty much the same.

WRIST RELIEF

Any time you've hurt your wrist and the pain doesn't start to get better within about a week or is really intense, get in touch with a doctor. It's always possible that a ligament or tendon (the tissue that connects bone to muscle) has been completely torn. In most cases, however, strains and sprains get better on their own. You'll probably notice quite an improvement within a few days if you follow these helpful tips.

Put your trust in RICE. Not the kind you eat, but a classic technique for treating sprains and strains. It stands for rest, ice, compression, and elevation, and it's the most effective way to reduce swelling as well as pain. As soon as you hurt your wrist:

• Rest the injured area. Don't put any kind of pressure on your wrist—and by all means, stop any-

---

soothing Salves

GRAB THE TIGER

A Chinese herbal salve called Tiger Balm, available in health food stores, reduces muscle stiffness by transmitting heat through the skin and into the injured tissues underneath, says John Nowicki, N.D. You can apply it several times a day.

R.I.C.E.

thing you've been doing that may have injured it in the first place.

• Ice your wrist for 24 hours. Apply a cold pack—a bag of frozen vegetables will work in a pinch—for about 20 minutes every few hours.

• Compress your wrist by wrapping it with a bandage. It should be snug, but not so tight that it cuts off circulation. If you can just barely slip a pencil between your wrist and the bandage, it's about right.

• Elevate your wrist. It should be level with or higher than your heart. This decreases swelling by causing fluids to drain away from the injured tissue.

Wait for the heat. People instinctively reach for the heating pad when they've hurt their wrists, but it's the wrong thing to do, at least right away. Heat stimulates circulation, which can bring more fluids to the injured area. After 24 to 48 hours, when the initial recovery phase is over, go ahead and heat the area with a warm compress or a heating pad set on low. The heat will flush away pain-causing chemicals and reduce stiffness.

Healing *Hands*

Tennis, anyone? You don't need fancy rehabilitation equipment when you've hurt your wrist; a tennis ball will do the trick. Simply take a few minutes each day to squeeze the ball as hard as you can for a second, relax, then squeeze it again, suggests John Nowicki, N.D. Repeat the exercise about 10 times. It shouldn't cause more than a tiny amount of pain, he adds. If it does, your wrist still has some recovering to do, so take it easy.

Put enzymes to work. Painkillers aren't the only pills to pop when you've hurt your wrist. Health food stores sell a variety of enzymes—bromelain, papain, and trypsin, to name just a few—that can cut healing time in half if you take them within the first 24 hours after an injury, says John Nowicki, N.D., a naturopathic physician in Issaquah, Washington. The recommended dose is one to three capsules three times daily for 5 to 10 days. Don't take them with food, however, as your digestive juices will make the enzymes ineffective.

Fill up on fish oil. Actually, all you need is 1 to 3 tablespoons daily. Fish oil is loaded with essential fatty acids that reduce inflammation and help injured tissues heal more quickly.

Take plenty of vitamin C. The Daily Value for this important nutrient is 60 milligrams, but you need a lot more—about 3,000 milligrams daily—following a wrist strain or sprain. Vitamin C mops up harmful body molecules that are produced in huge amounts following strains and sprains, and it promotes the repair of con-

Stretch Away

Muscles, tendons, and ligaments naturally get tight after injuries. That's what causes a lot of the pain, and it increases the risk of additional injuries. Wrist stretches are the best way to stay flexible—and you don't even need a yoga mat to do them. Just hold your arm in front of you and slowly flex your wrist all the way down. Hold for a moment, then gently bend it all the way up. Repeat this sequence about 10 times, rest for a while, then do it again.

STRETCHING

nective tissues. If you have kidney or stomach problems, however, don't take high amounts of vitamin C. Also, to prevent stomach upset or diarrhea, divide the dose and take smaller amounts at different times of the day. Taking it with food is also helpful.

Bend while you're on the mend. Don't baby your wrist after a strain or sprain, says Dr. Nowicki. By all means, rest the area for a few days, but resume your normal activities as soon as possible. As long as you can move your wrist with little or no pain, you'll get better faster if you keep the joint in motion.

Build the muscles. Doctors used to advise people to totally rest their wrists—sometimes for weeks—following minor strains and sprains. They now know that exercising the muscles promotes healing and helps prevent future injuries. As soon as the worst of the pain is gone, do the following workouts. But remember: If the pain gets worse while doing the exercises, take a day or two off before attempting them again.

• Find a large can of soup or vegetables that weighs about a pound. Holding the can, lay your forearm on a table with your palm up and your wrist and hand hanging over the edge. Bend your wrist and slowly raise and lower your hand about 10 times. Rest a minute, then do it again. Repeat the exercise once a day, every other day, until your wrist feels better.

• Using string, tie a 1-pound weight in the center of a broomstick so the weight hangs almost to the floor when you hold the stick at about chest height. Then hold the stick with both hands, palms facing down, and extend your arms. Using your wrists, wind the weight all the way up, then wind it down. Repeat the exercise once a day, every other day. To keep things interesting, change your hand position now and then: Have your palms facing down one time and up the next.

Pain in Your Chest

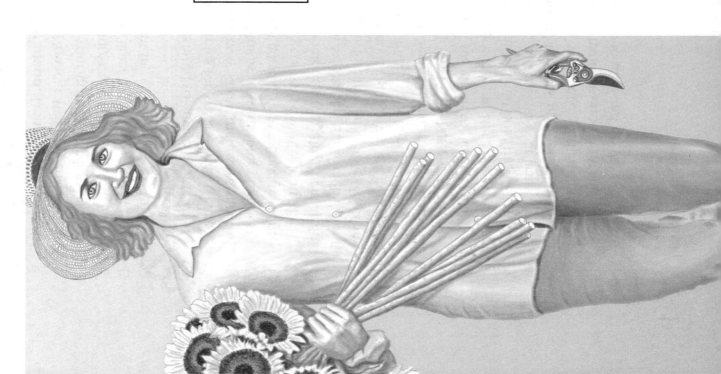

Angina
Breast Pain
Cough
Heartburn
Pneumonia

Angina

Healing Hints for Your Heart

My friend Joe's dad was worried when he started having intermittent chest pain, as anyone would be. But he put off going to the doctor, afraid of bad news and hoping the painful episodes would stop on their own. They didn't, of course, and after a few weeks, Joe convinced his father to have a checkup.

"When Dad finally did that, he ended up feeling so relieved," Joe says. His father found out that he didn't have to worry that he was having a heart attack every time his chest pain flared up. He had a condition that doctors call angina pectoris, and while it's a prelude to more serious problems, it's also a wake-up call to make changes for the better.

"Little by little, my dad changed his diet, changed his

It's an Emergency!

Although many people live with angina for decades, you should never take it for granted, especially if the pain comes on when you're not exerting yourself and doesn't stop when you rest. This is known as unstable angina, and it means you need emergency help because your coronary arteries may be almost totally blocked.

whole lifestyle," says Joe. "And now he's in better health than he's been in years."

THE HEART OF THE MATTER

Angina isn't a disease; it's a symptom that causes pressure or tightness in your chest—a squeezing pain that extends into your neck, jaw, or arm and sometimes even makes breathing difficult.

When your doctor talks to you about angina, you'll hear a lot of references to the coronary arteries, the blood vessels that carry oxygen-rich blood to your heart. If they are partly blocked by cholesterol and other fatty deposits, your heart doesn't get enough oxygen. You may not notice anything when you're resting, but when you're active, your heart needs more oxygen than usual. If it doesn't get enough, it lets you know with the sudden discomfort of angina pain.

MORE BLOOD, LESS DISCOMFORT

Angina is among the most serious symptoms you're ever likely to experience. It won't necessarily prevent you from living a full, active life, but it's definitely a warning—one that you have to take seriously in order to prevent a future heart attack.

See your doctor immediately if you have any kind of chest

A Cup of Comfort

Long before doctors developed nitroglycerine and other drugs for angina, herbalists were treating people with hawthorn. "I've had good results using it to prevent angina pain in my patients," says Andrew Parkinson, N.D. You can make hawthorn tea by steeping a tablespoon of the dried herb in a cup of boiling water for about 10 minutes. If you're taking any other drugs, check with your doctor before using hawthorn.

pain. You'll probably undergo a variety of tests to determine if the pain is caused by angina. If it is, your doctor will want to know which arteries are blocked and how severely. Angina that remains stable can often be managed with drugs that allow the coronary arteries to carry as much blood as they can handle. You may need surgery or angioplasty, procedures that help ensure that your heart gets enough blood to survive.

It's scary to know that your heart is in peril, but think of angina as a second chance: A warning and an opportunity to protect your heart before it's too late. Here's how.

Think like a tortoise, not a hare. Exercise is a double-edged sword for people with angina. Because it increases your heart's demand for oxygen, it can bring on an attack of angina. Over time, however, regular exercise improves blood flow and strengthens your heart. Nearly everyone with angina should be on some kind of exercise plan.

Definitely talk to your doctor to find out how much exercise you can safely do. Even if the angina is somewhat severe, your doctor will probably advise a daily program of mild exercise, such as walking or bicycling. You don't want to rush into anything. Like the fairytale tortoise who raced the hare, you're more likely to be a winner when you make slow and steady progress, says Andrew Parkinson, N.D., a naturopathic physician and faculty member at the Bastyr Center for Natural Health near Seattle.

Stop when it hurts. The quickest way to halt an angina attack is to stop what you're doing. The pain generally occurs during exertion, when your heart isn't getting enough blood and oxygen. As soon as you relax, your heart slows down and consumes less oxygen, and the pain will almost always go away within a few minutes.

Eat like a champion. Angina may have put your heart in a half-nelson, but the match isn't over yet. You can avoid getting pinned to the mat by switching to a heart-healthy diet, says Dr. Parkinson. "You want to avoid fried foods and animal fats, and replace them with fruits and vegetables," he says. This and other simple changes, such as getting more fiber in your diet and watching your weight, will lower cholesterol levels in your blood.

That way, your arteries won't become more clogged than they already are.

Here's another reason to eat a healthful diet: Fruits, vegetables, legumes, and other plant foods are rich in antioxidants, chemical compounds that help prevent cholesterol from sticking to artery walls.

Feed on fish. The natural oils in seafood have been shown to help elevate levels of high-density lipoprotein (HDL), the "good" cholesterol. This is important because HDL helps remove artery-clogging low-density lipoprotein (LDL), the "bad" cholesterol, from the blood.

Here's another reason to eat more fish: The natural oils, called omega-3 fatty acids, suppress the inflammation that contributes to the artery-clogging process. For optimal heart protection, eat fish three or four times a week or take a teaspoon of fish oil daily.

Put magnesium on the menu. This important mineral has a variety of critical functions, among them keeping the heart healthy and strong, says Dr. Parkinson. When you have angina, make an extra effort to get plenty of magnesium. He advises taking supplements; the recommended amount is 500 to 1,000 milligrams a day, divided into two or three doses. Check with your doctor first. This amount of magnesium may cause diarrhea in some people. If this occurs, reduce the dose.

Defend with C and E. Both of these vitamins are powerful antioxidants that help keep harmful oxygen molecules, called free radicals, from damaging artery walls. They also help prevent chemical changes in cholesterol that make it more likely to stick to artery walls.

Unless your doctor tells you otherwise, plan on taking at least 500 milligrams of vitamin C daily, preferably in two doses to prevent diarrhea or an upset stomach. For vitamin E, the recommended amount is 400 to 800 IU daily. Because angina is such a serious problem, be sure to let your doctor know that you're taking the supplements, since they can potentially interact with other drugs that you may be taking.

Put selenium in your sights. Many of us don't get nearly enough of this trace mineral. Like vitamins C and E, selenium is a powerful antioxidant that appears to play a role in keeping arteries clear. Nuts, whole grains, onions, and shellfish contain quite a bit of selenium, but you may want to take a supplement just to be safe, says Dr. Parkinson. He advises taking 200 micrograms daily.

Take a breath test. Does your breath have a strong garlic smell? It should if you have angina, because garlic

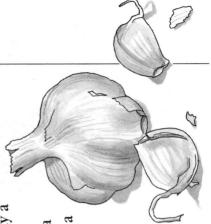

Grab Some Grapes

We can't be certain, but it seems likely that the ancient Romans didn't get angina very often. The credit may go to all those grapes they ate while lounging around the Forum. Grapes are loaded with pectin, a type of fiber that removes cholesterol from the blood. They're also rich in bioflavonoids, natural chemicals that have heart-protective effects. So take a tip from the Romans, and eat a bunch!

has been shown to lower cholesterol. The more raw or cooked garlic you eat, the more it will help. Just be sure to let the garlic rest on your cutting board for at least 10 minutes after you chop it. This allows the heart-healthy compounds to form.

If you prefer to get your garlic in capsule form, aim for 3 grams (3,000 milligrams) a day. "Even half a gram or a gram of garlic will be helpful," says Dr. Parkinson.

Don't forget the onions. Like garlic, they have a mild blood-thinning effect that can prevent blood clots—a serious risk for people with angina or other heart problems.

Eat alfalfa sprouts. Laboratory studies suggest that alfalfa sprouts may help dissolve the artery-blocking deposits that cause angina. Research hasn't been done with people, so it's not certain that alfalfa helps, but the evidence is compelling enough that you may want to give it a try. Two caveats: Since sprouts are known to frequently be contaminated with bacteria, buy from a local grower who takes care to keep his sprouts bacteria-free, and always wash them thoroughly.

Spice up your life. Keep some pungent ginger in the first row of your spice cabinet if you have angina. It contains chemical compounds that lower cholesterol and inhibit the formation of blood clots. Along with other spices, such as turmeric and red pepper, ginger also inhibits arterial inflammation that may lead to or worsen angina.

Breast Pain

Challenge Hormonal Changes

The women in my life aren't exactly shrinking violets. They talk about the kinds of things that would make the average man—and certainly me—blush. But even though I'm sure that they talk to each other about breast pain, I guess it's not the kind of thing that they share with their male friends. In fact, I never heard a thing about it until recently, and then I was shocked to discover how common it is.

Jana Nalbandian, N.D., a naturopathic physician and faculty member at Bastyr University near Seattle, told me that about half of women ages 25 to 50 sometimes experience breast pain during their monthly menstrual cycles. "It's probably the most common reason women go to their gynecologists," she says. After talking with Dr. Nalbandian, I asked some of my women friends if they suffered from breast pain and what they did about it.

Take a Poke at Relieving Pain

The herb pokeroot is an herbalist's favorite for relieving breast pain. Health food stores carry pokeroot tincture and oil. Whichever you use, put some on a cotton ball and rub it all over your breasts for relief.

Once again, I was surprised. Most said it bothered them sometimes, but none of them did anything about it because they thought there weren't any effective treatments. Nothing, however, could be further from the truth.

BLAME THOSE HORMONES

Breast pain that occurs in conjunction with a woman's period is known as cyclic mastitis. If the breasts also become lumpy or stiff, doctors may call it fibrocystic breast disease. But monthly breast pain isn't a disease in the usual sense. It's just an exaggeration of the normal changes that occur in the second half of a woman's cycle. "After ovulation, the breasts get ready for a possible pregnancy," Dr. Nalbandian explains. "There's increased circulation to the mammary glands, which causes fluid retention and possibly some discomfort."

While some fluid retention is normal, too much can be a problem. Women who produce large amounts of estrogen or who have breast tissue that's unusually sensitive to its effects tend to retain way too much fluid. Their breasts swell so much that they become tight and painful. At the same time, some of the breast glands fill up with fluid. At this point, they're called cysts, the lumps that women sometimes feel and that usually disappear after their periods. At least until the next cycle rolls around.

TAKE AWAY THE ACHE

Painful breasts aren't the easiest things to live with, but they're rarely something to panic about. Most women will do

---

Instant Ahhh...

Relax with Moist Heat

When your breasts are aching, you can get quick relief by draping them with a bath towel that's been soaked in hot water, says Jana Nalbandian, N.D. Heat promotes circulation and can help flush away excess fluid, she explains.

---

just fine once they discover a few useful tricks for dealing with the discomfort. This doesn't mean, however, that it's never a serious problem. "I once saw a woman whose breasts had become almost rock-solid," says Dr. Nalbandian. "The pain wasn't cyclical anymore—she had it all the time."

You'll want to stay in touch with your doctor and report any changes in your monthly symptoms. You'll definitely want to get help if the pain is severe or getting worse, affects only one breast, or is accompanied by signs of infection, such as redness, nipple discharge, a fever, or general aches. Otherwise, try these remedies to see which ones work best for you.

Eat light. I'm talking not about calories but about color: Some dark-colored foods seem to aggravate monthly breast pain. The worst offenders seem to be chocolate, black tea, cola, and coffee. "I advise women with breast pain to cut back on coffee, but because many of my patients live in Seattle (the corporate headquarters for Starbucks), that advice doesn't always go over too well," says Dr. Nalbandian.

Ease it with E. A number of scientific studies have shown that vitamin E supplements can help ease breast pain. The recommended dose is 400 to 800 IU daily. Be sure to get supplements that contain d-alpha toco-

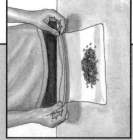

A Pain-Relieving Poultice

Long before there were doctors or corner drugstores, herbalists treated breast pain with a poultice made from green clay (available at health food stores) and cabbage. The mixture appears to soften breast tissue and reduce monthly breast lumps and discomfort. Combine 4 parts shredded cabbage with 1 part clay, mix well, and apply it to your breasts at bedtime. Cover the poultice with a moist cloth, then wrap a layer of gauze bandage around your body or wear a loose-fitting, soft cotton bra to hold it in place. Your breasts will probably feel a whole lot better in the morning.

pherols, which are thought to be more effective than other forms of vitamin E.

Fight back with omega-6.

Evening primrose is a traditional remedy for breast pain, and there's some evidence that it works. It's rich in omega-6 fatty acids, which inhibit the body's production of prostaglandins, natural chemicals that cause pain. Dr. Nalbandian advises women to take 1,500 milligrams of evening primrose oil in capsule form twice a day.

The problem with evening primrose oil supplements is that they're expensive. Some less costly supplements include borage oil, flaxseed oil, and black currant oil, all of which contain the beneficial omega-6 fatty acids.

Eat bright. Fruits and vegetables with bright red, yellow, or orange hues are loaded with beta-carotene, a plant pigment that appears to prevent breast pain in some women. Add as many to your diet as you can.

Keep fat to a minimum. You already know that dietary fat is loaded with calories. Here's one more reason to cut back: Red meat, rich desserts, fast-food burgers, and other foods high in fat stimulate estrogen production. High levels of estrogen can promote monthly breast pain, says Dr. Nalbandian.

Stay regular. Comfort isn't the only reason to eat more fiber, drink plenty of water,

---

Dig Dandelions!

Dandelion greens have a pleasant, slightly bitter taste, and they contain compounds that act as natural diuretics to reduce fluid retention. As long as you don't use pesticides on your lawn and you pick the leaves before the dandelion flowers bloom, you'll have the fixings for a fresh-tasting and wholesome salad that keeps breast pain at bay. Mix 'em up with spinach leaves, which also help reduce excess body fluid.

and exercise—the three best ways to prevent constipation. Having regular bowel movements also affects your body's estrogen supply.

Here's what happens: Your liver normally breaks down excess estrogen and ships it to your intestine, where it's carried out of your body in the stools. If you get constipated, however, bacteria in your colon can "reactivate" estrogen and return it to your bloodstream. "Studies show that women who have fewer than three bowel movements a week are more than four times as likely to have breast pain than those who stay regular," says Dr. Nalbandian.

Yogurt helps. It's loaded with beneficial organisms that slightly decrease the time that stools—and the estrogen they contain—stay in your intestine. Check the label to be sure the yogurt contains live cultures of *Lactobacillus acidophilus*, the helpful form of bacteria.

Toss the salt. It's especially important to eat fewer salty foods during the second half of your cycle, because less salt means less fluid retention and breast pain. "The best way to cut your salt intake is to eat more whole foods, such as fresh vegetables, fruits, and whole grains," Dr. Nalbandian says. Most of the salt in our diets comes from processed foods. When you replace them with fresh, wholesome foods, you'll almost automatically lower your salt intake to healthful levels.

Chase down chasteberry. "It's a classic herb for regulating hormones," says Dr. Nalbandian. She advises women with breast pain to take 250 milligrams daily. You can find the supplements at health food stores.

Wear a sports bra. Even if you're not an athlete, a sports bra is an important piece of equipment if your breasts are tender and sensitive. It will keep them in place so they don't rub against each other or your clothing. Also, avoid underwire bras, which can impede circulation.

Cough

Halt the Hack Attacks

Everyone coughs. Infants do it. Kids do it. The guy sitting in front of you at the movies does it. With all of this coughing going on, it's hardly surprising that drugstore aisles almost overflow with cough medicines. We'll do anything, it seems, to rid ourselves of this all-too-common nuisance.

NATURE'S PURGE

As annoying and uncomfortable as coughs can be, we should be glad for them. A strong cough is your body's equivalent of a bouncer. It tosses out all the potential troublemakers in the exclusive nightclub of your respiratory system.

Take germs. The longer they stay in your upper airways, the more likely they are to cause a lingering infection. Coughing is your body's way of getting rid of them before they settle in and leave you miserable with a cold or the flu. Coughs also help eliminate irritating substances, such as smoke, pollen, and clouds of cologne, from your lungs.

AXING THE HACKING

Many coughs are now-and-then affairs. Something tickles your airways, you cough, and that's the end of it. With upper respiratory infections, however, coughs really stick around, sometimes for a week or more—and all that hacking hurts.

Coughs can keep you up at night, and severe attacks have even left some people with broken ribs. If your cough really hurts or is getting worse instead of better after a week or so, check in with your doctor. You may have a hard-hitting infection that won't go away until you take antibiotics. Coughing can even be a symptom of heart disease, so don't wait too long before looking into it.

In the meantime, of course, you're going to need some relief. Over-the-counter cough suppressants aren't the best choice because they make it harder for your body to expel whatever's causing the trouble. What you want to do instead is soothe the irritated tissues in your throat and airways until the cough goes away naturally, plus boost your immune system so that any germs disappear as quickly as possible. Here's what may help.

Take thyme out. This familiar kitchen spice is great for fighting off a nagging cough. It inhibits bacteria and reduces cough-causing inflammation in your throat and other tissues. Thyme is also an effective expectorant: It makes mucus thinner, so you don't have to cough as hard to get rid of it. You can make thyme tea by steeping 1 teaspoon of dried herb in a cup of hot water. Or visit a health food store, pick up a bottle of thyme tincture, and take 10 to 20 drops up to four times daily.

Soothing Salves

A POULTICE THAT PLEASES

Traditional healers swear by herbal oil poultices for easing coughs. To make one, add a few drops of thyme or eucalyptus essential oil to a teaspoon of olive oil. Rub the mixture on your chest and the outside of your throat, and cover the area with an old towel or a piece of flannel so you don't stain your clothes. Leave the poultice on for about 20 minutes. The vapors will soothe your irritated airways and reduce the urge to cough.

Put your feet up. Since most coughs are caused by upper respiratory infections, your first approach should be to help your body heal. The best way to do this—one that most of us, with our too-busy schedules, don't do often enough—is to kick back and take it easy until you're feeling better, says Priscilla Natanson, N.D., a naturopathic physician in Plantation, Florida.

Watch some TV. Read a couple of novels. Shoot, take a day or two off from work. The more you relax and take it easy, the more energy your body will have to fight the infection and oust the germs.

Be a water lover. Your immune system doesn't work very well when you're dehydrated. Drinking lots of fluids not only helps keep your aggravated throat irrigated, it also supports your immune system in its fight against cold or flu germs. Most people need four to eight glasses of water a day; the exact amount depends on your size and how active you are. But you really can't go wrong drinking more rather than less. The best way to stay properly hydrated is to keep some H_2O nearby and sip it liberally as you go about your daily activities.

Take a multi. Even if you get all of the essential nutrients in your diet, your body needs extra vitamins and minerals when you're fighting an upper respiratory infection. Taking a daily multivitamin is an easy way to ensure that you get all the nutrients you need to heal quickly.

Drink your veggies. Fresh vegetable juice is packed with nutrients that will feed your immune system. The advantage of juices over solid foods when you're sick is that your body is able to absorb the nutrients quickly and easily. Unpack that juicer someone gave you for your birthday five years ago and crank it up. "Green leafy vegetables are the best choices for juicing," says Dr. Natanson. Be sure to use organic veggies so you don't ingest any unwanted pesticides.

Avoid forbidden fruit. While vegetable juices are great when you have a cold or the flu, fruit juices can hurt more than they help. They're loaded with sugar, and all that sweetness is just what germs need to flourish. Also, the acids in citrus fruit juices can aggravate your throat and make a cough worse. Stick with vegetable juice until you're well again.

Get extra vitamin C. This all-purpose nutrient is essential when you're sick because it strengthens your immune system and can help reduce cold symptoms, including coughs, in a hurry. Unless you have kidney or stomach problems, take 500 milligrams every few hours until you're feeling better. If you start having diarrhea, reduce the dose to a level you can tolerate.

Make nice with anise. The herb anise, which has a pleasant licorice flavor and fragrance, is another traditional cough remedy. You can buy anise tea bags at health food stores or raid your spice cabinet and steep a teaspoon of anise in a cup of

A Cup of Comfort

A good way to eliminate mucus—and the coughing that goes with it—is to drink hyssop tea. A traditional herb for treating coughs, hyssop makes mucus thinner and easier to cough up, says Priscilla Natanson, N.D. Buy dried hyssop at a health food store, then add 1 teaspoon to a cup of freshly boiled water. Steep for about 10 minutes, then strain out the herb. Drink it throughout the day.

hot water. It's also fine to use a tincture. The recommended dose for quelling a cough is about 20 drops up to four times daily.

Gulp down some grindelia. Despite the unappetizing name, this common herb, also known as gum weed, is a top-flight cough remedy. "It's great when you have a dry, raw kind of cough," says Dr. Natanson. She advises taking about 20 drops daily of grindelia tincture, available at health food stores.

Soften up with marshmallow. When mixed with hot water, the herb marshmallow (which was used to make the candy in the days before high-tech laboratories) forms a slippery liquid that coats and moisturizes a dry, raspy throat. Slippery elm has similar effects. You can buy both herbs in powdered form at most health food stores. Add a tablespoon of either to a cup of hot water and sip it slowly several times a day.

Look for trouble. A lot of coughs are caused by obvious things, such as upper respiratory infections, air pollution, or secondhand smoke. But if you can't figure out what's making you cough, you're going to have to be a bit of a detective. "It can be almost anything," says Dr. Natanson. "People can be sensitive to certain plants, to solvents in cleaning supplies, to detergents, to perfumes, to any number of things." The only way to find out for sure is to make notes about what you're doing and where you are when coughing fits strike. Sooner or later, you'll have a good idea of what's causing the trouble, and you'll be able to take steps to avoid it.

Heartburn

Turn Down the Heat

My grandmother was a fantastic Italian cook, and my dad always figured that heartburn was an unavoidable consequence of the big dinners she made. Did I say "dinners"? "Banquets" is more like it—feasts that went on for hours. Dad was renowned for his eating speed, and he'd be mopping up the last bit of manicotti while the rest of us were still on the antipasto. He'd put down his fork, shove himself away from the table, and moan, "Oh, my God," which meant that the after-dinner flames were already raging.

Over the years, Dad lost some weight and began eating fewer rich foods and more fruits and vegetables. Now, I can't remember the last time he let loose with that heartburn moan. But a lot of people aren't that lucky. Jana Nalbandian, N.D., a naturopathic physician and faculty member at Bastyr University near Seattle, told me about a patient who had heartburn every day for 19 years. *Nineteen years!*

I don't think I could take that much pain without going a bit nuts. I'm sure my dad couldn't have—and you probably can't, either. Well, guess what? You don't have to, because there are plenty of ways to take the burn out of heartburn.

FIRE IN THE HOLE

Nearly half of all Americans experience that miserable, burning feeling behind the breastbone at least once a month. Heartburn usually smolders after meals, and it can last for hours. UGH!

You probably already know that heartburn doesn't have anything to do with the heart. The source of the burning is stomach acid that surges upward into your esophagus, the tube that carries food from your mouth to your stomach. There's a valve at the bottom of your esophagus that's supposed to prevent this upsurge, but sometimes it doesn't work very well. When this happens, you'll know it because of the sudden, burning pain.

SMOTHER THE FLAMES

If you get heartburn only once in a while, don't give it a second thought. There are plenty of home remedies that will knock out the discomfort, and most of them work in just a few minutes.

If you have heartburn more often—say, at least once a week over a period of months—you need to check with your doctor. For one thing, heartburn is too painful to live with every day. For another, the irritation caused by persistent heartburn can lead to cancer of the esophagus. Chronic heartburn that's accompanied by weight loss, trouble swallowing, or visible blood when you cough or have a bowel movement can indicate that acid has already caused serious damage. So if you have

The Cabbage Cure

A head of cabbage will help you get ahead of heartburn. Cabbage is loaded with glutamine, an amino acid that appears to promote healing in the digestive tract. People who eat cabbage several times a week may be less likely to experience heartburn than those who never eat it.

I know, cabbage isn't to everyone's taste. An alternative is to buy powdered glutamine at a health food store, mix a teaspoon in a glass of water, and drink it once a day.

chronic heartburn, play it safe and see your doctor right away. If he thinks your health is in danger, he may use a lighted tube to take a look at the lining of your esophagus. Most likely, he'll simply recommend medications that cut down on acid production. The bottom line is: Less acid, less burn.

But heartburn medications aren't perfect. Some can cause diarrhea, while others can trigger constipation or even dizziness, so you'll want to do everything you can to make episodes less frequent and less painful. Heartburn, as it turns out, is very easy to treat yourself. Here's how to do it.

Take a big gulp. Water is one of the best remedies for heartburn because it dilutes the burning acid and flushes it back into the stomach, says Roy Orlando, M.D., chief of gastroenterology and hepatology at Tulane University Health Sciences Center in New Orleans. So chug it every chance you get.

Forget the milk myth. Milk has a reputation as a stomach soother, but it can actually make heartburn worse by increasing acid production. So avoid it like the plague.

Recognize the gravity of the situation. Everything that

It's an Emergency!

Emergency room doctors see a lot of people with heartburn who think they're having heart attacks. But don't laugh; even doctors can't always tell the difference right away.

The bottom line: Go to the emergency room immediately when you have chest pain, especially if you have a history of heart problems, or if you smoke or have other risk factors for heart disease. The doctor may chuckle and send you home with some antacids, but it's better to be a little embarrassed than to take chances with your life.

goes up has to come down. It was true for Isaac Newton's apple, and it's equally true for stomach acid that splashes upstream. To help gravity do its job, stand up at the first pangs of heartburn. You'll feel better when the acid drains back into your stomach.

Loosen up. Tight clothing presses on the stomach and literally pushes acid uphill. So get comfortable: Loosen your belt a few notches, untuck your shirt, or undo a few buttons. Less pressure means less heartburn.

Chew on it. It may not be polite at formal gatherings, but chewing on a stick of gum is a great way to stop heartburn fast. Chewing increases the flow of saliva, which acts as a natural acid neutralizer.

Ax the acid. Over-the-counter antacids will do the trick. There are dozens of brands, and they all work equally well at stopping heartburn. Liquid antacids work better than tablets because they neutralize more acid, says Dr. Nalbandian.

Eat less, more often. As my dad learned the hard way, eating gargantuan meals almost guarantees heartburn because all of that food in the stomach requires enormous quantities of digestive acids. You'll be much less likely to get heartburn if you eat five or six small meals a day instead of gorging yourself on two or three large ones.

Stand up to pain. I know how tempting it is to curl up on the couch and fall into a coma after a big dinner, but don't

A Cup of Comfort

Chamomile tea is an excellent heartburn remedy because it contains anti-inflammatory substances that soothe irritation. It also settles your stomach after heavy meals. Other soothing herbal teas include slippery elm, marshmallow, and plantain (look for them at health food stores). If you're allergic to ragweed, however, avoid chamomile.

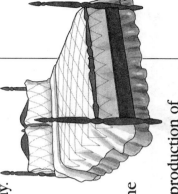

do it! Remember, gravity is your friend and heartburn's enemy. Taking a post-meal walk or simply remaining upright makes it harder for stomach acid to go where it shouldn't, and it allows acid that's already present to drain away.

Sleep on a slope. A lot of people get heartburn after going to bed because lying prone puts the stomach at the same level as the vulnerable esophagus. An easy solution is to raise the head of your bed a few inches by putting boards or sturdy, wide blocks under the legs.

Don't dine at nine. As you'd expect, the production of stomach acid peaks soon after meals. You're a lot more likely to get heartburn when you eat late and go to bed within an hour or two. If you can, eat earlier in the evening so that most of the food is digested by the time you hit the hay.

Cut back on heartburn culprits. Caffeine, alcohol, and chocolate are notorious for causing and aggravating heartburn. You don't necessarily have to quit drinking coffee or alcohol, and I would never tell anyone to give up chocolate, but a little moderation may be all that's needed to bring blessed relief.

Nix the mints. I've always wondered why restaurants often keep a big bowl of after-dinner mints by the cash register. Peppermint, spearmint, and other mints may freshen your breath, but they also trigger heartburn by relaxing the muscle in the esophagus that's supposed to keep acid out.

Switch to lean cuisine. When my dad started eating healthier and quit eating cheeseburgers and other fatty foods, his heartburn disappeared almost completely. This makes sense because fatty foods stay in the stomach for a long time and trigger the release of more acid. So drop the fat.

Pneumonia

Clear Out the Pain

Almost from the time I was old enough to pull on my own parka and knitted cap, my mom confronted every winter outing with the same warning: "Dress warmly or you'll get pneumonia!"

I suspect a lot of us heard this growing up, and perhaps most of us believed it. But when I recently looked into the causes of pneumonia, I learned that cold has very little to do with it.

HARD ON THE LUNGS

Pneumonia is the general term for any infection of your lungs. Like other infections, it can be caused by bacteria, a virus, or even a fungus or parasite. As you might guess, your lungs are protected by some pretty sophisticated defense mechanisms.

But when those defenses are weaker than they should be—because of smoking, for example, or the natural decline in

---

It's an Emergency!

Pneumonia kills more than 40,000 Americans each year, so it's important to get medical help if you develop a high fever, difficulty breathing, or severe chest pain, or if you begin coughing up blood. If you have any one of these symptoms, go to an emergency room or urgent-care center right away.

---

immunity that occurs as we get older—germs are more likely to proliferate.

The symptoms of pneumonia are pretty much the same as those of a bad cold or the flu. You may have a fever, chest pain, coughing, chills, and fatigue. In addition, you'll find it increasingly difficult to breathe as the illness progresses. Your lungs simply can't function well when you have infection-related inflammation and fluid buildup.

BREATHE EASIER

Even though many people with pneumonia naturally recover on their own, the fact remains that your lungs are pretty crucial pieces of equipment, and severe pneumonia is life-threatening. It doesn't pay to take chances: You must see a doctor if you even suspect you have pneumonia.

Antibiotics and other medications can knock out most serious cases of pneumonia pretty quickly, but severe pneumonia requires ongoing care, either at home or in the hospital, to ensure that your lungs make a full recovery. While you're recuperating, or if you have only a minor case, here are the best ways to bounce back again.

Stay well watered. You should never be more than arm's length from a glass of water while you're recovering, says

Soothing Salves

PACK IT WITH MUSTARD

Chest pain is probably the most uncomfortable symptom of pneumonia. A quick way to ease the ache is to use a mustard pack, says Christian Dodge, N.D. "It will increase circulation and ease the pain."

Crush some mustard seeds and add enough warm water to make a paste. Spread the paste on your chest and cover it with plastic wrap, then top that with a cloth moistened with warm water. Mustard oil can burn, so keep the compress in place for no longer than 5 to 10 minutes. Repeat the treatment two or three times a day for as long as you're hurting.

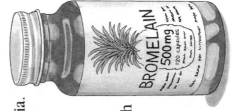

Norman H. Edelman, M.D., scientific consultant for the American Lung Association and dean of Stony Brook School of Medicine in New York. "We suggest that people drink plenty of fluids, at least eight glasses a day," he says.

Drinking lots of water dilutes all the mucus your lungs produce when you have pneumonia. You'll breathe easier, and your lungs will recover more quickly.

Stay off your feet. Your immune system needs every ounce of energy it can muster to defeat pneumonia, so it's important to get as much rest as you can. Pneumonia will clear up much more quickly when you take it easy, says Dr. Edelman.

Slurp lots of soup. For one thing, it increases the amount of lung-cleansing fluid in your body. In addition, soup provides an abundance of healing nutrients, and it's easy to eat when you're sick and your appetite is low.

Soup has some other benefits. The warmth helps loosen mucus in your chest, and the high protein content of chicken or other meat-based soup helps your body recover. There's also some evidence that chicken soup increases the activity of immune cells that help mop up infections.

Bet on bromelain. This natural enzyme from pineapple can help your body overcome pneumonia. "It's an enzyme that helps break up mucus and reduce inflammation," says Christian Dodge, N.D., a naturopathic physician and faculty member at Bastyr University near Seattle. Bromelain also helps your body absorb antibiotics more efficiently, which is important if you're being treated for bacterial pneumonia.

Bromelain is available in health food stores and most drugstores. Follow the directions on the label, and be sure to take it on an empty stomach, Dr. Dodge advises. Taking bromelain with meals will inactivate the beneficial enzyme. Also, let your doctor know you're taking it.

Clobber it with garlic. If you like your food on the pungent side, you're in luck: Garlic is one of the best herbs for strengthening immunity and fighting infections, says Dr. Dodge. He advises eating two raw garlic cloves a day until the infection is completely gone. "If that's too intense, you can lightly bake the garlic," he adds.

Sniff some saltwater. Your nose and throat will probably feel intensely irritated when you're battling pneumonia. Sniffing saltwater is a quick way to ease the discomfort because it draws fluid from the tissues and encourages the inflammation to clear up, says Dr. Dodge.

You can buy ready-made saline solution at drugstores, or you can make your own by mixing a few teaspoons of salt in a few ounces of warm water. Cup some of the solution in your hand, sniff it into your nostrils, then swallow it or blow it out.

Cough it up. The chest-racking cough that accompanies pneumonia can be agonizing, but you don't necessarily want to

A Cup of Comfort

All liquids are helpful when you have pneumonia, but warm echinacea tea is in a class by itself. It reduces chest congestion and soothes your throat and lungs while also boosting the ability of your immune system to fight the infection. Steep a teaspoon of dried herb in a cup of hot water for about 10 minutes, then sip. Plan on drinking two or three cups of echinacea tea a day until the infection is gone and you're feeling better.

block it with a cough suppressant. Coughing is your body's way of expelling the gunk that's clogging your lungs. The more mucus you cough up, the better you'll feel and the more quickly you'll recover, says Dr. Dodge.

Of course, there are times when a cough is so severe that it interferes with sleep or causes intense pain; people have even broken ribs during attacks. If your cough is really bad, go ahead and use an over-the-counter cough suppressant, following the label directions. (See page 154 for more tips on easing coughs.)

Humidity helps. A dry environment causes mucus to dry and thicken, impeding your recovery. Keep the surrounding air moist with a humidifier or bedside vaporizer, but be sure to get some fresh air at the same time. "If you have a window in the bedroom or wherever you're spending most of your time, keep it cracked open," Dr. Dodge suggests.

Do away with dairy. Milk, cheese, and other dairy foods are loaded with beneficial calcium and protein, but they also tend to thicken mucus—the last thing you need when you're recovering from pneumonia. Once the infection is gone, you can go back to the dairy aisle and stock up again.

Take all your medicine. Antibiotics are extremely effective at combating pneumonia. They're so effective, in fact, that many people feel better within a day or two, and then they quit taking the drugs because they're convinced that they're cured. In a word: Don't!

That's about the worst thing you can do, says Dr. Edelman. The only way to knock out pneumonia is to take the full course of antibiotics. Stopping treatment early will allow some germs to survive, and the infection could come roaring back with a vengeance.

Pain in Your **Back**

Disk Pain
Lower-Back Pain
Sciatica

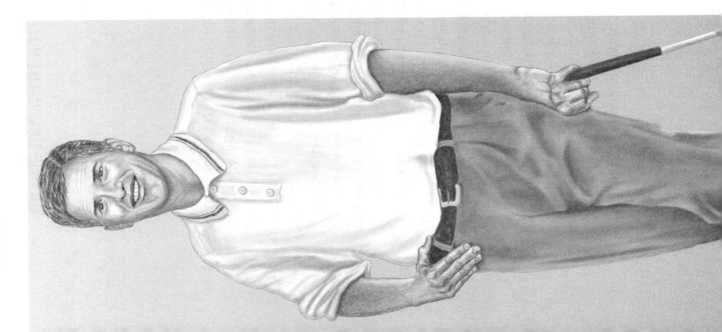

Disk Pain

Soothing Strategies for a Sad Spine

Recently, I was surprised to learn that my fiancée's brother, Bobby, has disk problems. He's the kind of guy who's always up at the crack of dawn, on the move all day, and early for every appointment. I would never have guessed that he has such a serious problem—and that when the pain flares up, his busy schedule grinds to a total halt.

I talked to Bobby about his back problems, and I could hear the frustration in his voice. There are a lot of times he can't play golf or ride his bike—the two activities he loves most—because the pain is so intense. In fact, when he's having "back days," just getting around can be a challenge. Fortunately, it's possible to keep those days to a minimum with an ounce of prevention and a few tricks to minimize the twists and strains most of us subject our backs to.

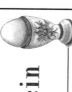

Power Protein

Fish and beans are nearly perfect foods when you have disk pain. They're jam-packed with protein, the nutrient that your body needs to repair damaged disks and ligaments. Unlike meat, dairy products, and some other high-protein foods, beans and fish don't stimulate the production of inflammatory chemicals in your body.

A SPINE-TINGLING TALE

Your spine is a wonder of engineering. It combines structural strength with a surprising degree of flexibility. Think about the construction: If it were solid bone, it would be strong, but not flexible; if it had more soft tissue, it would be flexible, but not strong. Nature hit on the perfect compromise by combining both of these characteristics.

Alternate segments of tough bone, or vertebrae, and soft, flexible disks make up your spine. The disks act as shock absorbers: If you didn't have them, you'd feel a jarring tremor with every step. They also keep the bony vertebrae from rubbing against one another.

The disks are normally held in place by strong ligaments, but the ligaments can stretch or tear, usually after a sharp movement or an accident of some kind. When that happens, one or more of the disks slip or bulge out from between the vertebrae. What happens next depends on where the disk goes. If it moves or bulges into a harmless place, you may feel nothing at all. If it happens to shove against one of several spinal nerves, however, you're going to know it. The pain can be excruciating!

FIX A FLOPPY DISK

Some people with severe disk damage have few or no symptoms. For others, even a minor problem can cause dis-

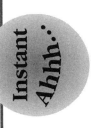

Press Your Point

Here's a disk pain remedy that you can use no matter where you are: Place your finger and thumb on the depressions on either side of your Achilles tendon, right at the back of your ankle. Press firmly for about 30 seconds, relax, then press again. According to Traditional Chinese Medicine, putting pressure on this area can block the transmission of pain signals and help ease disk pain almost right away.

abling back pain or even shooting pains down one or both legs. Only your doctor, with the help of a CT scan or MRI, will be able to tell you what's going on. Although you may need surgery to remove portions of the damaged disks, in the vast majority of cases (probably more than 90 percent), you can treat the problem with simple home remedies. Disk problems can be very slow to heal, but there's a lot you can do to minimize discomfort as they do. Here's how to get going.

Get up and about. When it comes to disk pain, the road to recovery isn't traveled in bed. "It's important not to stay in bed too long," says Lanika Buchanan, N.D., a naturopathic physician in the Puget Sound area of Washington. "Activity facilitates the healing process, so I don't recommend spending more than two days in bed for back pain."

Studies have shown, in fact, that extended bed rest causes supporting muscles in your back to get weak and stiff, which makes the pain worse. You certainly don't want to do any activity that aggravates the pain, but try to stay as mobile as you can.

Hit it with ice. It's far and away the fastest-acting treatment for disk pain. As soon as the pain strikes, put an ice pack on the spot for about 20 minutes. Take a break for 20 or 30 minutes, then apply the ice again. Keeping the area good and cold will help prevent post-injury inflammation.

Use heat, then cold again. This cold-heat cycle, known as contrast hydrotherapy, is a simple and effective way to speed healing and reduce disk pain. Soak a washcloth in hot water, wring it out, and apply it to the sore area for 3 minutes. Replace it with a cold, moist cloth and keep that in place for 30 seconds. Then start over by applying heat again. Repeat the cycle two or three times, always ending with the cold application. "This increases blood flow in the injured area, which drives out inflammatory products that can damage the tissues," says Dr. Buchanan.

Pop a pineapple in a pill. A natural enzyme called bromelain, extracted from pineapples, quickly stops inflammation and helps disk or muscle injuries heal faster. You should take a bromelain supplement as soon as possible after the injury. The recommended dose is 400 milligrams two or three times daily, taken on an empty stomach. If you take bromelain with food, the active ingredient will be destroyed by your digestive juices.

Smear and soothe. There are plenty of topical ointments in drugstores that can help ease the muscle aches that accompany disk pain. Look for products that contain camphor or menthol, which produce a cooling sensation and decrease pain and inflammation in the area, advises Dr. Buchanan.

Strike oil. A light massage using herbal essential oils can soothe and relax stiff muscles produced by a slipped disk. Two oils to try are arnica and St. John's wort. Gently rub the oil onto the sore area and leave it on for 20 to 30 minutes.

Hug your knees. One reason that slipped disks are so painful is that the surrounding muscles tighten and go into spasm. Stretching the muscles will help them relax, in turn reducing pain and helping speed recovery, says Dr. Buchanan.

Sit upright on the floor with your feet on the floor and your knees bent. Grip one leg below the knee and pull it toward your chest. Hold the stretch for a few seconds, then relax. Repeat with the other leg, then stretch both legs at once. Remember, the stretches shouldn't be painful. If they are, you're pulling your knee too far. "You don't want to push through the pain," she says.

Walk, don't run. Once you've started having disk problems, there's a good chance they'll keep coming back. One way to keep return appearances to a minimum is to avoid jarring types of exercise. Running is the worst for people with disk pain because it puts too much pressure on the spine, says Dr. Buchanan. Walking, cycling, and swimming are better choices. "You want activities that will stimulate your back muscles, but are gentle," she says.

Eat to beat inflammation. Controlling inflammation is key to healing disk pain. "Inflammation breaks down tissues, and you need to stop the process to let your body heal itself," says Dr. Buchanan. Foods such as meat and dairy foods promote inflammation, while vegetables, fruit, and fish suppress it.

Make magic with cal-mag. Supplements that contain both calcium and magnesium will encourage your tense back muscles to loosen and relax. Look for combination supplements that provide 500 to 800 milligrams of each of these important minerals. This amount of magnesium may cause diarrhea in some people. If this occurs, reduce the dose. Capsules tend to work better than tablets because they're easier for the body to break down, says Dr. Buchanan.

Healing Hands

Almost nothing feels better than a massage when you have a slipped disk. It's most effective when someone massages your entire back, not just the area where it hurts. "All the muscles in the back, as well as in the shoulders and neck, are involved in the pain," says Lanika Buchanan, N.D. Ask the person doing your massage to hit all of these areas equally, she advises, and you'll feel much better.

Lower-Back Pain

Stop the Back Attacks

I've talked to many people who, like me, remember their dads moaning in pain and rubbing their lower backs when they came home from work. Men of my father's generation worked so hard for such long hours that it seemed that back pain was just part of being a dad.

These days, now that he's retired, my dad hardly ever complains about back pain, and I think I know why his problem never progressed to a serious disability. Dad isn't the kind of guy who lies around and waits for things to get better. Whenever his back pain flared up, he rested only long enough for the pain to subside. Then he'd go back to his usual routine.

BACK OUT OF WHACK

There are few muscles that work as hard and long as the muscles in your back. From the moment you get out of bed to the moment you turn in for the night, these muscles are on the job. Even when you're not moving, they're constantly flexing and relaxing to keep you upright or properly aligned. Every now and then, the muscles simply get tired. Sometimes they get strained, inflamed, or even torn. Back pain is second only to sore throat as the most common condition doctors treat.

BACK IN ACTION

Few conditions are more painful than persistent back pain. The pain, paradoxically, is part of the healing cycle. When muscles are tired, weak, or strained, they sometimes say "No more!" and lock into spasms. These spasms hold the muscles immobile and prevent further damage, but boy, do they hurt!

The vast majority of people who experience back pain will get better in a few days—or in extreme cases, maybe a few months. Back pain that doesn't improve within a week or two always needs to be checked by a doctor. Chances are you'll just need pain medication or perhaps a prescription drug to help your muscles relax. If there's damage to the nerves around your spine, that's a different matter altogether—one that always requires a doctor's care. Most of the time, though, a few simple strategies will get you on your feet and back in action in a hurry. Here's what they are.

Don't be a bed bug. Doctors used to advise people with back pain to get plenty of bed rest—weeks' worth, in fact. But the latest studies show that it's better to get up and moving as soon as you can. "I tell people they have one day to baby themselves," says Dennis Dowling, D.O., chairman of the department of osteopathic and manipulative medicine at the New York College of Osteopathic Medicine in Old Westbury. After your day of rest, get moving. It increases circulation, which brings

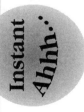

Instant Ahhh…

Get in the Swim

Swimming is one of the fastest ways to take the kinks out of aching back muscles. For one thing, merely submerging yourself in warm water will help reduce muscle tension. More important, the water supports your weight, which allows you to exercise without putting additional strain on your back, says Dennis Dowling, D.O.

healing nutrients to damaged muscles. It also keeps them loose and limber. Lying in bed, on the other hand, can make your beleaguered muscles weaker and tighter.

Play it cool. It seems that the only time hot water bottles or heating pads come out of the closet is when back pain makes an appearance. There's nothing wrong with using heat after a few days of pain, but don't use it right away, because it increases inflammation. As soon as your back starts hurting, apply a cold pack or ice cubes wrapped in a towel to your sore muscles. Cool the area for about 20 minutes every few hours. Keep at it for the first 24 hours after the pain starts. Cold constricts, or narrows, blood vessels and reduces blood flow, in turn reducing pain in the first day or two after an injury.

Get comfortable. Everyone with back pain can find at least one position, and possibly more than one, that puts the least strain on their overworked muscles. For some people, the best position is leaning slightly forward when walking. For others, it may be standing straight. Experiment a bit to find the

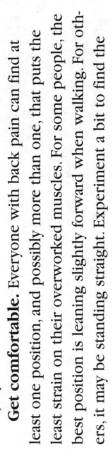

Healing Hands

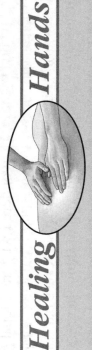

Massage is strong medicine for back pain. The pressure from firm hands loosens and relaxes strained muscles. Massage also stimulates your circulatory system and brings healing fluids and nutrients into your muscles while carrying out pain-causing substances such as lactic acid. It's important, however, to wait a day or two after your back starts hurting to have a massage. If you do it too soon, the pressure may only increase your discomfort.

position or positions that cause you the least pain. The less strain you put on your back muscles, the more quickly the injury will heal.

Take an anti-inflammatory. Studies have shown that aspirin, ibuprofen, and similar drugs often work as well for back pain as more powerful prescription drugs. They help in two ways: They're analgesics, which means they work directly on pain, and they have anti-inflammatory effects, which reduce painful swelling. Acetaminophen is fine for pain, but it has little or no effect on inflammation.

Sleep on your side. "I encourage people with back pain to lie on their sides with a pillow between their knees," says Dr. Dowling. If you're comfortable only when you sleep on your back, at least put a pillow under your knees to reduce the arch in your back and relieve some of the strain.

Get a leg up. Have you ever wondered why traditional pubs have foot railings that run the length of the bar? It's because bar owners want you to stand there—and buy drinks—as long as you can. Standing with one foot raised greatly reduces pressure on back muscles, so it's a good position when your back is hurting. When you're standing for more than a few minutes, look for any raised surface—a curb, a chair rung, or anything else that's at least a few inches off the ground—that you

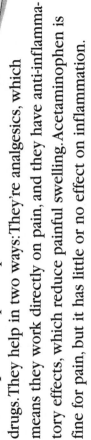

It's an Emergency!

Back pain almost always gets better on its own, and it's fine to wait a few weeks before seeing a doctor. The one exception is when the pain is accompanied by other symptoms, such as shooting pains, weakness, or tingling in one or both legs. These are common symptoms of sciatica, a nerve injury (see page 181). Another, more serious symptom of sciatica is loss of bowel or bladder control. If you experience any of these symptoms, get to a doctor immediately.

can use to keep one foot higher than the other.

Sit up straight. Slumping when you sit is a bad habit that puts most of your weight on your tailbone rather than on your stronger pelvic bones. Your back will feel a lot better—and will be less likely to get hurt—if you make it a point to sit with your knees bent and pulled in close to the edge of the chair.

See what's afoot. Sorry, ladies, but high heels are terrifically hard on your back. What you may not know is that even flats can be back breakers if they don't provide adequate support. When your back is hurting, wear shoes that have plenty of cushioning. You should be able to walk on a hard floor without feeling the impact, says Dr. Dowling. Running shoes are too lightweight to provide optimal cushioning, so you'll do better with cross-training or walking shoes.

Stretch it out. Back pain goes away more quickly when you gently stretch your injured muscles. It's not enough merely to stretch your back, however. You also need to loosen muscles in your legs, which will ease muscle tightness in your back, says Dr. Dowling. Here's a stretch that can help. Once or twice a day, stand on one leg next to a sturdy table and extend your other leg in front of you, with the heel resting on a chair or low table. Lean forward at your hips and try to touch the toes of your outstretched foot. Don't go too far, just to the point at which the pain starts. Hold the stretch for a moment, relax, then repeat the movements with your other leg. Use the table to steady yourself if you need to.

Do the psoas stretch. Another important muscle to stretch is the psoas, which reaches from your leg to your lower and middle back. Stand on your right foot, with your right hand on sturdy chair, table, or countertop for balance. Bend your left leg at the knee and grab the foot with your left hand. Pull upward, hold the stretch for a moment, then relax and repeat with your other leg.

Relax your back. Here's an all-around stretch that will really loosen and relax your back muscles: Stand with your back straight and pretend that you're in the middle of a compass, facing north. Slowly bend forward at your hips as far as you comfortably can. Hold the stretch for a moment, then return to the starting position. Repeat the same movement, this time bending backward, to the south. Then do the same thing to the left and right (or west and east, if you prefer). Each time you stretch, move your body in one compass direction only, without twisting. If you feel the least twinge of pain, stop immediately.

Strengthen your abdomen. For long-term protection from back pain, crunches—exercises that firm your abdominal muscles—are indispensable. The reason is simple: When your abs are strong, your back muscles don't have to work as hard. Here's the proper way to do abdominal crunches: Lie on your back with your hands crossed over your chest, your knees bent, and your feet flat on the floor. Raise your shoulder blades just a few inches off the floor and hold the stretch for a moment, then lower yourself back to the floor. Repeat the exercise as often as you comfortably can. Remember to keep your lower back on the floor. The goal isn't to do full sit-ups, just to make your abdominal muscles more taut.

Bend your knees. Improper lifting is a major cause of back pain, and you don't have to lift something heavy to knock your back out of whack. Just bending over to reach for a pencil or paper clip on the floor can do it. No matter what you're lifting, use the proper technique: Bend your knees, not your back, and let your leg muscles bring you back up.

STRETCHING

Sciatica

Say No to Nerve Pain

Anyone who's had back problems is all too familiar with the term *sciatica*, a type of nerve pain that's irritating if you're lucky—and devastating if you're not. Sciatica is the main reason that people have back surgery, but most folks who have it don't necessarily need to book an appointment with a surgeon. It turns out that the most qualified person to cure your sciatica is you.

"The body has an inherent capacity to heal itself," says Boyd R. Buser, D.O., associate dean at the University of New England College of Osteopathic Medicine in Biddeford, Maine. Once you eliminate some of the factors that interfere with healing and do more of the things that help it along, sciatica will often disappear on its own.

YOU'VE GOT SOME NERVE

Sciatica gets its name from the sciatic nerve, a major conduit of your nervous system with branches that run from your lower back all the way down to your feet. Anything that pinches or irritates your sciatic nerve has the potential to cause real trouble. Sciatica can produce symptoms as mild as a slight backache or as severe as shooting pains through your buttocks and legs.

Sciatica is often caused by muscle injuries. When muscles tighten or become inflamed, they can put painful pressure on this all-important nerve. It can also occur when one or more of the spinal disks, the shock absorbers between the vertebrae, squeeze out of the spinal column and jam against the nerve. The spinal bone spurs that occur with age can cause sciatica as well.

KNOCK OUT NERVE PAIN

Nerve pain is always potentially serious, so it's essential to see a doctor at the first sign of symptoms. Surgery is one of the main treatments for sciatica, and for good reason: Anything that's pressing against the nerve has to be removed before permanent damage occurs. In the majority of cases, however, the pressure and the pain will go away on their own. Here's the catch: Nerves are very slow to heal, so it may be weeks or months before all the pain is completely gone.

Do your best to be patient. For one thing, you don't want to have surgery unless you have to. More important, there are many things that you can do to reduce discomfort and protect the nerve from future damage. Here's a look at a few of them.

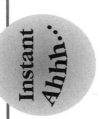

Instant Ahhh...

Uncan Those Hams

Stretching is always good for sciatica, but don't focus on just your back muscles. It's just as important to stretch your hamstrings, the muscles at the backs of your thighs that often press on the tender nerve, says John Nowicki, N.D. Here's a good stretch: Lie on your back with your knees slightly bent. Grab your right thigh above the knee with both hands and gently pull your leg toward your head. Raise it as close to vertical as you comfortably can, hold for a moment, then relax. Repeat with your other leg.

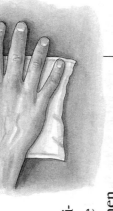

Ice it fast. Even in this age of high-tech medicine, ice is still one of the best treatments for back and nerve pain. When you apply ice immediately after an injury, there's a lot less swelling and inflammation, which means there's less pressure on the vulnerable nerve.

At the first sign of sciatica, apply a cold pack to your lower back, as close to the origin of the pain as you can get. Hold it there for 20 minutes, remove it for 20 minutes, then repeat the cycle. Keep applying cold for at least 24 hours, says Dr. Buser.

Turn up the heat. After applying cold for a day or two, use a warm compress or a heating pad set on low. "Heat's very helpful for relieving pain and relaxing those tight muscles," says John Nowicki, N.D., a naturopathic physician in Issaquah, Washington. Another benefit is that it increases blood flow, which helps flush pain-causing chemicals from the area and promotes the flow of healing nutrients to the injury.

Reach for the aspirin. To keep painful swelling to a minimum, take aspirin or ibuprofen at the first hint of sciatica, then keep taking it for at least the first week or two. Along with similar over-the-counter analgesics, these drugs inhibit the production of prostaglandins, body chemicals that cause pain as well as nerve-irritating inflammation, says Dr. Buser. Acetaminophen isn't your best bet for sciatica because, although it eases pain, it doesn't have significant anti-inflammatory effects. If you're sensitive to aspirin, talk to your doctor before using it.

Spice up your life. People with sciatica who like spicy foods should definitely seek out recipes that contain turmeric.

This fragrant herb has powerful anti-inflammatory effects that help counteract sciatica flare-ups. You'd have to eat a lot of turmeric to get enough of the active ingredient, though, so a more practical approach is to get turmeric in capsule form at a health food store. Check with your doctor first, then start with about 250 milligrams three times daily, preferably with food.

Be a switch sitter. People with sciatica are liable to be uncomfortable standing or sitting for long periods of time. "For most people, prolonged sitting is a problem, although some people have trouble with standing," says Dr. Buser. One way to keep pain at a minimum is to change positions frequently. If you're taking a long drive, for example, stop at least once an hour to get out and stretch. If you're working at a desk, set the alarm on your watch or clock to remind you to get up and walk around.

Make your moves. As with other types of back pain, sciatica heals more quickly if you don't subject yourself to prolonged bed rest. "You want to limit strenuous activities, but you should keep up with your usual walking and other daily activities," says Dr. Buser.

It's okay to take a day or

Soothing Salves

PENETRATING HEAT

Castor oil is a traditional remedy for muscle tightness, inflammation, and sciatica. Don't worry, though; you don't have to drink it. Just add it to equal parts St. John's wort oil and arnica oil, then apply the whole slick mess to the painful area of your back. Cover it with plastic wrap and warm it with a warm compress or a heating pad set on low for about 20 minutes. The heat will penetrate deeply into the muscles and help them relax.

two to recoup after the initial injury. In fact, a little rest is a good thing. After that, try to stay as active as the pain allows.

Don't twist, and you won't shout. You don't want to do anything to increase pressure on the irritated nerve. Obviously, this means no heavy lifting and a minimum of bending. In addition, try not to twist your torso too much so you don't increase muscle spasms, which can put a lot of pressure on the injured nerve.

Load up on minerals. Supplements that contain both calcium and magnesium are like a magic bullet for sciatica because they help tight muscles relax. Check with your doctor first, then look for a supplement that provides 500 to 800 milligrams of each and take it daily until the pain is gone. Magnesium may cause diarrhea in some people. If this occurs, reduce the dose. Capsules tend to work better than tablets because they're easier for the body to break down, doctors say.

Take a C cruise. Along with its many other health-promoting functions, vitamin C has been shown to help repair muscle damage that can lead to tightness as well as nerve pain. Unless you have stomach or kidney problems, you'll want to take up to 5,000 milligrams of vitamin C a day when you have sciatica. That's a lot more than the usual daily dose, so it's a good idea to take it in several smaller doses throughout the day to help

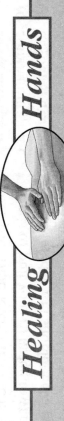

Healing Hands

Sometimes it's a good idea to let someone grab your butt. No kidding: When you have sciatica, massaging your buttocks can reduce muscle ten- sion that puts painful pressure on the nerve, says Lanika Buchanan, N.D., a naturopathic physician in the Puget Sound area of Washington.

prevent diarrhea or stomach upset. Taking it with food also helps.

Feed on fish oil. The essential fatty acids in fish and fish oil block your body's production of chemicals that promote pain and

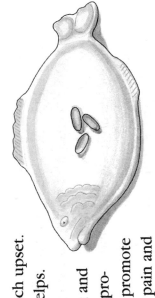

inflammation. You can get plenty of these fatty acids by eating fish several times a week. If you're not a fish fan, try some ground flaxseed. It's loaded with fatty acids, and you can sprinkle it on cereal or salads for a pleasantly nutty crunch.

Try a sciatic stretch. There are two main muscle groups, called the gluteal and piriformis groups, that contribute to sciatica pain. One of the best ways to ease sciatica—and to prevent it—is to keep those muscles long and limber by stretching.

Lie on your back on the floor with your knees bent and your feet flat on the floor. Put your left ankle over your right knee, then use both hands to pull your right leg toward your shoulder. You should feel a good stretch on your left side. Then switch legs and stretch your other side.

Rub, don't walk. It's okay to have a back rub if you have sciatica; in fact, it will probably help you feel better. Just make sure you tell your massage therapist where you hurt.

It's an Emergency!

Although most people with sciatica are terribly uncomfortable, it's unlikely that they have really serious problems. In some cases, however, there is severe nerve damage. Call your doctor immediately if your sciatica pain is accompanied by loss of bowel or bladder control, numbness around your rectum, or noticeable weakness or tingling in your back, legs, or feet. You could have a serious condition called cauda equina syndrome, in which the nerves coming out of the lower part of your spinal cord are being crushed. "It is an emergency," says Boyd R. Buser, D.O. "The pressure on those nerves has to be relieved surgically as soon as possible." So don't delay!

Pain in Your Abdomen

Constipation
Diarrhea
Gallstones
Gas Pain
Irritable Bowel Syndrome
Kidney Stones
Menstrual Pain
Side Stitches
Stomachache
Ulcers

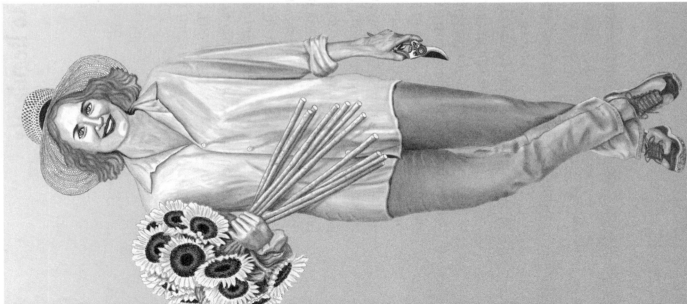

Constipation
The Route to Regularity

Like many people, I had always thought of constipation as a minor inconvenience. Then I talked to a friend, Phil, whose older brother had severe constipation when he was a kid that caused him all kinds of problems.

The poor kid was only 12 years old when all this was going on. Can you imagine how constipation, that "minor" problem, affected his school life, his social life, and his self-image? Luckily, Phil's brother had a supportive family who worked with his doctors to come up with an appropriate diet. That, along with improvements in his bathroom habits, eventually turned things around.

So I'm happy to say that there is hope. More than hope, actually. Nearly everyone who has to deal with constipation can reverse it—and more important, prevent it—with some very basic changes.

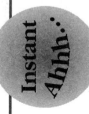

Instant Ahhh…

Sit and Soothe

The abdominal cramps that often accompany constipation can be excruciatingly painful. A fast way to get relief is to soak in a warm bath for 15 to 20 minutes. The warm water relaxes the muscles and helps reduce painful pressure and spasms.

WHEN THE GOING GETS ROUGH

Everyone experiences constipation in different ways. For someone who's accustomed to having a bowel movement every day, a reduction to three or four a week could be a sign of constipation. For others, having three bowel movements a week is normal, but having fewer than that is a problem.

GET MOVING

Since there's so much individual variation, doctors offer this advice: If there's been any change in your usual bathroom habits, get professional advice. There are literally hundreds of things that can cause constipation. Sometimes, it's a side effect of medications. Lack of exercise can cause it, or drinking too little water, or not eating enough fiber. The list goes on and on.

Constipation is rarely serious, although if it goes on for too long, stools can get so hard and impacted that they simply won't budge without a heavy-duty enema or other medical help.

In most cases, however, things don't have to go that far. There are a number of ways to help your large intestine work more efficiently as well as more regularly. Here are some tips

Healing Hands

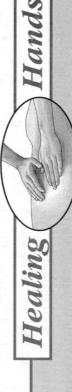

To encourage movement in sluggish bowels, try a simple belly-button rub. Use your favorite massage oil and lightly massage your stomach with the tips of your fingers, starting at your belly button and moving in small clockwise circles. Gradually expand the circles until you're massaging your entire abdomen. If you do this for 10 to 15 minutes every morning, you may find that your daily routine will be a bit more regular.

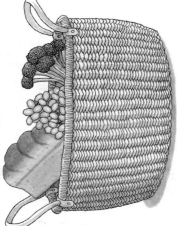

you may want to try.

Eat fresh from the garden.
The best diet for beating constipation is the same one that doctors recommend for preventing heart disease, cancer, and dozens of other serious health problems: a lot of plant foods and very little, if any, junk food.

In other words, eat as though processed foods had never been invented. "You want a diet that's high in fiber and complex carbohydrates," says Rob Dramov, N.D., a naturopathic physician in Tigard, Oregon. That means lots of fruits and vegetables, whole grains, and legumes every day, as well as high-fiber cereals such as oatmeal and oat bran.

Supplement your fiber. It's best to get fiber into your system by eating high-fiber foods, but there's nothing wrong with taking a fiber supplement to help you along. Unlike high-powered laxatives, they're safe enough to use every day. For example, products that contain psyllium, such as Metamucil, can be very helpful. "Try different kinds of supplements until you find the one that works best for you," says Michael P. Spencer, M.D., a colon and rectal surgeon and assistant professor of surgery

Soothing Salves

THE CASTOR OIL CURE

One way to gently encourage things to move along when you're bound up is to use a castor oil pack. Soak a small towel in castor oil and drape it over your abdomen. Cover the towel with plastic wrap and put a heating pad set on low on top. Keep the pack on your abdomen for about 20 minutes. "The treatment helps stimulate digestive contractions," explains Rob Dramov, N.D.

at the University of Minnesota, Twin Cities.

Relax a bit after meals. It's the best way to encourage your digestive tract to kick into gear. If you're the type who likes to eat and run, you're diverting blood to other parts of your body and leaving your intestine shortchanged. "The old adage, 'rest and digest' is just as true today as it ever was," says Dr. Dramov.

Don't drink and dine. Even though we traditionally drink water or enjoy a glass of wine with meals, it's best to take it easy. Taking in too much liquid when you eat will dilute the digestive juices in your stomach, which can interfere with normal digestion and can lead to constipation.

It's fine to drink a little bit with meals, of course, but plan on limiting yourself to one glass of water, for example, or a single serving of wine or beer.

When nature calls... If you're reluctant to use a public restroom no matter how urgent the need, you're setting yourself up for trouble. Resisting the urge to have a bowel movement—whether at home or anywhere else—can make it difficult to go later on.

In fact, delaying bowel movements can make your large intestine lazy, Dr. Dramov says. Essentially, you're teaching your body to resist its natural urges. You'll be a lot more regular if you go as soon as possible when you feel the need.

Drink lots of water. It's one of the best ways to treat and

Berries and Weeds

Strawberries are sweet treats, and they're full of the soluble fiber that helps keep your large intestine in fine fettle. Try eating several fresh strawberries every day while coping with constipation.

Dandelion is another natural constipation fighter. You can make an anti-gridlock tonic by pureeing dandelion leaves with some water, but be sure to use leaves gathered from an area that hasn't been chemically treated. Try drinking two or three glasses daily.

prevent constipation. If you don't drink enough, stools passing through your digestive tract will get harder and smaller and be more difficult to pass.

As a general rule, plan on drinking at least eight full glasses of water daily, and more if you smoke or drink alcohol, both of which can deplete your body of fluids.

Set aside morning time. Most people find it easiest to have a bowel movement in the morning, usually after breakfast or a cup of coffee. Take advantage of this time. Even if you're not sure you can go, plan on spending 5 to 10 minutes in the bathroom. This will help "train" your bowels to move at that time.

Exercise daily. Any kind of physical movement—walking, lifting weights, riding a bicycle—helps the intestine work more efficiently. In fact, it's not uncommon for people who have been constipated for years to get completely better once they start exercising for 20 to 30 minutes daily.

Check out vitamins. The mineral magnesium helps soften stools and make bowel movements easier, says Dr. Dramov. Talk to your doctor about starting the day with 500 milligrams of supplemental magnesium or taking 1,000 to 2,000 milligrams of vitamin C a day, split into two or three doses. Relatively high doses of this vitamin often soften stools, he explains. If either supplement causes diarrhea, though, reduce the dose.

Medications matter. Constipation is among the most common side effects of medications. Antacids are common culprits, as are pain medications. It's worth making a list of all the drugs you're taking to review with your pharmacist. If it turns out that one of them may be responsible, your doctor shouldn't have any trouble finding an acceptable alternative.

Diarrhea

Slow the Flow

When I was in college, I had a prolonged episode of diarrhea that was unusually wretched. It lasted for nearly a week, and I was so sore and crampy that I could barely bring myself to climb out of bed, let alone cook meals or go to classes. Looking back, I realize that most of the things I did to treat it weren't very helpful—and I didn't know about the handful of useful remedies that really would have made a difference.

For example, I quit eating solid foods because someone told me that it's better to eat nothing but soup and broth. I've since learned that this particular approach isn't much help. I've also learned that I should have been drinking more water to make up for all of the fluid I'd lost, and I certainly should have put the brakes on my cravings for coffee and sugar-laden sodas.

Probably the worst mistake I made was not seeing a doctor. Fortunately, the problem went away on its own despite my mistakes, but a doctor could have evaluated my condition and given me the advice I needed to recover more quickly.

GUT REACTION

We all get diarrhea from time to time. Loose stools occur when the large intestine isn't able to absorb the usual amount of fluid from wastes on their journey out of the body. All sorts of things can make this happen. Mild infections are the main cause, but eating too much junk food and even emotional stress can make stools looser than they should be.

Unfortunately, loose stools aren't the only symptom of diarrhea. The underlying problem irritates the intestine and causes painful abdominal cramps, along with sudden "emergencies" that send you running to the bathroom.

BACK ON SOLID GROUND

Although diarrhea is among the most common intestinal ailments, don't make the mistake of treating it lightly. True, it's usually a result of garden-variety infections that make you miserable for a few days and clear up on their own, but there are plenty of exceptions.

For example, diarrhea is sometimes triggered by heavy-duty infections that require prompt treatment with antibiotics. It can also be a symptom of a serious intestinal disorder, such as inflammatory bowel disease, or even a warning sign of cancer.

That's why you should always call your doctor when diarrhea doesn't go away within two days. Don't wait even that long if you have a fever, are nauseated or vomiting, or notice that your stools are black and tarry-looking.

A Cup of Comfort

A pleasant-tasting way to ease the abdominal cramps that accompany diarrhea is to drink two or three cups of chamomile tea a day—unless you're allergic to ragweed. This herb reduces painful abdominal spasms, and the tea helps replace the fluid that you lose with diarrhea. Peppermint tea is another good choice. To make either tea, steep a tea bag or fresh herbs in a cup of hot water for 10 minutes.

Apart from these exceptions, it's pretty easy to get through a short bout of diarrhea. Here's what the experts advise.

Stay away from sugar. This means not only sugary sweets but also simple carbohydrates such as honey. Bacteria that invade your digestive tract like sugar just as much as you do. The more you give them to eat, the more likely they'll be to stick around, says Rob Dramov, N.D., a naturopathic physician in Tigard, Oregon.

Get plenty of fiber. There's a good reason that doctors advise people with diarrhea to eat plenty of fresh fruits and vegetables, along with whole-grain cereals and breads. These foods are loaded with fiber, which absorbs water in the intestine and makes stools firmer and less watery. Most doctors recommend that you get 30 to 35 grams of fiber a day.

Drink to your health. Most people don't drink as much water as their bodies need. If you're also losing fluid from diarrhea, it's easy to see how your water levels can dip dangerously. Dehydration is the reason that doctors take diarrhea seriously. Your body simply can't function without adequate fluid, especially because dehydration invariably results in low levels of essential minerals called electrolytes, which control everything from muscle movements to normal nerve functions.

When you're coping with diarrhea, be sure to drink about half your body weight, in ounces, of water daily.

Bring on the bacteria. Diarrhea often occurs when harmful bacteria set up camp in your digestive tract. Actually, your

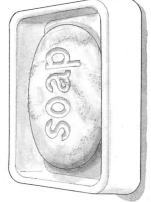

intestine is normally chock-full of bacteria, the good along with the bad, but the bad bugs are usually kept in check by the microscopic good guys. Anything that changes the usual balance—taking antibiotics, for example—can allow harmful germs to proliferate.

A quick way to restore the normal balance is to have one or two daily servings of live-culture yogurt. It's packed with *Lactobacillus acidophilus*, a type of beneficial organism that makes it harder for diarrhea-causing germs to thrive.

Load up on vitamins and minerals. Even if you don't usually supplement your diet with multi-nutrients, you should certainly take them when you have diarrhea. A once-a-day supplement is all you need. It's a fast way to replace the essential nutrients that diarrhea takes out of your body.

Keep 'em clean. We're surrounded by bacteria all the time, and usually our immune systems keep them in check. But there are times in life—when stress levels are high, for example—when your natural immunity can't keep up with bacterial marauders. An easy way to prevent problems is simply to wash your hands with soap and water several times a day. Studies have shown that many of the common infections that cause diarrhea could be

Quick Kitchen Cures

For a homemade diarrhea treatment, try mixing 1 teaspoon of carob powder with 1/4 cup of applesauce. The combo will give you plenty of natural fiber to absorb excess water and firm up loose stools. Try two or three doses of the mixture throughout the day, and eat it slowly.

Another kitchen cure for diarrhea is rice water. Boil 1/2 cup of brown rice in a quart of water for 15 to 20 minutes, stirring constantly, then strain. Drink the liquid throughout the day to soothe your digestive tract and replace lost fluid.

prevented just by keeping your hands clean, says Dr. Dramov.

Nix a quick fix. When diarrhea is taking the wind out of your sails, it's tempting to reach for an over-the-counter drug to stop it. There's nothing wrong with "drying up" diarrhea when you absolutely have to—if you're going to spend the day on an airplane, for instance—but for the most part, these products do more harm than good.

Diarrhea is one of the body's ways of eliminating unsafe substances, including harmful germs. Letting diarrhea run its course is often the quickest way to expel whatever it is that's making you sick in the first place.

Watch what you're eating. If you get diarrhea fairly frequently, it's possible that something in your diet is behind it. Some people, for example, are sensitive to fatty foods. Others react to artificial sweeteners. It's worth taking the time to keep track of everything you eat long enough to figure out what may be upsetting your intestine.

Recoup Your Losses

Because diarrhea can quickly deplete your body of essential fluid and electrolytes, it's essential to replace both as soon as possible. Drinking water or sports drinks is one way to do it. It's also helpful to drink soup, broth, or fruit or vegetable juice.

Another option is to buy packets of powdered electrolyte replacement formulas, available at drugstores and supermarkets. Mix the contents of the packet with water and drink the formula once or twice a day, following the directions on the label.

Gallstones

Relief from the Rocks

Old-timers used to say that the smallest dog has the most painful bite, and there seems to be some truth to it. If you're knocked in the eye by a baseball bat (as I once was), it will hurt like the dickens, but you'll probably be laughing about it an hour later. But no one laughs at gallstones. They can be smaller than grains of sand, but they cause such intense pain that they've been known to make strong men cry.

When I talked to Rowan Hamilton, Dip.Phyt., professor of botanical medicine at Bastyr University near Seattle, about gallstones, he said, "It's some of the worst pain you've ever dreamed of in your life." He says that many women compare the pain to that of childbirth. With childbirth, though, once the labor pains are over, at least you have a new tax deduction to show for it. Not so with gallstones.

ROLLING STONES

Bile, a digestive fluid that your body uses to digest fats, is stored in a small pouch called the gallbladder. Bile usually stays in liquid form, but sometimes one of the substances it contains, such as cholesterol, forms a hard little crystal, or gallstone, that floats around in your gallbladder. Most gallstones don't cause symptoms; you can have them for your entire life without ever knowing it. Sometimes, however, a stone lodges in one of the ducts leading out of the gallbladder. When that happens, you're going to experience a world of hurt.

The crazy thing about gallstone attacks is that they're totally unpredictable. You may be in agonizing pain for a few minutes or a few hours. You may have three attacks a day for three weeks, then never have another. There's just no way to tell.

SAFE FROM STONES

There's some good news and some bad news about gallstones. The good news is that as long as you're not having symptoms, you don't have to worry about them. The bad news is that the main—and by far the best—treatment for symptomatic stones is to have your gallbladder removed. It's a fairly simple "band-aid" procedure, and most people are back on their feet in a day or two. But who wants surgery if it can possibly be avoided? Not me!

If you've had gallstones in the past, your doctor may give you a medication that helps dissolve them in the gallbladder. Another approach involves using painless sound waves to break up the stones. Yet another option, the one doctors often recommend first, is to make some simple lifestyle changes that can help prevent stones from recurring. Here's what they suggest.

Eat leaner. The more fat in your diet, the more bile your

Garden-Variety Cocktail

Because the liver and gallbladder are intimately involved with digestion, it makes sense that food therapies can help them work a little better. A traditional way to help the gallbladder work more efficiently is to drink vegetable-juice cocktails that include celery, parsley, beets, carrots, radishes, and lemon. Mix and match the ingredients to suit your taste and drink about two cups a day, says Rowan Hamilton, Dip.Phyt.

liver will generate to digest it—and the greater your risk for gallstones. Studies have shown that people who get no more than 30 percent of calories from fat are less likely to get gallstones than those who eat more fat.

"Look for foods that have less than **5** grams of fat per serving," suggests Leslie Bonci, R.D., a Pittsburgh dietitian and spokesperson for the American Dietetic Association.

Split your squares. Most of us were raised on three square meals a day. If you divide the same amount of food into smaller, more frequent meals, though, you'll be less vulnerable to gallstones because the gallbladder won't secrete as much bile at once, Bonci says. "You should eat something every 3 to 4 hours," she adds. "For instance, instead of eating a sandwich, a bowl of soup, and a piece of fruit for lunch, you might have a cup of soup and half a sandwich, then eat the rest later on."

Avoid crash diets. We've all seen those ads for diet plans that promise to change us from Titanic to Twiggy in a few weeks. But crash diets are bad news for the gallstone prone. "Rapid weight loss increases the risk of gallstones," says Michael F. Leitzmann, M.D., Dr.PH., an epidemiologist in the department of nutrition at the Harvard School of Public Health. "If you're planning a weight-loss program, it's a good idea to con-

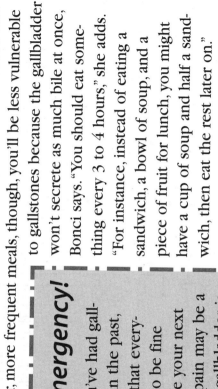

It's an Emergency!

Even if you've had gallstone attacks in the past, don't assume that everything's going to be fine when you have your next one. Extreme pain may be a sign that your gallbladder is infected, which can be life-threatening without immediate treatment. Don't take chances: Go to an emergency room at the first sign of pain, especially if your skin or eyes have turned slightly yellow or you have chills, fever, or a sudden change in stool color.

tact a health care provider for advice on how to lose weight gradually," he says.

Soothe it with castor oil. A quick way to help ease the pain of gallstone attacks is to relax with a castor oil pack. Rub castor oil over the painful part of your abdomen. Cover it with a layer of plastic wrap, then put a heating pad set on low on top of the wrap. Relax for an hour or two, then remove the pack and wash off the oil. The soothing warmth won't eliminate gallstone discomfort, but it will make it a lot easier to live with until you can get in to see your doctor.

Flood 'em out. Small gallstones can often be flushed from the gallbladder if you drink enough water, says Richard Kitaeff, N.D., a naturopathic physician and director of the New Health Medical Center in Edmonds, Washington. "I recommend drinking six to eight glasses of water a day, and more is probably better," he says.

Eat exotic. If you enjoy the cuisines of India, you're in luck. The spice turmeric, commonly used in Indian cooking, is a traditional gallstone remedy. If you don't care for the taste of turmeric but still want the benefits, you can take 50 to 100 milligrams in capsule form three times a day, preferably with meals.

A Dandy Remedy

You may consider them weeds, but dandelion greens are good as gold for your gallbladder. They contain chemical compounds that stimulate bile flow, and the more often your gallbladder empties of bile, the harder it is for stones to form.

You'll get some of the benefits by eating fresh dandelion leaves, but herbalists usually advise using dried leaves to make a tea. Add a teaspoon to a cup of hot water, steep for 10 minutes, then drink it down. You can get dried dandelion at a health food store.

Lighten up with lecithin. Lecithin is a nutrient that helps prevent gallstones from forming and keeps existing stones from getting bigger. Some doctors advise taking 1 gram of lecithin in divided doses with meals.

Go natural. Studies suggest that processed foods, especially refined sugars, may be associated with an increased risk of gallstones. You'll be less likely to have trouble if you replace processed foods in your diet with fresh fruits, vegetables, whole grains, and other wholesome, natural foods.

Be a moving target. Doctors aren't sure why, but people who exercise regularly get gallstones less often than those who are sedentary, says Dr. Leitzmann. He recommends exercising—including walking, swimming, biking, and even dancing—for 20 to 30 minutes three to five days a week if you can.

Check your medicine cabinet. If you're taking cholesterol-lowering drugs, you may be on the gallstone A-list. These drugs cause the gallbladder to excrete excess cholesterol, which in turn can raise the risk of stones. Don't stop taking the medicine, of course, but talk to your doctor. Together, you may be able to come up with a plan that will lower cholesterol without the need for medications.

Gas Pain

Fight the Fumes

As I write this, Thanksgiving is about a month away. That means I'll be sharing some big, delicious meals with various relatives. It also means that I'll be sharing a table with one relative who has the unfortunate habit of concluding his meal with an ungodly burst of post-digestive vapors.

I'm sure you know what I'm talking about, and maybe you have a relative who does the same thing. In any event, my research into the not-so-delicate subject of flatulence has persuaded me that no one has to live with it.

UNFORTUNATE FUMES

Gas is a natural by-product of digestion, so you can't avoid it entirely. Flatus, as gas is known among doctors, is a result of swallowed air and the fermentation process triggered by intestinal bacteria. Food that enters your digestive tract provides nourishment for enormous colonies of bacteria, which emit clouds of smelly chemicals. Basically, their gas becomes your gas, and that's where the problem starts.

THE SWEETER SMELL OF SUCCESS

Excess gas isn't only socially embarrassing; it's also uncomfortable because it puts painful pressure on your intestine. If you've suddenly noticed an increase in gas or it seems more painful than it should be, talk to your doctor. While flatulence itself isn't a disease, it may be a symptom of other digestive problems.

Of course, there are times when we all generate more gas than we would like. While you can't get rid of it altogether, there are a number of strategies for keeping it at manageable levels. Here are a few tips you may want to try.

Eat politely. Believe it or not, most people release about 2 pints of gas a day. "Half of that is swallowed air," explains Sean Sapunar, N.D., a naturopathic physician and clinical faculty member at the Bastyr Center for Natural Health near Seattle. There would be a lot less swallowed air—and expelled gas—in the world if everyone would eat the way their mothers told them: Take small bites, don't talk while you're eating, and eat slowly. "Hurried eating increases the amount of air you swallow," Dr. Sapunar explains.

Ax the antacids. Low stomach acid can cause gas problems because it may interfere with normal digestion, says Dr. Sapunar. If you need antacids to control heartburn, but you'd just as soon do without the extra gas, see "Heartburn" on page 159. You'll learn ways to relieve heartburn without suppressing stomach acid.

Sit up straight. It may be comfortable to eat from a TV tray while you're sprawled in the recliner, but you're more likely to contribute to diminished air quality if you dine that way. Eating in a reclining position changes the angle at which your stom-

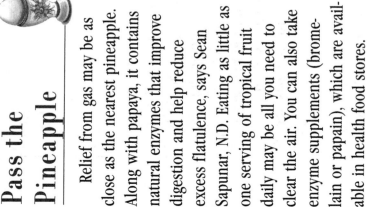

Pass the Pineapple

Relief from gas may be as close as the nearest pineapple. Along with papaya, it contains natural enzymes that improve digestion and help reduce excess flatulence, says Sean Sapunar, N.D. Eating as little as one serving of tropical fruit daily may be all you need to clear the air. You can also take enzyme supplements (bromelain or papain), which are available in health food stores.

ach and esophagus (the tube that carries food to your stomach) meet. "Swallowed air gets trapped if you're leaning backward," says Dr. Sapunar. And swallowed air, remember, has to go somewhere.

Make time for mealtimes. Stressful, hurried meals are among the leading causes of poor digestion and its related gas.

For good digestion, your body can't be in "fight or flight" mode, so give yourself time to eat in a calm, comfortable way. Turn off the TV. Forget about the day's troubles. And after the meal, sit back and relax for a while.

Bet on bitters. Bitter herbs have been used for thousands of years to improve the digestive process, but you don't have to eat pounds of arugula or dandelion to get the benefits. "I advise patients to sip a little Angostura bitters," says Dr. Sapunar. This classic after-dinner drink is available in most supermarkets.

Don't drink and eat. Once food is served, the bar should be closed. Drinking any kind of liquid, including water, while you eat dilutes digestive juices and can cause an increase in gas. Quench your thirst before or after you eat, but don't quaff while you're dining.

Chew on sweet seeds. You'll often see a bowl filled with aniseed or fennel seeds at Indian restaurants, and there's a good reason for this: The aromatic seeds are excellent digestive aids. "They help calm the digestive tract when you're feeling bloated or gassy," Dr. Sapunar says.

A Cup of Comfort

Lemon water slips your stomach into gear and helps your digestive system work more efficiently. When you're having trouble with gas, squeeze the juice from a slice of lemon into a glass of water and drink it before and after meals.

Take the Gas Out of Beans

On the scale of gas-producing foods, beans, along with broccoli, cauliflower, and other high-fiber foods, are almost off the chart. But what you may not know is that these foods cause trouble mainly for people who don't eat them very often. Adding beans to your menu more frequently will often cut down on the excess emissions. And that's good news for everyone!

You can further disarm those little gas grenades by soaking dried beans overnight. This causes the beans to germinate and produce enzymes that help break down the gas-causing compounds. Before cooking, drain off the soaking water and replace it with fresh water. When cooking with canned beans, rinse them thoroughly in a colander to remove some of the gas-producing compounds.

Here's another helpful hint: The Japanese seaweed kombu reduces beans' odoriferous by-products, thanks to a chemical compound called glutamic acid. Add a little kombu to beans or other gas-producing foods while they're cooking.

Don't be a soda jerk. We all have gas to spare, so the last thing you want to do is pump more gas into your system by drinking carbonated beverages. It's fine to enjoy a soft drink or soda water now and then, but the more you drink, the gassier you're going to be.

Decrease the dairy. Millions of Americans lack an enzyme to digest lactose, a sugar in milk, cheese, and other dairy foods. One of the main symptoms of this condition, called lactose intolerance, is gas. Try avoiding dairy products for a week or two to see if your problem clears up. If that seems to help, gradually add dairy foods back into your diet to find out just how much your system can tolerate. "Everybody's different. Some people have problems with just a little milk; others can

Teas That Turn Off the Gas

For centuries, people of many cultures have used natural gas-fighting, or carminative, herbs to tame the effects of poor digestion. You can take advantage of these herbal gas busters by whipping up an after-meal tummy-taming tea. Just mix equal amounts of caraway seeds, fennel seeds, and aniseed. Crush 1 teaspoon of the mixture and add it to a cup of freshly boiled water. Steep for about 20 minutes, strain out the seeds, and sip.

Other natural gas fighters include cinnamon and bee balm. To make cinnamon tea, steep a cinnamon stick in boiling water for 10 minutes. Let it cool, then remove the stick and sip the tea after eating. For bee balm tea, mix 1 tablespoon of dried bee balm with 1 teaspoon of powdered marshmallow root (both are available at health food stores). Put the mixture in a tea ball and steep in hot water for 5 to 10 minutes. Add 1 teaspoon of honey or maple syrup to a half-cup of tea and drink it before meals.

Best herbs to use:
- Caraway seeds
- Fennel seeds
- Aniseed
- Cinnamon
- Bee balm
- Marshmallow

drink two or three glasses a day," says Dr. Sapunar. You can also try some of the dairy products available in supermarkets to which the lactose-digesting enzyme has been added.

Anticipate with antibiotics. When you take antibiotics for an infection, you can plan on having an increase in gas. Besides attacking harmful bacteria, these medications also kill beneficial bacteria in your digestive tract, often causing an increase in discomfort. Adding yogurt to your diet on a daily basis should help reduce the problem.

Irritable Bowel Syndrome

Fast-Acting Intestinal Protection

Have you ever had one of those "Aha!" moments, when a lot of seemingly unrelated information suddenly falls into place? Mine came when I was reading about irritable bowel syndrome (IBS). I realized that the symptoms—abdominal pain, cramping, and the urgent need to find a bathroom—are nearly identical to those described by a friend of mine, who often finds herself overwhelmed by work and taking care of her three kids.

She's been living with this problem for years, and sometimes it seems that her digestive discomfort—and the unpredictable nature of the attacks—controls her life. I hope she tries some of the suggestions below because I'm convinced they'll help—but only time will tell.

A MYSTERIOUS MALADY

Even though IBS is among the most common conditions treated by doctors, they still don't know what causes it. For

Pain in Your Abdomen

some reason, people with IBS have intestines that are, well…irritable. They seem to have abnormal electrical activity that causes frequent, uncomfortable muscle contractions, or spasms.

Everyone with IBS has a slightly different pattern of problems. Some people have mainly cramps, some have episodes of diarrhea and/or constipation, and others are afflicted with gas and bloating. The symptoms may occur daily for years, or they may disappear for a while, then come roaring back without any warning.

PUT IBS TO REST

Irritable bowel syndrome is a frustrating condition because there aren't any one-size-fits-all treatments. It isn't dangerous in the long run, but it can make it impossible for people to live normal lives, not only because of the discomfort but also because of insecurity about being too far from a bathroom.

If your symptoms are so severe that they interfere with your day-to-day life, you should see a doctor right away. For one thing, there are a number of other conditions that cause similar symptoms. Also, the doctor may be able to prescribe med-

Count on Castor Oil

For rapid relief from abdominal pain and cramps, use a castor oil pack. Moisten a washcloth with the oil, drape it over your abdomen, and cover it with plastic wrap. Put a heating pad set on low on top of the plastic and leave it on for 20 minutes. The combination of oil and plastic traps the heat and helps reduce spasms and cramping.

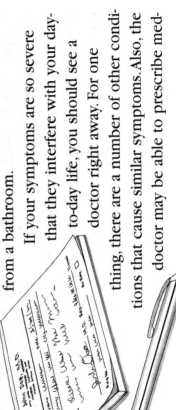

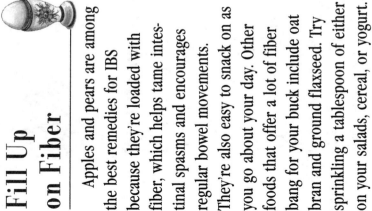

ication to reduce the intensity and frequency of intestinal contractions. If it turns out that you have IBS, lifestyle changes may be just as important as medical care. Here's what doctors advise.

Say "so long" to sugar. If you have IBS, sweets are a one-way ticket to disasterville. Sugary foods appear to interfere with the normal muscle contractions that propel food through the intestine. "Cutting back on sugar is an important change for people with IBS," says Michael A. Visconti, N.D., a naturopathic physician in Orlando, Florida.

Get fiber from fruit and veggies. You should have five daily servings of fruit and vegetables. While that's good advice for everyone, it's especially important if you have IBS. The fiber in these foods is very effective at reducing symptoms.

"Five servings a day is a good start," says Dr. Visconti. But more is even better. The more fiber you eat, the less painful—and frequent—your symptoms are likely to be.

Eat less, more often. Many people with IBS find that it helps to split their day's calories among five or six small meals, rather than following the traditional breakfast-lunch-dinner schedule. Eating less food at one time puts less strain on the large intestine.

Chew each bite. When you have IBS, your goal should be

Fill Up on Fiber

Apples and pears are among the best remedies for IBS because they're loaded with fiber, which helps tame intestinal spasms and encourages regular bowel movements. They're also easy to snack on as you go about your day. Other foods that offer a lot of fiber bang for your buck include oat bran and ground flaxseed. Try sprinkling a tablespoon of either on your salads, cereal, or yogurt.

to make life as easy as possible for your digestive system. If you eat slowly and chew food thoroughly, your intestine has less work to do, which can reduce or even eliminate some of the discomfort.

Five-alarm alert! While some people with IBS have painful flare-ups when they eat spicy foods, others find that a little culinary heat makes them feel better. "The right kinds of spices seem to help," says Dr. Visconti. Hot foods, such as chile peppers and ground red pepper, contain capsaicin, a chemical compound that may make your intestine less sensitive.

Fight fire with fish. Some foods can help quell the intestinal inflammation that contributes to IBS symptoms. For example, salmon and other cold-water fish, as well as ground flaxseed, contain omega-3 fatty acids, which help your body suppress inflammation.

Pop a peppermint pill. Peppermint is a traditional treatment for gastrointestinal problems. Look for enteric-coated peppermint capsules, available in health food stores. The coating allows the capsules to break down in your intestine rather than in your stomach. Follow the label directions.

Load up on yogurt. Not all germs are bad germs. In fact, we couldn't get along without certain types of bacteria that live in the intestine and aid digestion. Live-culture yogurt contains beneficial *Lactobacillus acidophilus* organisms, which

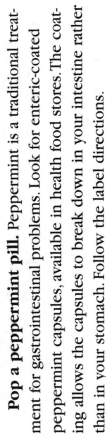

A Slick Solution

Many digestive ailments respond well to the herb slippery elm, and IBS is no exception. You can buy the powdered form at health food stores and drugstores. Mix a teaspoon of powder in a cup of warm water, stir well, and drink. It will coat and soothe your irritated digestive tract.

appear to reduce IBS symptoms. Plan on having at least a few servings of live-culture yogurt a week.

Imagine less stress. For many people with IBS, the best way to ease discomfort is to change the ways in which they respond to stress, says Dr. Visconti. "You have to learn to manage stress without sending it to your digestive tract," he explains.

A technique called imagery is a great way to manage stress. Every day, set aside a few minutes to relax in a quiet place. Fill your mind with peaceful thoughts—the sights, smells, and sounds of a garden, for example—and simply relax for 10 to 15 minutes. "It really works," he says.

Take a hike. You may not be up to it when your symptoms are in high gear, but 15 to 20 minutes of exercise every day is an important IBS-stopping strategy. Physical activity helps in two ways: It reduces levels of emotional stress, and it helps your bowel work more regularly. "People who exercise have a significant reduction of symptoms," says Dr. Visconti.

Turn off the tube. If you watch TV during meals, you could be setting yourself up for an IBS attack. Disquieting news programs and annoying commercials tend to ratchet up stress levels, which invariably makes symptoms worse, says Dr. Visconti. You'll also tend to eat too quickly because you're not paying attention to your food. His advice: Turn off the TV and enjoy your meals in peace and quiet.

Kidney Stones

Pass On the Pain

If you don't know anyone who's had kidney stones, be patient; the odds are very good that you or someone you know will have to deal with these miserable little buggers sometime soon.

According to the National Institutes of Health, about 1 in 10 of us will get kidney stones at some point in our lives. Yet when I talked to Amy Turnbull, N.D., a naturopathic physician at the Bastyr Center for Natural Health near Seattle, I was surprised to find out that experts aren't sure why some people are prone to this all-too-common ailment, or why men get kidney stones more often than women. "These are the million-dollar questions," Dr. Turnbull says. "I wish we knew the answers, because it would make kidney stones easier to treat."

NO-PASSING ZONE

Here's what we do know: Chemicals and minerals that are normally present in urine sometimes solidify and form hard little crystals, or stones. Most of the stones are so tiny that they pass harmlessly through your body without making you aware of their existence. Larger stones are more of a problem. They can get stuck in the narrow tubes, called ureters, that connect your kidneys and bladder. Or they can irritate the urethra, the tube that carries urine out of your body.

The excruciating pain of a kidney stone usually occurs in your lower back or groin. The pain can come and go as the stone moves through your body. Many people also experience nausea, blood in the urine, or an increased urge to urinate.

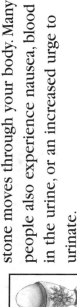

Orange You Glad?

Anyone who's concerned about kidney stones will want to start the day with an orange or a tall glass of juice, then continue to eat oranges or quaff orange juice throughout the day. The citrus fruit raises your body's level of citrates, natural chemicals that keep new stones from forming and existing stones from getting worse. Discuss this with your doctor first, however, since not all types of stones are affected by citrates.

ROLL WITH 'EM

If you were experiencing kidney stone pain right now, you wouldn't be reading this book. You'd be on the floor, curled up in agony. A kidney stone isn't something to handle on your own; you need to see a doctor immediately. You'll probably need x-rays or other tests to determine exactly where the stone is. Once your doctor knows its location and size, there are a number of treatment options. He may recommend "watch-ful waiting"—giving the stone a little time to exit your body on its own—or give you medication to dissolve it. If the problem is severe, however, you'll probably need surgery to remove the stone.

Your body is usually pretty good at getting rid of kidney stones. The usual strategy is to hang in there until the stone works its way out. But if you get kidney stones frequently, you'll need to find ways to minimize the pain—and more important, to keep stones from recurring. Here's what doctors advise.

Add heat—or cold. During a kidney stone attack, one of

the best things you can do is apply an ice pack or a heating pad to your abdomen, lower back, or wherever you're feeling the pain. Either will take the edge off until you can get professional help.

Drink lots of water. Staying well hydrated should be a top priority for those who are stone-prone. Keeping enough water flowing through your system reduces the concentration of stone-forming minerals. Water can also help dissolve small stones that have already formed.

Fill up on fiber. You'll do yourself a big favor by adding more fiber to your diet. "People who have

high-fiber diets are less likely to get stones," Dr. Turnbull says. You can get loads by filling up on fresh fruit and vegetables, as well as legumes, whole grains, and high-fiber cereals. You want to get at least 20 grams of fiber a day, but 30 to 35 grams is even better.

Be a teetotaler. Avoid alcohol and caffeine when you're coping with a kidney stone. Alcohol's dehydrating effects will interfere with your body's ability to dissolve and flush the stone. Caffeine has diuretic properties and can be dehydrating as

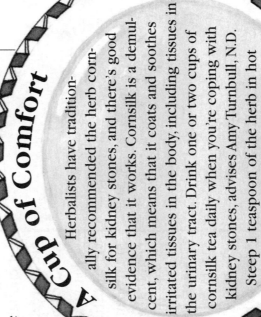

A Cup of Comfort

Herbalists have traditionally recommended the herb cornsilk for kidney stones, and there's good evidence that it works. Cornsilk is a demulcent, which means that it coats and soothes irritated tissues in the body, including tissues in the urinary tract. Drink one or two cups of cornsilk tea daily when you're coping with kidney stones, advises Amy Turnbull, N.D. Steep 1 teaspoon of the herb in hot water for about 10 minutes, then strain and sip.

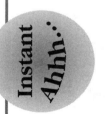

well. It will make you feel a lot more uncomfortable when your system is trying to eliminate one or more stones. "Caffeine increases activity in the nervous system, which can aggravate the pain," Dr. Turnbull explains.

Relax with magnesium. The mineral magnesium relaxes muscles throughout your body, which can reduce pain during kidney stone attacks, says Dr. Turnbull. "Take 600 milligrams a day," she advises. This amount may cause diarrhea in some people. If this occurs, reduce the dose.

Beat them with B_6. It hasn't been proven, but there's some evidence that people who don't get enough vitamin B_6 in their diets are more likely to get kidney stones, says Dr. Turnbull. If you've had kidney stones in the past, an easy preventive strategy is to take a daily multivitamin that contains 100 percent of the Daily Value B_6.

Get the correct calcium. Some types of kidney stones are composed mainly of calcium. In the past, people who got these kinds of stones were advised to cut back on the mineral. Doctors now believe that the calcium you get from foods actually helps prevent kidney stones, although the calcium in supplements may make you more prone to them.

When you talk to your doctor, find out if your stones are the calcium variety. If they are, ask whether

Soak That Stone

Your doctor will probably advise you to take an over-the-counter or prescription painkiller during kidney stone attacks. While you're waiting for it to work, add a cup or two of Epsom salts to a warm bath and soak for a while. The warmth of the water will ease stress as well as discomfort. In addition, the magnesium in Epsom salts may help relax muscles in your urinary tract and further reduce the pain.

Instant Ahhh...

he recommends increasing or cutting back on calcium in your diet.

Widen the road. The herb viburnum is a muscle relaxant that makes it easier for stones to move through your body. It's available at health food stores in many forms, including capsules, tinctures, and teas. Each product contains different amounts of the active ingredient, so follow the label directions to be sure you're taking the proper amount.

Dissolve and conquer. Also check the shelves at the health food store for gravelroot, stoneroot, and pellitory-of-the-wall. These herbs have long been used by herbalists as kidney tonics for people who are prone to developing stones. Make a tea by adding 1 tablespoon of each herb to 1 quart of hot water. Steep for 20 minutes, then let cool and drink throughout the day for up to one week. Once again, check the label directions before taking any of these herbs. If you plan to use them for more than a few days, consult a naturopathic physician, who can advise you about their benefits and risks.

It's an Emergency!

Don't assume that everything's going to be fine if you've been diagnosed with kidney stones. While pain is normal, you shouldn't have fever, nausea, or vomiting, nor should the pain get significantly worse. If you experience any of these symptoms, call your doctor immediately. There's a good chance that the stone has caused an infection, and you may need antibiotics right away to keep it from getting worse.

Menstrual Pain

Ride a Smoother Cycle

There's a whole constellation of things that can plague a woman during the second half of her monthly cycle, and—despite the impression given by some made-for-TV movies—none of them involve howling at the moon!

Some of the most common discomforts include body aches, fatigue, headaches, bloating, and mood changes. Then, once the menstrual period begins, there may be painful cramping, which doctors call dysmenorrhea. The discomfort usually doesn't last longer than three to five days, but it can make your life pretty miserable in the meantime.

SHIFTING HORMONES

Cramps are caused by uterine contractions, and many of the other symptoms are thought to be due to an imbalance of the hormones estrogen and progesterone. Usually, progesterone is the dominant hormone after ovulation. An excess of estrogen or a deficiency of progesterone can trigger discomfort.

BEAT THE PRE-MENS BLUES

Just about every woman experiences some type of premenstrual or menstrual discomfort. The intensity of that discomfort, however, varies widely. Some women barely notice their symptoms, while others are all but disabled by them.

If your symptoms are so extreme that you can't function normally, talk to your doctor. You may need prescription drugs to quell the discomfort. Most women, however, don't need cutting-edge medical technology to feel better. There are plenty of strategies for handling the pain, and many of them have been working for women for centuries. Here are a few of the best.

Eat like Eve. The more fresh fruits, vegetables, and whole grains you eat, the less room there will be in your diet for packaged and processed foods. That means you'll cut a lot of sodium out of your diet, which will reduce the discomfort of water retention and bloating. It also means that you'll eat fewer

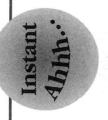

animal-based saturated fats, which have been linked to pain and inflammation. Plus, you'll get plenty of complex carbohydrates, which will keep your blood sugar levels steady and your mood on an even keel. So consider your supermarket's produce department to be your personal garden of eatin'.

Feel better with B$_6$. "The big vitamin for premenstrual problems is vitamin B$_6$," says Jana Nalbandian, N.D., a naturo-

Take Up Belly Dancing

If you've ever had an urge to explore the culture of the Middle East, here's your excuse: The movements taught in belly dancing are great for stretching your pelvis and keeping cramps at bay. "Belly dancing can be very helpful," says Jana Nalbandian, N.D. "Any exercise that gets you moving and rocking your pelvis will help."

pathic physician and faculty member at Bastyr University near Seattle. It seems to have a positive effect on levels of serotonin, a feel-good chemical in the brain. Most women can take up to 50 milligrams of B_6 daily for four or five days when premenstrual problems flare up. Talk to your doctor first, though, since high doses of B_6 can cause nerve problems in rare cases.

Call on the dynamic duo. The minerals magnesium and calcium are the Batman and Robin of pain relief. They can rescue you from a whole rogue's gallery of symptoms, including muscle aches, cramps, headaches, water retention, and food cravings. Talk to your doctor about taking 300 to 500 milligrams of each daily when you're having premenstrual or menstrual discomfort. Magnesium may cause diarrhea in some people. If this occurs, reduce the dose.

Overpower pain with pumpkin seeds. They're loaded with fatty acids that lower levels of body chemicals responsible for muscle aches and menstrual cramps. You can get the same oils by eating ground flaxseed or cold-water fish, such as salmon and tuna. Plan on having at least one of these foods daily when your symptoms are flaring

A Cup of Comfort

Raspberry leaf tea is a traditional remedy for menstrual cramps. It appears to strengthen the uterus and makes it less likely to contract too vigorously. "Three cups a day for a month or so will tone the uterus," says Jana Nalbandian, N.D. "I'd add some ginger to increase circulation—and it makes the tea taste better." You can find the tea at health food stores, but don't use it if there's a chance you may be pregnant.

up. Or, for convenience, take fatty-acid capsules or liquids, available in health food stores.

Run hot and cold. You can unkink menstrual cramps with compresses made by soaking washcloths in hot and cold water. First, place a hot compress on your abdomen for about 3 minutes. Replace it with a cold compress and leave it in place for 30 seconds. Repeat the cycle two more times, always ending with cold. This simple technique is a very effective way to increase blood flow, which in turn reduces cramps.

Consider castor oil. A castor oil pack is a traditional way to ease the pain of menstrual cramps. Spread castor oil on the skin of your abdomen and cover it with a layer of plastic wrap. Then heat the area with a warm, moist towel or a heating pad set on low. The gentle heat penetrates deeply into your abdomen and relaxes muscles as well as cramps.

Butt out. Smoking is a notorious contributor to painful menstrual cramps. "It can decrease the flow of blood and oxygen to the uterus," says Dr. Nalbandian. It's just one more reason to quit.

Shift gears. Studies show that exercise eases premenstrual and menstrual symptoms, but a high-impact workout may be uncomfortable if you're cramping. Take it easy for a few

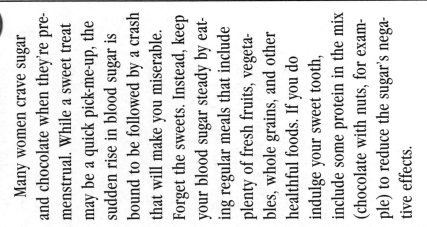

The Chocolate Crash

Many women crave sugar and chocolate when they're premenstrual. While a sweet treat may be a quick pick-me-up, the sudden rise in blood sugar is bound to be followed by a crash that will make you miserable. Forget the sweets. Instead, keep your blood sugar steady by eating regular meals that include plenty of fresh fruits, vegetables, whole grains, and other healthful foods. If you do indulge your sweet tooth, include some protein in the mix (chocolate with nuts, for example) to reduce the sugar's negative effects.

days and stick to low-impact forms of exercise such as yoga, swimming, or tai chi.

Take advantage of analgesics. Aspirin, ibuprofen, and similar over-the-counter painkillers are very effective at quelling menstrual cramps. They inhibit the body's production of prostaglandins, chemicals that cause pain as well as increased uterine contractions. While acetaminophen can ease your discomfort somewhat, it isn't as effective because it has little effect on prostaglandins.

Act like a cat. "Yoga's great for menstrual problems because it's relaxing and it increases circulation," says Dr. Nalbandian. One yoga stretch in particular, called The Cat, is especially helpful because it targets the abdominal area. Get on the floor on your hands and knees. Moving slowly and gently, tilt your pelvis and tailbone toward the floor while arching your back toward the ceiling. Hold the stretch for a few moments, then go the opposite way: Tilt your pelvis upward and let your spine curve toward the floor.

Try the Child's Pose. This is another yoga move that's good for menstrual discomfort. Kneel on the floor and sit back on your heels. Lean forward, gently lowering your chest until it's resting on your thighs. Extend your arms in front of you until your palms touch the floor. Hold the pose for as long as you're comfortable, then slowly return to the kneeling position. It's very relaxing—and good for you, too!

STRETCHING

Side Stitches

Fast Fixes

I hang out with a few athletes, so I thought it would be easy to find people who could tell me about side stitches. You know, those nasty, pinching pains that occur during exercise and can make you feel as if you've been stabbed in the ribs with a salad fork.

But I was wrong. No one I knew got them, and I soon found out why. Side stitches are a problem mostly for beginning runners or people who haven't been working out for very long. Some of the athletes I spoke to seemed almost offended that I raised the subject. Maybe they've forgotten what a burden side stitches can be to those of us who aren't in top shape.

Doctors, on the other hand, are very familiar with the problem. As it turns out, there's a lot you can do to stop them fast—and keep them from coming back.

Instant Ahhh...

Breathe Deep

The quickest way to stop a side stitch may be simply to take a deep breath. But don't just fill your lungs—let your abdomen expand as you breathe in. This technique, called belly breathing, seems to stretch the diaphragm and make side stitches less intense.

SIDE-SPLITTING PAIN

Most of us have experienced side stitches at one time or another—while running to catch a bus, for example, or taking an extra lap around the track. The painful, cramp-like sensation does indeed feel as if a tight stitch has been sewn into your side. The pain doesn't last very long, but it can sure slow you down until it goes away.

Side stitches are something of a mystery to doctors, since no one really knows what causes them. It could be a cramp in your diaphragm, the muscle that moves up and down to fill and empty your lungs as you breathe, or perhaps a muscle cramp in your side or somewhere in your respiratory tract. Other theories are that side stitches are caused by gas bubbles in your intestine or even the weight of your liver pulling on your diaphragm.

SAVE YOUR SIDE

For reasons that aren't clear, side stitches occur more often on the right side than on the left. They never last very long, and they're never serious. The one sure cure is to rest, but there are a few other things you can do to make the pain go away more quickly.

Slow down, hands down. If you don't want to stop exercising when a side stitch strikes, you can often cut it short just

---

Healing Hands

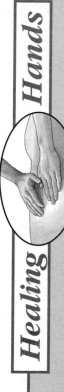

One way to deal with a side stitch is to rub it out, according to John Nowicki, N.D. "Deep pressure on the affected area can help," he says. Just press against the painful spot for several seconds, then release. Repeat the pressure until the side stitch is gone.

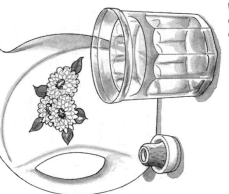

by slowing down, taking some deep breaths, and letting your hands drop to your sides.

"This helps stretch the diaphragm, which often helps relieve the pain," says John Nowicki, N.D., a naturopathic physician in Issaquah, Washington. Once the stitch is gone, you can ease back up to full speed.

Reach for the sky. Stretching the side of your body that's stitched will often bring relief. If the stitch is in your right side, for example, raise your right arm over your head and bend your torso to the left. Hold the position (called a side stretch) for about 30 seconds, then switch and do the other side. By the time you've finished, the stitch will probably be gone.

Lighten up. Decreasing the intensity of your workouts is a fairly reliable way to cut down on the frequency of side stitches, Dr. Nowicki says. "No one knows exactly what a side stitch is, so I can't say for sure that it's a clear sign that you're working too hard. But decreasing the intensity does seem to help."

Shun the bubbly. Your favorite carbonated beverage is best left in the fridge if you're trying to avoid side stitches. The bubbles tend to cause excess gas, which some experts think leads to side stitches or cramps. Stay away from fizzy drinks immediately before or right after your workout.

Drink lots of water. If your body is properly hydrated, you're less likely to get cramps of all sorts, side stitches included. On average, you need between 64 and 80 ounces of water a day. "Add 8 to 16 ounces of water for each hour of exercise," says Dr. Nowicki.

Stomachache

Quit Your Belly-Achin'

One of my neighbor's kids used to get terrible stomachaches when he was in fourth grade. His parents tried everything they could think of: They changed his diet, they talked to his teachers, and they even had him checked for allergies. But the stomachaches kept coming.

Then one day, when his mom was volunteering in the lunchroom, she noticed something interesting. Her son, who had always been the gregarious type, spent most of his lunch period chatting and goofing around with his many friends. Just before lunchtime ended, he wolfed down almost all of his meal. And sure enough, that was the cause of his afternoon stomach woes. It took some doing, but eventually he learned to eat at a more reasonable pace, and his stomachaches became a thing of the past.

THE GUT REACTION

Most stomachaches don't occur in your stomach at all, even though that's

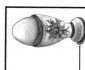

Lemon Aid

To prevent stomachaches from getting started, squeeze a little lemon juice into a glass of water and sip it before meals. It will stimulate digestive secretions and get your stomach ready for business.

where the trouble usually begins. For various reasons, your stomach doesn't always do a great job of digesting its contents. When undigested food travels into the intestine, you're likely to experience cramps or painful gas. Thus, a stomachache is really an intestine ache—one that occurs when your bowel has to deal with your stomach's unfinished business.

TAMING TENDER TUMMIES

A stomachache isn't always a routine problem. In fact, there's a long list of medical conditions that cause pain somewhere in the belly, and some of them are serious. The basic rule is this: A stomachache that

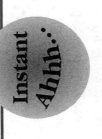

clears up within a day or two probably isn't anything serious. If the pain lingers, is accompanied by fever or vomiting, or keeps coming back, see your doctor. You're probably going to need some tests to find out exactly what's going on. For ordinary stomachaches, though, here are a few things that are sure to help.

Have a dandy salad. Dandelion greens are a traditional remedy for stomach problems of all kinds. Eaten before a meal, the pleasantly bitter greens stimulate digestive secretions and reduce cramping.

Be sure to pick dandelions from an area that hasn't been treated with chemicals. The leaves are most tender when they're picked just before the flowers bloom.

Instant Ahhh...

Move Along

It's tempting to curl up on the couch after a big meal, but making a beeline from the kitchen to the sofa could leave you with a stomachache. A walk, combined with the effects of gravity when you're standing up, will prevent many stomachaches from getting started, says Andrew Parkinson, N.D.

Supplement your enzymes. If your stomach doesn't do an effective job of digesting your meals, you're sure to get heartburn or a stomachache. Supplemental digestive enzymes can help, says Andrew Parkinson, N.D., a naturopathic physician and faculty member at the Bastyr Center for Natural Health near Seattle.

Many different digestive enzymes are available at health food stores, including bromelain and papain. It doesn't really matter what kind you get; they're all helpful. Take them before you eat, following the directions on the label. "They're particularly good for reducing that bloated, after-meal feeling," says Dr. Parkinson.

Eat, don't drink. If you tend to get stomachaches after eating, you may want to give up drinking water or other liquids with your meals, because they dilute the stomach's acid secretions, says Dr. Parkinson. The acid, of course, helps you digest food.

Bring on the bacteria. Your gut is loaded with beneficial bacteria that break down and digest food. Sometimes, these bacteria get depleted—if you've been taking antibiotics, for example—resulting in painful abdominal cramps.

A Cup of Comfort

Chamomile is one of the world's most popular teas, and for good reason: It's been used as a stomach soother for centuries. Just be sure to wait 15 minutes after meals before drinking it. Otherwise, the liquid will dilute the acids needed for proper digestion. As long as you're not allergic to ragweed, you can make tea by adding a tea bag or a teaspoon of dried herb to a cup of freshly boiled water. Steep for 10 minutes, remove the tea bag or strain and drink.

An easy way to boost their numbers back to healthful levels is to take supplements that contain acidophilus. One or two acidophilus capsules is often all you need to calm the upset feeling.

Just say Yo! A serving of yogurt is another great way to load your gut with more beneficial bacteria. Look for brands that contain live cultures. "It's not something you need on a daily basis, but it's a good idea to try to replenish those bacteria from time to time," says Dr. Parkinson.

Have an aperitif. If you're a wine lover, you may know this already: A glass of dry white wine before a meal is good for digestion. In fact, a trip to the liquor store will reveal many aperitifs and "bitters" traditionally used to jump-start the digestive process. These liquid appetizers contain natural chemicals that stimulate digestion.

Count on catnip. Everyone knows what catnip does to our feline friends. In humans, however, the herb is actually quite soothing. "It has a mild sedating quality, calms the gastrointestinal tract, and decreases cramping," says Dr. Parkinson.

He recommends taking catnip in capsule form when you have a stomachache, following the directions on the label. Or make a tea by adding a teaspoon of the dried herb to a cup of freshly boiled water. Steep for 10 minutes, strain, and drink. Both forms are available at health food stores.

Spice up your menu. Many pungent spices can help relieve stomach problems. "Ginger, turmeric, cumin, coriander,

Settle Your Stomach with a Scented Sniff

Sometimes, all it takes to calm an upset stomach is the right scent. The next time your gut's in a knot, scratch the peel of an uncut lemon and take a few whiffs, or open a bottle of peppermint essential oil and take a deep sniff. The odors travel to your brain and appear to help keep your stomach from going topsy-turvy.

clove, cinnamon, and garlic all promote good digestion," says Dr. Parkinson. And you don't have to eat tons of these herbs to get the benefits: Just look for recipes that already include them.

Walk, don't run. An after-dinner stroll is a good idea, but you don't want to be too active after eating. If you are, your body won't have enough energy for proper digestion—and cramps and gas may result.

Forget the antacids. While they're great for occasional bouts of heartburn, antacids won't do you any good when you have a stomachache. In fact, they can cause side effects, including constipation or diarrhea, that will make you feel even worse.

Drop the dairy. If you tend to get stomachaches after drinking milk or eating other dairy products, it's probably because you don't produce enough of the enzyme needed to digest lactose, a sugar found in dairy products.

One solution, of course, is to give up dairy altogether. Another is to buy reduced-lactose dairy foods at supermarkets. In addition, having small servings—say, half a glass of milk instead of a full pint—may allow your stomach to handle dairy foods without discomfort.

Ulcers

Soothe Internal Sores

Whenever I have reason to think about ulcers, the first thing that jumps into my mind is *The Odd Couple*. As you may remember, one of the recurring themes of this classic 1970s sitcom was poor Oscar Madison's ongoing struggle with ulcers. He was always getting them, mainly (he thought) because of his terrible diet, constant cigar smoking, and the stress of living with his obsessively neat roommate, Felix Unger.

I've watched reruns, and while the show is as funny as ever, its whole premise about ulcers is obsolete. Today, Oscar would be treated with antibiotics to eradicate the true cause of his never-ending discomfort: not Felix, but tiny, screw-shaped organisms that were living in his digestive tract.

Of course, this is nowhere near as amusing as watching

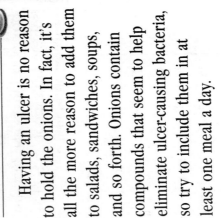

More Onions, Less Pain

Having an ulcer is no reason to hold the onions. In fact, it's all the more reason to add them to salads, sandwiches, soups, and so forth. Onions contain compounds that seem to help eliminate ulcer-causing bacteria, so try to include them in at least one meal a day.

Oscar throw Felix out of the apartment for the 17th time. But that's the price of progress.

PAIN IN THE PIT

The digestive acids in your stomach are strong enough to dissolve the heaviest meal into a digestible soup of nutrients. In fact, these acids are nearly as strong as battery acid. I've often wondered why they don't digest the stomach just as efficiently as they break down a serving of my mother's pasta.

Nature, it turns out, designed the stomach to withstand constant acid onslaughts by giving it a thin, protective lining that prevents the acids from damaging the tender tissue underneath. Of course, this system works only if the protective barrier is intact.

That's where germs come in. *Helicobacter pylori*, a type of bacterium that commonly inhabits the stomach and intestine, digs into this protective lining. If you're infected with *H. pylori*, the lining may be pitted with tiny holes that permit stomach acid to leak through. The result: small, painful little sores known as ulcers. Ulcers can also be triggered by the prolonged use of pain relievers, including aspirin and ibuprofen. You need to stay in touch with your doctor if you take these drugs on a regular basis.

BUILD UP YOUR BELLY

Most people with ulcers experience a burning sensation from time to time, usually between meals, when their stomachs

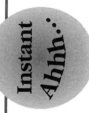

Instant Ahhh...

Beat It with Baking Soda

For a handy way to neutralize acid that may be aggravating your ulcer, reach to the back of your fridge for that box of baking soda. Just dissolve a tablespoon in a glass of water and imbibe.

are empty. Don't ignore the pain; see your doctor. Ulcers that aren't treated can bleed, and sometimes they bleed a lot. It's not uncommon, in fact, for people with ulcers to become anemic because of blood loss.

Severe ulcers sometimes need to be treated surgically, but that's rare. Most often, they can be eliminated with a relatively simple, two-part treatment: Antibiotics to kill the bacteria and medications to lower levels of stomach acid. Along with treatment, however, there are a few lifestyle approaches that do make a difference. Here's what doctors recommend.

Antacids aren't always the answer. When the burning pain of ulcers flares, your natural instinct is probably to pop a few antacids. There's certainly nothing wrong with this approach in some cases, but some doctors suspect that quenching stomach acid with antacids may make ulcers worse in the long run.

"You need stomach acids to obliterate microorganisms," says Christie C. Yerby, N.D., a naturopathic physician in Sanford, North Carolina. "Lowering the acidity of the stomach makes it easier for ulcer-causing bacteria to survive."

If you're taking antacids, but they don't seem to help, make an appointment to see your doctor. You may be doing yourself a lot more harm than good.

A Cup of Comfort

Tea made with slippery elm forms a sticky, soothing coating on the lining of the digestive tract. This protects small ulcers from further acid damage and may help them heal more quickly. Slippery elm tea is available in powdered form at health food stores. Add a teaspoon of powder to a cup of freshly boiled water and steep for 10 to 15 minutes. Drink one to two cups daily when ulcers flare up.

Tame your sweet tooth. Most of us love sugar—but we're not the only ones. The bacteria that cause ulcers are also extremely fond of sweets. "The more sugar you consume, the more you're feeding the bacteria that cause ulcers," says Dr. Yerby. Her advice: Give up sweets, or at least save them for very special occasions.

Say hello to aloe. Aloe vera is one of nature's great healers, and it's especially good for ulcers because it coats irritated tissues and may promote faster healing. You can buy aloe juice at health food stores, or if you grow aloe at home to treat minor injuries, just break open a leaf and squeeze some juice into your mouth, Dr. Yerby suggests. You can take aloe up to a couple of times a day.

Supplement your diet. If you don't eat a lot of fruit, vegetables, and other plant foods, you may not be getting enough of a few key nutrients—mainly vitamins A, C, and E—that are needed to repair damaged tissue throughout your body, including the stomach lining. If you have a history of ulcers, it's a good idea to take daily supplements that provide the recommended daily amounts of each of these important nutrients.

Pop a fish pill. Doctors and nutritionists almost beg Americans to eat more fish, in part because it's a rich source of essential fatty acids that help quell inflammation. If you have ulcers, however, eating too much fish may cause an increase in stomach acid—and pain, says Dr. Yerby. So instead of eating fish, she recommends that people with ulcers take fish-oil supplements, which are available at drugstores and health food stores. Follow the directions on the label.

Lick it with licorice. This sweet-tasting herb (not the candy) is powerful medicine. It reduces inflammation and appears to help ulcers heal more quickly. You can buy licorice-root tea bags or powder at health food stores. As long as you don't have high blood pressure, you can drink two or three cups of tea a day to ease the pain of ulcers and help keep them from coming back.

Also look for chewable DGL tablets, which are made from licorice that's had the blood pressure–raising compound removed. Chewing these tablets between meals will speed pain relief and aid in healing an ulcer. Follow the package directions.

Eliminate alcohol. And while you're at it, give up cigarettes if you're a smoker. Alcohol and tobacco tend to make ulcer pain worse, and they inhibit your body's ability to heal the damage. People who smoke and drink are also more likely to get ulcers than those who don't indulge.

Enjoy peaceful moments. Even though emotional stress doesn't cause ulcers, it does increase levels of stomach acid, which can make the pain worse. Stress reduction should be part of every anti-ulcer strategy, says Dr. Yerby.

When you feel your stress level rising, close your eyes, breathe deeply, and visualize a peaceful scene from nature, she advises. Keep the scene in your mind for 15 to 20 minutes. You'll find that you feel a lot more relaxed afterward— and you'll have less discomfort.

Pain in Your Nether Regions

- **Anal Pain**
- **Childbirth**
- **Hemorrhoids**
- **Painful Intercourse**
- **Penis and Testicle Pain**
- **Urinary Tract Infection**
- **Yeast Infection**

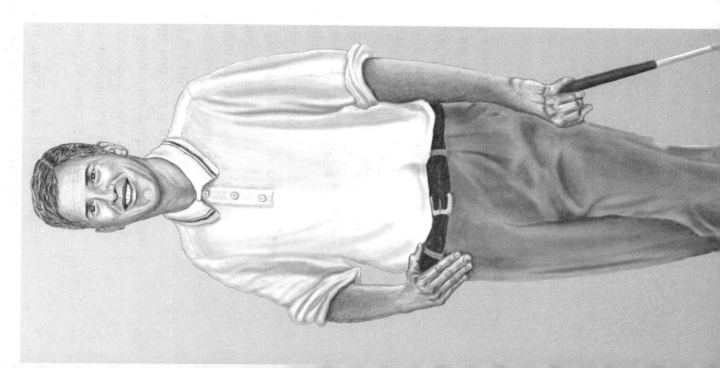

Anal Pain

Rear-Guard Actions

Since I started writing this book, I've begged, pestered, and cajoled my friends and acquaintances to share stories about their various ailments. But friendship goes only so far. When I asked around for accounts of pain in the rear end, my storytellers were suddenly silent.

That doesn't surprise Michael P. Spencer, M.D., a colon and rectal surgeon and assistant professor of surgery at the University of Minnesota, Twin Cities. "There's embarrassment about it," he says. "People are reluctant even to tell their doctors."

His final words of advice make good sense: Pain is pain, and there's no reason to suffer in silence just because it occurs in an "embarrassing" part of your body. If the discomfort is more than you can handle, don't keep it a secret. Get some help.

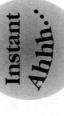

Instant Ahhh...

Sit and Soak

No matter what's making your bottom hurt, soaking in a warm bath for 10 to 20 minutes will almost certainly make you feel better. "It helps soothe the area and relaxes tight muscles," says Michael P. Spencer, M.D.

WHAT GOES WRONG

The anus is the last link in the digestive chain, and for the most part, it's pretty tough. But it's not invulnerable to problems, and some of them are pretty painful.

Consider anal fissures, which are small tears in the tissue. They're rarely serious, but they can be excruciating for the one to two weeks it takes them to heal. An anal abscess, an infection of a gland inside the anus, can make the area sore and tender. Then there are hemorrhoids, those pesky protuberances that can make sitting an agonizing experience (see page 248).

PUT THE PAIN BEHIND YOU

It's not a pleasant prospect, but anal pain generally requires a trip to the doctor. Without professional attention, there's really no way to tell what's causing the problem.

Consider anal abscesses.

Sometimes, they go away on their own, but other times, the infection gets worse, and the abscess has to be surgically drained. An untreated abscess can also progress to a dangerous, tunnel-like growth called a fistula, which also requires surgery.

Even anal fissures, which almost always heal on their own, can cause so much pain that they require a doctor's care. So here's the bottom line: Call your doctor if you have anal pain accompanied by fever, chills, sweating, or other signs of infection, or if it hurts so much that you can't have a bowel movement.

A Cup of Comfort

A daily cup of slippery elm tea will help keep your digestive tract, including the back end, running smoothly. It also soothes aggravated tissues throughout the intestine. Mix a teaspoon of slippery elm powder, available at health food stores, in a cup of hot water and steep for 10 minutes. Drink several cups of tea a day.

In the meantime, here are some easy solutions that will make your life a lot more comfortable.

Sit on some heat. A little gentle heat makes everything feel better, and your rear end is no exception. Cover a heating pad with a towel, set the heat on low, and sit and relax for as long as it feels comfortable.

Pop a pain reliever. Don't ignore the benefits of common pain relievers, such as aspirin and ibuprofen. They block chemicals in the body that cause pain, and they help control inflammation.

Pile on the produce. Fruit, vegetables, and other plant foods are loaded with fiber, which absorbs water in the intestine and makes stools softer and easier to pass. This helps in two ways: It makes bowel movements a lot less painful when you're having anal grief, and it reduces the risk that you'll have problems in the first place.

"People need to get at least 30 grams of fiber a day," says Dr. Spencer. That may sound like a lot for one day, but it's not. If you start the morning with a breakfast of bran cereal or shredded wheat, make your lunchtime sandwich with whole grain bread, and have several servings of vegetables and fruit throughout the day, you'll easily get all the fiber you need.

Supplement your fiber. If you can't seem to get adequate fiber from foods, take advantage of the fiber supplements that are available at drugstores and health food stores. Just follow the directions on the label. Products that contain psyllium, for example, are loaded with fiber and can help prevent those hard, painful stools that fre-

Fixes for Itches

Pruritus ani is a fancy term for anal itching, and it has all sorts of causes: too much perspiration, a bout of diarrhea, spicy foods, or even yeast infection. The itch can be maddening—and sometimes it lasts for days or even weeks.

Itching that lasts too long needs a doctor's care, but there's a good chance that you can treat it yourself. Here are some tips you may want to try.

Wipe without soap. A natural response to itchiness is to clean the area thoroughly, but it's important not to use soap of any kind. "We recommend that people keep clean with baby wipes or a moist washcloth," says Michael P. Spencer, M.D. Damp toilet paper is fine, too. The problem with soaps is that they tend to dry and irritate the skin, making the itching worse.

Be gentle. Don't be too rough after bowel movements or when quently cause anal pain.

Just be sure not to confuse fiber supplements with stimulant laxatives. They do different jobs, and powerful laxatives should be used only under the supervision of a doctor.

Drink lots of water. No kidding: By the time you're feeling thirsty, your body is already running low on water, which means that you're more likely to suffer from hard stools or other causes of anal pain.

Most people need about 6 glasses of water daily, says Dr. Spencer. If you're active or live in a warm climate, drink 8 to 10 glasses, and don't wait until you're parched. Keep water nearby and sip it throughout the day.

washing. Gently blot or pat the area clean.

Dry thoroughly. Moisture is your enemy, so be sure you stay dry. After you shower or bathe, you may want to towel off, then dust on a little cornstarch powder to absorb moisture.

Forget hydrocortisone. This anti-inflammatory cream is generally an excellent itch fighter, but you don't want to apply it to your anal area. You could get an allergic reaction that will only make matters worse.

Watch what you eat. Some people find that certain foods and beverages trigger or aggravate itching. Common culprits include chocolate, fruit, tomatoes, nuts, popcorn, milk, citrus fruit juices, alcoholic beverages, and drinks containing caffeine.

In fact, you should avoid any foods that can throw your bowel habits out of whack. "It's not the time to go out and drink a lot of beer or eat hot tamales," says Dr. Spencer.

Check your prescriptions. Unfortunately, some prescription drugs increase the risk of constipation, which can cause or aggravate anal pain. Among the likely suspects are prescription analgesics, antidepressants, tranquilizers, blood pressure drugs, iron and calcium supplements, and antacids. If you've noticed any change in your usual bowel habits or you're constipated more than occasionally, ask your doctor or pharmacist if any of your medications could be to blame. (See "Constipation" on page 188.)

Childbirth

Take the Pain Out of Labor

I recently attended a family reunion, and boy, there were babies everywhere. For each baby, it seemed, there was a different story about the birth. One mother had a quick but painful delivery. Another chose natural childbirth. My sister, Suzanne, had a relatively easy delivery, but her recovery was somewhat difficult.

When I talked to doctors about the wonders—and discomfort—of childbirth, they all said the same thing: It's amazing that women are willing to go through it more than once. But for me, the most amazing thing is that no two births are exactly alike.

NO WONDER THEY CALL IT LABOR!

Having a baby is painful. In fact, whenever we want to describe an unusually painful condition, we'll say

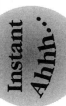

Instant Ahhh...

Power of the Press

A fast way to ease pain in your back during labor is to firmly press the area on either side of your sacrum, or tailbone. Pressing on both sides simultaneously appears to blunt the flow of pain signals from your lower back.

something like, "It hurts as much as giving birth."

But pain is only a tiny part of the entire miracle of childbirth. It's reasonable for women to mentally prepare themselves for the discomfort, but they shouldn't let their worries and misgivings overshadow what should be a joyous, exhilarating experience.

"The fear of pain makes a big difference in how labor progresses and how well women deal with labor," says Donielle Wilson, N.D., a naturopathic physician at Sea Change Healing Center in New York City. "Take classes and do a lot of reading," she advises. And while you can't take away the pain of childbirth, there are a lot of ways to make it much more bearable.

SPECIAL DELIVERY

Obviously, different women experience labor in different ways. The doctors I talked to agreed that there are a number of techniques that can make the entire process go more smoothly, but only you and your doctor are aware of the relevant factors in your particular case. With that in mind, here are some approaches that have been shown to work.

Head back to school. Childbirth classes are a routine part of pregnancy these days. They're a great way to learn what to expect, and the instructors give a lot of practical advice on ways to ease the process. Your doctor or health care provider can refer you to classes in your area.

Accentuate the positive. It's natural to talk with other women about their experiences, but don't encourage them to share their war stories. "When women hear stories from family members and friends, and most of the stories focus on pain, they get even more frightened," says Dr. Wilson. Encourage

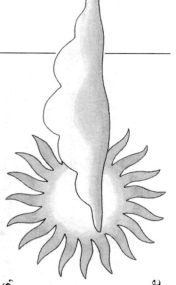

Breathe Away Pain

The natural breathing that you do in day-to-day life isn't the same kind of breathing that you need to do during labor. Here's what doctors advise.

- Take slow, deep breaths in the early stages of labor to ensure that you're breathing regularly. Some women tend to hold their breath when they're in pain.

- When you feel a contraction, take a good, deep "cleansing" breath to ride it out.

- As contractions get more frequent, prevent hyperventilation with "patterned" breathing. You can take two or three short breaths, then one longer one, for example.

- Once you start pushing, hold your breath to make it easier. Your doctor may advise you to take a breath and hold it while you push for 10 seconds. Then you'll breathe, hold your breath, and push again.

your friends to discuss all of the things that went right with their deliveries, not just the difficult aspects.

Build some muscle. Women who have strong pelvic muscles tend to have easier deliveries. A quick way to build these muscles is with Kegel exercises, in which you contract your pelvic area as if you're trying to stop the flow of urine. Squeezing and relaxing these muscles throughout the day—when you're watching TV, for example, or even when you're standing in line at the supermarket—can make a lot of difference when the important day comes.

To do Kegels, tightly clench your pelvic muscles, hold for a count of 10, then relax. Repeat the sequence 10 to 20 times two or three times a day. You should continue to do these exercises throughout your pregnancy.

Stay active. Doctors used to advise women to be sedentary in the latter part of pregnancy. They now know, however, that regular exercise will not only make you feel better, it will also help labor proceed more smoothly.

Talk to your doctor about how much exercise is appropriate for you. Exercise is almost always safe during pregnancy, as long as you aren't at risk for premature labor.

Work out with other mothers. It's not hard to find prenatal exercise classes; most health clubs offer them. There are yoga classes, dance classes, and so on. Many women find that it's less intimidating and more comfortable to exercise with other moms-to-be.

Prep your perineum. Massaging your perineum—the area below the vaginal opening—prepares the area for the delivery and makes it less likely to tear. "A perineal massage gets that tissue ready to be stretched, and it also gets you ready for the sensations that you'll experience during labor," says Dr. Wilson.

Starting a month before your due date, give the area a daily massage by gently rubbing it with your fingers or thumbs. The massage will be more comfortable if you use a little oil. "Almond and wheat germ oils are good choices," says Dr. Wilson. "You can even use olive or vegetable oil."

Don't take it lying down. There's no reason to stay flat on your back during labor. Getting up and about can ease some of the discomfort. "Especially when you're early in the labor process, moving around is great because it encourages labor to progress," says Dr. Wilson. "You should be able to take a walk, stand up, squat, or kneel. Try every possible position that you can think of to make yourself more comfortable."

Moving around during labor will help you find the optimal position for your pelvis. Just do whatever feels comfortable.

You'll also find that moving around regularly will help the time pass more quickly.

Press the point. Acupressure, which is like acupuncture without the puncture, can help take the edge off painful contractions. During labor, press against the sides of your wrists, in line with your pinky finger, for 10 to 15 seconds.

A warm reception. Another way to ease the pain of labor is to put a heating pad or hot water bottle on your abdomen or waist. Stores that carry massage and relaxation products sell long, rice-filled pads that fit around your body under your belly. After being heated in the microwave, they can help. Check with your doctor to see if it's advisable for you to use one.

Chill the pain. Back pain is very common during labor. Some women apply hot water bottles or heating pads to soothe their lower backs, but ice is often better because it acts as a local anesthetic. If you opt for ice, wrap it in a small towel or a washcloth and hold it right where the pain is. Keep the cold in place for about 20 minutes. Let your back warm up for a while, then apply the ice again.

Take a mental vacation. "It's amazing how the mind can take us away from where we are," says Dr. Wilson. "If you're anxious or fearful or in pain, using imagery can be very effective."

In its simplest form, imagery involves focusing your mind on something that you find relaxing: a flower, a blue sky, or a calm ocean. Or you can have a friend or your spouse describe a relaxing scene—including the setting and all the sounds, colors, and sensations—such as walking on the beach or relaxing in a garden.

Depend on a doula. "One thing that helps a lot of women who are dealing with the pain of childbirth is using a doula," says Dr. Wilson. A doula (pronounced *DOO-la*) is essentially a pregnancy coach—a woman who's trained to provide physical and emotional support during labor.

"She's there the whole time," says Dr. Wilson. "A doula will help you with position changes or remind you to breathe or take a drink of water."

Doulas help husbands get through the process as well. If your husband becomes anxious because you're in pain, for instance, the doula can give him suggestions and remind him what to do to help you.

To find a doula in your area, contact Doulas of North America at 888-788-DONA. The Web address is www.dona.org.

Hemorrhoids

Put the Pain Behind You

I don't know about you, but even saying the word *bemorrhoid* makes me blush a little. We all get these annoying (and uncomfortable) anal nuisances from time to time, but it's not the type of thing that you chat about with your next-door neighbor. Let's face it, that's an intimate area back there.

Actually, our embarrassment about hemorrhoids is entirely uncalled for, not to mention unhealthy. Apart from the fact that hemorrhoids are nearly universal, the reluctance to talk about them—even with pharmacists or doctors—means that a lot of folks aren't getting the advice and treatment they may need.

PAIN IN THE VEINS

Forget the fancy name: Hemorrhoids are simply the anal equivalent of varicose veins—blood

---

Wash with Witch

One of the fastest ways to ease itchy hemorrhoids is to apply a little witch hazel. Pour some on a washcloth or tissue, then gently apply it to the tender area. Witch hazel evaporates quickly and leaves a cool, soothing sensation.

Instant Ahhh...

---

vessels in the anus or rectal area that are swollen or inflamed. Straining during bowel movements is the main cause, but sitting for a long time can also contribute to them. So can lack of exercise or not getting enough fiber in your diet.

Doctors divide hemorrhoids into two main types. *Internal* hemorrhoids occur inside the rectum, an inch or more beyond the anal opening. These hemorrhoids sometimes bleed, but they don't hurt, because there aren't many nerve endings in the area. Chances are that you'll never know you have them unless you happen to notice a little blood in the toilet bowl.

External hemorrhoids, on the other hand, definitely make their presence known. These are the little bulges that you can sometimes feel protruding from your anus. There are plenty of nerves in this area, which is why external hemorrhoids can often hurt or itch like the dickens.

A REAR-GUARD ACTION PLAN

For the most part, hemorrhoids aren't serious. They almost always go away on their own, usually within a few days. But there are a few things you need to be aware of. While it's common for hemorrhoids to bleed a little, it's impossible to know for sure if blood in the toilet bowl is from a hemorrhoid or something a lot more serious, such as colon cancer. Never ignore blood in the stool—see your doctor right away.

Also, it's not uncommon for little blood clots to form inside hemorrhoids. The clots aren't serious health threats, but they

A Cup of Comfort

The next time you have hemorrhoids, go to a health food store, pick up some powdered marshmallow, and brew a cup of tea by adding a teaspoon of powder to a cup of freshly boiled water. A traditional herbal remedy for digestive discomfort, marshmallow tea has a slightly thick, gummy texture that coats irritated tissues and reduces pain as well as itching.

can be excruciatingly painful. If your hemorrhoids are making you miserable, your doctor may advise cutting out any clots. It's a simple office procedure that just takes a few minutes and eliminates the pain immediately.

Most hemorrhoids don't require medical attention. It's almost always possible to ease the pain and, just as important, prevent them from coming back. Here's what doctors advise.

Soak and soothe. A soak in the bathtub is just the ticket for hemorrhoid pain. It doesn't have to be lengthy, either. A 10-minute bath will relax the muscles surrounding the hemorrhoids and reduce irritation and discomfort, says Rajesh Vyas, N.D., a naturopathic physician in Morgan Hill, California.

Sit in a sitz. If you don't have the time or inclination to take a long bath, a sitz bath is a good compromise. Fill the tub with 3 to 4 inches of water or however much it takes to submerge the irritated area, then soak for a few minutes. Taking two or three sitz baths a day is often all you need to make hemorrhoids more bearable until they go away.

Maintain regular movements. It's among the best ways to prevent constipation, which in turn prevents vein-damaging straining. For starters, get in the habit of having bowel movements at the same time every day. For most people, nature's call comes early, usually after breakfast or

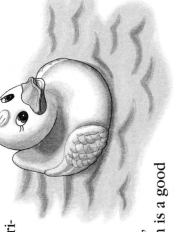

Okra Is A-OK!

Even if you're not a big fan of okra, it's one of the best foods for soothing as well as preventing hemorrhoids. For one thing, it's loaded with fiber. It also has a naturally "slimy" texture that augments the natural mucous coating in the intestine, says Rajesh Vyas, N.D. "It's a good excuse to eat lots of gumbo," he adds.

a cup of coffee. Don't ignore your body's signals. If you wait until later to go, your intestines will have to work harder than they should. (For more tips on dealing with constipation, see page 188.)

Get off the can. Since straining to have bowel movements aggravates hemorrhoids, don't try to force the issue. "Your body knows when it's time to go," says Dr. Vyas. "If you miss your regular time, let your body decide when it's ready."

His advice: If you don't get results within 10 minutes, it's time to get off the throne. There's no prize for success and no penalty for coming back later to try again.

Lose the magazines. That's right, get those *National Geographics* and Jerry Baker catalogs out of there. They only encourage you to spend too much time on the toilet.

Sip some aloe juice. Available in health food stores, this mild-tasting beverage is a traditional remedy for digestive problems because it soothes your system right where it counts. Drink a glass a day until the hemorrhoids are gone.

Fill up on fiber. The indigestible fiber in fruit, vegetables, legumes, and whole grains soaks up water in the intestine like a sponge. A high-fiber diet makes stools softer and easier to pass. The result is less straining—and less pressure on tender hemorrhoids.

Doctors advise getting 30 to 35

Soothing Salves

AHHH...ALOE

Aloe gel is one of the most soothing treatments for hemorrhoid pain. Apply a little to your finger and dab it directly on the tender spots. It may help the tissue heal more quickly, and it will lubricate the area so there's less irritation. You can buy the gel at health food stores or simply squeeze some from a freshly cut aloe leaf.

Soothing Spuds

A potato poultice will ease the pain of hemorrhoids and reduce uncomfortable swelling. Simply grate a tablespoon or two of raw potato, wrap it in cheesecloth, and apply it to the affected area, using a strip of gauze to hold it in place. Apply the poultice before bed and keep it on overnight.

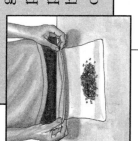

grams of fiber daily, but you don't have to put your produce on a scale to be sure you get the right amount. When you fill your plate, salads or vegetables should take up about a quarter of the space. Also, snack on vegetables or fresh or dried fruit during the day.

Drink lots of water. Getting enough water throughout the day will go a long way toward making stools softer and easier to pass. Everyone needs different amounts of water, but a good goal is at least 5 full glasses daily; 8 to 10 may be even better.

Here's a good way to tell if you're getting your fill: Urine that's mainly clear, with just a slight hint of yellow, means that you're drinking enough to stay well hydrated.

Keep active. People who exercise regularly are a lot less likely to get hemorrhoids than those who spend most of their time lounging. Twenty minutes of exercise a day, even if it's no more than a slow walk, helps your intestines work more efficiently and with less straining.

Nix the spices. Even if your taste buds cry out for Tabasco or other fiery hot sauces, you may want to avoid them until your hemorrhoids heal. Spicy foods contain oils that can irritate tender tissues on the way out of your body.

Painful Intercourse

Banish the Bedroom Blues

If you experience any pain during intercourse, please, please talk to your doctor right away. It's understandable that there's so much silence about this very common, yet very troubling condition. Most of us hesitate to discuss sexual issues, especially with strangers. But painful intercourse can have a profound impact on your body, your self-esteem, and your relationship with the person closest to you.

"I knew a woman who had been unable to have sex for three years because of vaginal pain," says Mary Bove, N.D., a naturopathic physician in Brattleboro, Vermont. "But she never told her partner what was going on. All he knew was that she seemed to be getting increasingly distant, and their anger and frustration continued to grow."

All of that anguish turned out to be unnecessary, because the woman simply had an infection. Once it was treated, the pain disappeared. "Her discomfort was gone, and their relationship flourished," says Dr. Bove.

So I'll say it again: Don't let embarrassment get in the way of your own happy ending.

WHEN LOVE HURTS

Pain during intercourse can be frightening, but the causes usually aren't all that serious. Vaginal infections can be to blame, and so can muscle spasms. Dryness can cause discomfort, especially after menopause, when a woman's estrogen levels decline.

Doctors estimate that about 1 in 10 women will experience painful intercourse at some time in their lives. Even though the causes are usually easy to treat, keep in mind that it's never normal. You certainly shouldn't keep silent and simply live with it.

SMOOTH SAILING AGAIN

Seeing your doctor is a good first step in addressing the problem. If your family physician can't figure things out, the next move is to see a specialist, probably a gynecologist, for a thorough exam.

In some cases, doctors don't find any obvious physical problems. That doesn't mean that the pain is imaginary, just that counseling may be an integral part of other treatments you may receive.

The doctors I talked to agreed that finding the cause of painful intercourse can be challenging in some cases. Most of the time, however,

---

Soothing Salves

E'S THE ANSWER

Vitamin E oil is effective for restoring vaginal flexibility. To try it, prick a vitamin E capsule with a pin and insert the capsule into your vagina before bed. Try it nightly for two weeks, then three times a week. Keep up the treatment if it seems to help.

the treatments are pretty straightforward. In addition, there's a lot you can do yourself to eliminate some or even all of the discomfort.

Rub and relax. Sometimes, intercourse is painful because the muscles at the entrance of your vagina go into spasm. While all sorts of things can cause this, some—such as memories of childhood abuse or simply a fear of sex—call for counseling, says Dr. Bove. Often, however, it's a purely physical problem.

Many women find it helpful to use massage oils externally to help those muscles relax prior to intercourse. "Almond and avocado oils can be very relaxing," says Dr. Bove. Adding certain herbs to the mix makes a good thing even better. "Oils made with cramp bark or valerian root tend to be the most helpful," she says, "Or use St. John's wort oil, which is a wonderful muscle relaxant."

You can make herbal massage oils yourself by adding 6 to 12 drops of herbal essential oil to an ounce of olive, hazelnut, or almond oil. Most health food stores, along with some salons and health and beauty stores, offer these oils for sale.

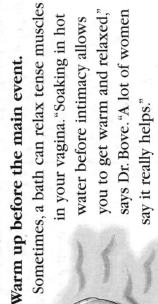

Warm up before the main event. Sometimes, a bath can relax tense muscles in your vagina. "Soaking in hot water before intimacy allows you to get warm and relaxed," says Dr. Bove. "A lot of women say it really helps."

Give nature a hand. Over time, your vagina's natural lubrication tends to diminish. Even slight dryness can make intercourse irritating or downright painful. An easy solution is to use a lubricating ointment made specifically for sex. Common brands include Astroglide, Very Private, and KY Jelly. You can also use olive, avocado, and other natural oils. "Aloe gel also works well, and coconut oil can be very lubricating and softening," says Dr. Bove.

Stay away from mineral-based or petroleum-based lubricants such as petroleum jelly. "Anything that has added colorings or alcohol-based ingredients could be irritating to the vagina," Dr. Bove explains.

Since each woman will have different impressions of lubricating creams and oils, consider buying small samples of several kinds. Remember, you may have to reapply a lubricant several times during sex. You can also try Replens, which you apply every three or four days to continually improve lubrication.

Plan an oily menu. Believe it or not, the oils in your diet can play a direct role in how comfortable intercourse feels. Fish, for example, is loaded with essential fatty acids that can help reduce vaginal dryness. Plan on having a few servings a week. If you don't care for fish, have a daily tablespoon of ground flaxseed, which contains the same essential oils. As a bonus, the oils in fish and flaxseed will also help improve vaginal tone.

Get less stress. Most of us have no shortage of stress in our lives. Just as it causes muscle tension in your neck and shoulders, stress also tightens muscles in your vagina.

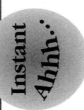

Instant *Ahhh...*

Sit in a Sitz

Just about any kind of vaginal pain can be helped by a sitz bath—a shallow bath that allows you to soak the vaginal area, says Annette Fuglsang Owens, M.D., Ph.D.

Soaking in lukewarm water for 15 minutes before or after intercourse can prevent or relieve pain, she explains. If you suspect it's a muscle spasm that's causing the trouble, add 1/2 to 1 cup of Epsom salts to the water. Or add 10 to 15 drops of comfrey essential oil to soothe any inflammation or irritation.

"People run around all day and don't have time to relax," says Annette Fuglsang Owens, M.D., Ph.D., founder of the Charlottesville Sexual Health and Wellness Clinic in Virginia. She advises doing everything possible to incorporate more downtime in your day. The more you relax during the day, the better prepared you'll be for sex later on.

Less rush, more foreplay. Just as men need more time to get erections as they get older, women need more time to achieve proper lubrication. Don't rush into things; give yourself time for plenty of foreplay. It will make intercourse feel more natural and less painful.

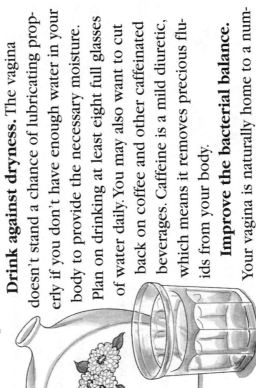

Drink against dryness. The vagina doesn't stand a chance of lubricating properly if you don't have enough water in your body to provide the necessary moisture. Plan on drinking at least eight full glasses of water daily. You may also want to cut back on coffee and other caffeinated beverages. Caffeine is a mild diuretic, which means it removes precious fluids from your body.

Improve the bacterial balance. Your vagina is naturally home to a number of types of harmless or even beneficial bacteria. But sometimes a change in the vagina's ecosystem causes an overgrowth of less benign organisms (such as yeast) that can cause dryness or pain.

You can tilt things back in your favor by taking probiotics, supplements that contain colonies of healthful bacteria. The most common type, *Lactobacillus acidophilus*, is available in health food stores. Follow the directions on the label.

The squeezes that please. You may be able overcome vaginal muscle spasms by doing exercises called Kegels, in which you contract and relax the muscles. Simply tighten the pelvic muscles that you would use to stop the flow of urine. Hold the tension for a moment, then relax. Do the exercise 10 or 20 times.

Change positions. If you and your partner try some different sexual positions, you may find that your pain diminishes considerably. One position that often helps is the man lying on his back with the woman sitting on top of him. "I often advise this for women who are sore from giving birth recently," Dr. Owens says. "It allows the woman to have better control of the depth and rhythm of penetration. It can also help her relax, since she knows she can pull back if she needs to."

Go beyond the body. It's not only physical problems that can lead to painful sex. "When physical solutions don't work, there may be other routes," says Gina Ogden, Ph.D., a certified sex therapist in Cambridge, Massachusetts, and author of *Women Who Love Sex.*

Counseling involves more than discussing deep-seated problems, she adds. Therapists can also help couples learn simple techniques—including sexual techniques—for restoring pleasure and getting beyond the pain. "It doesn't always take a lot of sessions to get results," Dr. Ogden adds.

Penis and Testicle Pain

Pamper the Family Jewels

I wasn't sure where to start when I first started doing research on the types of pain that only men get. My thinking got a lot more focused, though, when I talked to Harry Adelson, N.D., a naturopathic physician in Layton, Utah, who told me this wince-inspiring story.

Dr. Adelson helped arrange an outdoor rock-climbing competition for a local health club. On the day of the competition, John, one of the gym employees, showed up with a truckload of ice to keep the drinks cool. "I suggested that we form a human chain to transport the ice," says Dr. Adelson. "I'd chuck the bags about 15 feet from the truck to John, he'd toss them another 15 feet to the next guy, and so on."

Just as Dr. Adelson was getting ready to throw the sixth bag, he saw John stagger, then drop face-first to the ground. "The last bag nailed me in the 'nads," John gasped.

"Well, at least you got ice on it right away," Dr. Adelson retorted.

He was able to joke because he knew that John wasn't seriously hurt. Most men have had the experience of taking a hit to the groin and enduring a flash of gut-wrenching pain. It certainly isn't a pleasant experience, but most guys won't be any the worse for it.

BELOW THE BELT

There are two types of genital pain that men tend to experience. One, of course, is caused by trauma—a sudden blow to the groin that causes excruciating pain, along with painful swelling in some cases, that lasts anywhere from a few hours to a few days.

The other cause of pain is infection. Men sometimes get infections in their testicles, prostate gland, or urethra, the tube through which urine flows. Any infection that affects the genitals can make it painful to urinate or have intercourse. Infections can also cause fever or other whole-body symptoms if they happen to get into the bloodstream.

BACK IN THE SADDLE

Any hint of infection, such as redness or tenderness, is always a signal to see your doctor. Most infections that affect the genitals can be knocked out by a simple course of antibiotics. It's worth treating them right away, because you don't want those germs to spread.

Trauma to the genitals is a little more complicated. As long as you don't have serious bruising, swelling, or bleeding, the

Instant Ahhh...

Get Extra Support

One of the quickest ways to ease the pain of groin injuries is to wear an athletic supporter for a few days. At the very least, wear snug-fitting briefs instead of boxers, says Martin Resnick, M.D. Supporting your genitals will reduce pain and make it easier to move while you're healing.

best thing is to simply wait it out. On the other hand, a fractured penis—sometimes caused by an accidental "collision" during intercourse—does have to be checked out to prevent it from healing at a curious and potentially painful angle.

The basic advice is this: Serious genital pain or pain without a known cause has to be checked by a doctor. You can usually treat mild injuries yourself. Here are a few strategies for feeling better and reducing the risk of long-term problems in that area.

Put it on ice. If you take a shot to the groin, the best treatment is also the simplest: Apply cold—either a cold pack or ice wrapped in a washcloth or small towel—to the area that hurts. The ice will numb the pain and restrict blood flow that could cause swelling.

If you can stand it, apply the cold pack with a little pressure to further counteract swelling. Keep it in place for about 20 minutes every hour until you're feeling better.

Bring on the heat. Applying cold is the best way to start treatment, but about 24 hours after the injury, start using heat as well. Soak a towel in hot water and apply it where you hurt. Keep it there for 3 minutes, then replace it with a cold cloth for about 30 seconds. Repeat the cycle two more times, ending with the cold.

A Cup of Comfort

If you're trying to oust an infection, make time for thyme. The popular kitchen spice contains a compound that kills germs. Add a tablespoon of dried thyme to a cup of boiling water and steep for 10 minutes. Strain out the herb, let cool slightly, and drink. Try drinking a few cups a day until the infection is history.

Alternating heat and cold gets your blood vessels to open and close. It increases circulation through the area to bring in more nutrients and flush out wastes. It's helpful not only for injuries but also for infections, says Dr. Adelson. "The increased blood flow helps your immune system do its thing," he says.

Take a pain pill. Over-the-counter analgesics are surprisingly effective at easing groin pain. Aspirin, ibuprofen, and acetaminophen can all help, says Martin Resnick, M.D., a urologist at the Cleveland Clinic in Ohio and president-elect of the American Urological Association. Ibuprofen and aspirin tend to be your best bets because they stop swelling as well as pain.

The arnica answer. Homeopathic arnica is good for healing and pain relief from any kind of blunt trauma, says Dr. Adelson. You can find it where most natural remedies are sold; it comes as pellets that you dissolve on your tongue. Check the label for dosage directions.

Stay active. Admittedly, you may not be able to do very much at first, "but the more activity you can do without further injury, the better," says Dr. Adelson. Exercise and other forms of activity, such as cleaning house or working in the yard, stimulate the release of chemicals that reduce pain and help the circulatory system flush pain-causing substances from the area.

Beat it with bromelain. This natural chemical extracted from pineapple acts like nature's ibuprofen, says Dr. Adelson. "It's been

It's an Emergency!

Most groin injuries heal on their own, but if the swelling seems severe, you notice blood in your urine, or you're having trouble urinating, get to an emergency room. Damage to nerves or blood vessels in the penis can lead to permanent problems, including impotence, without immediate treatment, says Martin Resnick, M.D.

shown to reduce swelling, and it aids in the cleanup of cellular debris after trauma."

Bromelain supplements are sold in health food stores and some drugstores. Follow the dosage directions on the label and take it three times daily until the pain is gone, says Dr. Adelson. And remember to take bromelain on an empty stomach; otherwise, the digestive acids that are released when you eat will make it less effective.

Soak in Epsom salts. For rapid relief from pain and swelling caused by infection or injury, add about 4 cups of Epsom salts to a warm bath and soak in it for about 20 minutes.

Zap infections with zinc. When your privates are waging war against infection, the mineral zinc should be brought to the front lines, Dr. Adelson says, because "it aids the function of your immune system and is highly concentrated in testicular tissue." Take 50 milligrams of zinc three times daily for at least a week but no more than two weeks, he advises.

The vitamin C solution. Vitamin C stimulates your immune system and makes it better able to combat infections, says Dr. Adelson. As long as you don't have kidney or stomach problems, he advises taking 2,000 milligrams daily, divided into two or three doses to prevent diarrhea or stomach upset.

Cheers for Cherries

If you've been laid up by a blow below the belt, keep a bowl of cherries within reach. These tasty treats are rich in bioflavonoids, natural chemicals that will help your body repair the delicate blood vessels that were damaged. Try to eat a cup of cherries every day. Other good choices include blueberries and blackberries.

Urinary Tract Infection

Natural Germ Protection

Urinary tract infections are among the most common—and the most annoying—health issues that women deal with. About a third of American women will get a urinary tract infection (UTI) at some point in their lives, and some women get them over and over again.

The infections can occur anywhere in the urinary tract, but they usually affect the urethra, the tube through which urine leaves the body, or the bladder. The main symptom is a burning sensation, along with urinary urgency—the sudden, overwhelming need to go to the bathroom.

"I used to have five or six infections a year," says Crystal Abernathy, N.D., a naturopathic physician in Charlotte, North Carolina. "It's a very irritating thing to deal with."

It took some time, but Dr. Abernathy eventually discovered how to keep the pesky infections under control. She hasn't had an infection in years—and the advice she shares here will work just as well for you.

THOSE PESKY GERMS

Most UTIs occur when bacteria that normally live in the area surrounding the anus make their way inside the urethra. Once they get into that warm, moist environment, they quickly multiply, and sometimes they even work their way up to the bladder.

Men sometimes get UTIs, but their extra inches of anatomy make it harder for bacteria to get inside. Women don't have that protection, so they're a lot more vulnerable.

BEAT THE BUGS

If you think you have a UTI, or even if you're sure you do (women who get them know the symptoms all too well), see your doctor right away. You're going to need antibiotics to knock out the germs and relieve the symptoms.

You don't want to wait too long to get help. The longer you have an infection, the greater the risk that it will spread all the way to the kidneys, possibly causing a much more serious infection called pyelonephritis.

With quick treatment, however, most UTIs disappear after a course of antibiotics. You usually have to take the drugs for a week, although three-day treatments are available.

In the meantime, now's the time to think about ways to

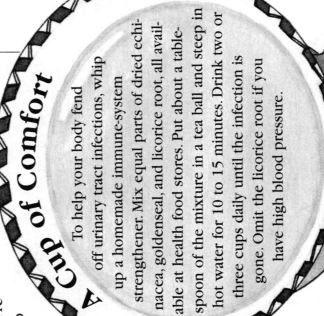

▷ Cup of Comfort

To help your body fend off urinary tract infections, whip up a homemade immune-system strengthener. Mix equal parts of dried echinacea, goldenseal, and licorice root, all available at health food stores. Put about a tablespoon of the mixture in a tea ball and steep in hot water for 10 to 15 minutes. Drink two or three cups daily until the infection is gone. Omit the licorice root if you have high blood pressure.

prevent future infections and take steps to keep your current discomfort to a minimum. Here's what you need to do.

Lose the sugar. Sweets can be a real problem if you get frequent UTIs. Sugar encourages the growth of bacteria, and it reduces the ability of your immune system to battle infection. "It's sort of a double whammy," says Dr. Abernathy.

And remember, it's not just sweets like candy that cause problems, but all sources of sugar, including the sugar in packaged foods. Read labels so you know what you're getting.

Vote for prohibition. The bacterial colonies that cause UTIs love alcohol because it's converted into sugar in your body. Give up the drinks until the infection is gone.

Be pro-protein. You need plenty of protein to keep your immune system healthy. To make sure you're getting enough, divide your weight by 2.2 to get your weight in kilograms, then eat 1 gram of protein daily for each kilogram of body weight. As long as you eat a healthy diet that includes plenty of whole grains, legumes, and lean meat and fish, you're almost guaranteed to get enough protein to boost your defenses against UTIs.

Take lots of C. "Vitamin C is helpful because it supports the immune system," says Dr. Abernathy. When you have a UTI, plan on taking 500 milligrams of vitamin C every 2 hours, she suggests.

Vitamin C in large amounts may

cause diarrhea. If you're having problems, cut back on the dose until you find a level that works for you. If you have kidney disease or stomach problems, discuss vitamin C with your doctor before giving it a try.

Take an herbal combo. "I use a combination of four different herbs to treat urinary tract infections," Dr. Abernathy says. "It tends to be pretty effective; people usually start getting relief in 1 to 4 hours."

The herbs she uses are uva-ursi (sometimes called bearberry), buchu, echinacea, and goldenseal, which are available at health food stores. Take 200 milligrams of each three times daily for a week, she advises.

Quaff cranberry juice. One cure for UTIs that both folk healers and main-

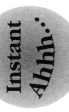

stream medical practitioners agree on is cranberry juice. The natural chemicals in the juice make it harder for bacteria to attach to the inside walls of your bladder. Rather than sticking around and causing trouble, they're more likely to be washed out of your body in the urine. Stock up on sugar-free cranberry juice from a health food store, then drink at least three glasses a day when you have a UTI.

Drown your sorrows. The more water you drink, the more bacteria will be flushed from your bladder. "Drink at least

---

More Heat, Less Pain

To quickly ease the localized discomfort of UTIs, apply a warm compress to the urethral opening and the surrounding area, suggests Crystal Abernathy, N.D. Moist warmth can reduce muscle spasms that result in pain, she explains. A long soak in a warm bath will have similar soothing effects.

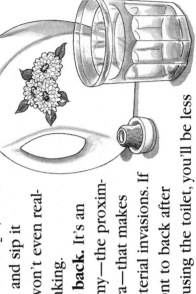

2 quarts of water a day," Dr. Abernathy suggests.

That may seem like a lot of H$_2$O, but if you carry water with you and sip it throughout the day, you won't even realize how much you're drinking.

Clean from front to back. It's an unfortunate fact of anatomy—the proximity of the anus and urethra—that makes women vulnerable to bacterial invasions. If you always wipe from front to back after using the toilet, you'll be less likely to push bacteria somewhere where they can cause problems.

Urinate after sex. Some women find that they get UTIs after sex because intercourse can push bacteria where they shouldn't go. Urinating after intercourse can flush out any germs that may have worked their way into the urinary tract.

Go when called. When your body tells you that it's time to find a restroom, do it. Holding urine in the bladder for too long gives bacteria the chance to multiply.

Shop for citrate supplements. If you take supplemental magnesium or calcium, be sure to get the citrate form, says Dr. Abernathy. Citrates are easier for your body to absorb, and they make the urine more alkaline, which can help prevent UTIs.

Shop for 'shrooms

Most supermarkets offer several tasty varieties of gourmet mushrooms. You should definitely stock up on them when you have a UTI, because they boost the ability of your immune system to combat infections. "Different mushrooms stimulate different aspects of the immune system, so it's good to combine them and get a broad spectrum of effects," says Crystal Abernathy, N.D. The types to look for include shiitake, reishi, and maitake.

Yeast Infection

Fight Back Against Fungi

Most infections occur when germs from the outside world somehow go where they shouldn't, such as into your throat or a cut in your skin. But germs that naturally live inside your body can also cause problems, at least some of the time—and that's the case with vaginal yeast infections. They occur when a fungus that's always present suddenly multiplies out of control. It doesn't happen all the time because other microorganisms keep the fungus in check, but when the overall balance is disrupted in some way, the "bad guys" may get the chance to whoop it up.

OUT OF CONTROL

The organism that causes most vaginal yeast infections, *Candida albicans*, does quite well in that warm, humid envi-

The Sex Link

Some women tend to get yeast infections after intercourse. It's not really the man's fault, it's just that semen is a bit alkaline and can alter the acidity of the vagina. Less acid means more yeast. To help restore a normal chemical balance after sex, either urinate soon afterward or take a quick shower and flush out the area.

ronment. Under normal circumstances, there's not enough of it for you to notice. When something upsets the body's internal ecosystem, though, candida may grow out of control. Thus, you can think of vaginal yeast infections as a sign that something's not quite the way it should be. Changing levels of hormones can allow candida to thrive. So can changes in acidity. Women who take antibiotics often get yeast infections because the drugs kill beneficial organisms that normally keep the fungus in check.

BACK IN BALANCE

Most women are all too familiar with the symptoms—usually pain, itching, or a bad odor—that accompany yeast infections. If you've never had one before and you experience any of these symptoms, check with your doctor just to be sure that what you have is really a yeast infection.

For the most part, your body is pretty good at getting this all-too-common problem under control, and most infections will clear up even if you do nothing. But why suffer? There are many over-the-counter treatments, and they're very effective. Drugs don't work instantly, however, and they won't prevent future problems, so take a look at the following remedies.

A Cup of Comfort

The herb echinacea is a powerful ally when you're fighting infections. To reap the benefits of this immune-boosting herb, drink it as a tea once or twice a day. You can buy echinacea tea bags at most drugstores and supermarkets, or use bulk herb from a health food store. Steep a tea bag or 1/2 teaspoon of dried herb in a cup of hot water for about 10 minutes. Sweeten with honey if you like, then sip and enjoy.

Unlike drugs, these strategies can help you get to the root of the problem and keep infections from recurring.

Switch pills. If you use oral contraceptives, they may be triggering yeast infections, says Jana Nalbandian, N.D., a naturopathic physician and faculty member at Bastyr University near Seattle. "Birth control pills are at the top of the list for causing vaginal yeast infections," she says.

You're more likely to have trouble with contraceptive pills that contain a high percentage of estrogen, she says. Ask your doctor if you should try a different type of pill or even switch to a different form of birth control.

Get the right antibiotic. If your doctor prescribes antibiotic treatment for an illness, be sure to let her know if you're prone to yeast infections. She'll be able to choose a drug that's less likely to cause problems.

Say yes to yogurt. Whether you want to prevent a yeast infection or relieve an existing one, the solution may be as close as your refrigerator. Eating a cup or two of live-culture yogurt daily will replenish your body's supply of healthful bacteria, which will help keep the bad bugs under control. "The bacteria make it difficult for the yeast to grow," says Dr. Nalbandian.

Overhaul your diet. Recurring, recalcitrant, or unre-

The Garlic Fix

"Garlic, garlic, and more garlic." That's yeast-fighting advice from Jana Nalbandian, N.D., who explains that garlic has powerful anti-fungal properties.

Raw or lightly cooked garlic delivers the biggest kick. "I tell people to toss the garlic in after the food's off the stove," says Dr. Nalbandian. "Just chop it up and throw it in."

sponsive yeast infections may require even more drastic dietary changes. Eliminate all refined starches, such as bread and pasta, from your diet. Avoid foods that contain yeast or fungus, such as beer, leavened pastry products, aged cheeses, and mushrooms. You'll also want to give up fermented foods, such as vinegar, pickles, and sauerkraut.

Take a blood test. Women who get frequent yeast infections sometimes have an underlying blood sugar problem, Dr. Nalbandian says. Elevated blood sugar levels caused by diabetes can greatly increase the risk of infections, so if you keep getting them, ask for a diabetes test just to be sure.

Spice it up. Many common kitchen spices, including oregano, thyme, and rosemary, have fungus-fighting properties. Use these spices liberally when preparing meals for as long as you're fighting off a yeast infection.

Strike oil. Peppermint and tea tree oils are also powerful fungus fighters. You can buy capsules at a health food store, then follow the label directions. Use oils that are meant for internal use, and don't put them anywhere but in your mouth.

Fungus-fighting herbs. Herbs that contain the chemical compound berberine are good at wiping out the offending fungus. Two of the best are barberry and goldenseal, available in

---

Instant Ahhh…

Soak Away the Itch

A quick way to ease the discomfort of a yeast infection is to soak in warm water. Fill your bathtub, add a handful of colloidal oatmeal, and relax for a while.

If you don't have colloidal oatmeal, it's fine to sprinkle in some baking soda, says Jana Nalbandian, N.D. Plain oatmeal also works. Just fill an old sock with a cup or two of oatmeal, fasten the open end to the faucet with a rubber band, and let the water run through it as the tub fills up. Oatmeal "softens" the water and helps soothe irritation.

health food stores. If you'd like to try them, taking capsules is easiest; just follow the label directions.

Use cooler water. "Heat and hot water will aggravate a yeast infection," says Dr. Nalbandian. You may want to shower in lukewarm water until the infection is gone.

Dress cool and natural. Summer's heat always makes yeast infections more uncomfortable, but even in winter, panty hose or tight clothing can trap heat and increase itching and other symptoms. It's a good idea to wear loose clothing made from cotton or other natural fibers, at least until the infection is gone.

Men and Yeast

It doesn't happen often, but men, especially those who aren't circumcised, sometimes get genital yeast infections. Symptoms may include a rash as well as itching or burning at the tip of the penis. The same treatments that work for women also work for men.

Pain in Your Legs and Feet

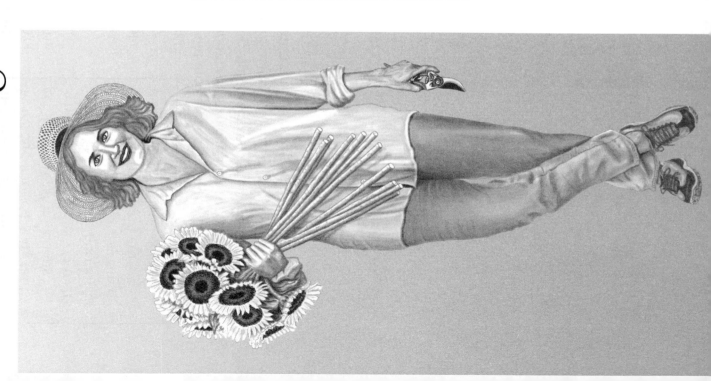

- Ankle Sprain or Strain
- Bunions
- Calf Pain
- Charley Horse
- Corns
- Foot Soreness
- Heel Pain
- Ingrown Toenail
- Intermittent Claudication
- Knee Pain
- Restless Legs Syndrome
- Shinsplints
- Stubbed Toe
- Varicose Veins

Ankle Sprain or Strain

Walk Away from Pain

I still remember one particular Thanksgiving, when all the dads in the neighborhood were celebrating with a game of touch football. My cousin Lou, who had been playing football almost since the time he left his crib, wasn't expecting to come out of the game with anything worse than grass stains. But a leap for a long pass proved him wrong: He landed awkwardly on his foot, and the next thing he knew, he was grounded.

"I literally felt something snap," he told me. "Then I was down for the count." Ordinarily, even if his foot had fallen off, Lou would have just tied it back on with a shoelace and gone back into the game. Fortunately, there was an orthopedic physician in the neighborhood, and he made sure Lou spent the holiday off his feet, with his ankle wrapped, iced, and elevated.

STRETCHED AND SORE

If you've ever sprained, strained, twisted, or otherwise abused one of your ankles, you have lots of company. The

American Academy of Orthopedic Surgeons reports that 25,000 people do it every day.

It's not surprising that there's so much ankle pain out there. With every step you take, the bones, muscles, ligaments, and tendons of your ankle joint have to cope with a tremendous amount of force—and one misstep can deliver more force than they can handle. When there's damage to the ligaments or tendons, as in Lou's case, it's called a sprain; muscle damage is known as a strain.

The difference doesn't matter all that much, however; pain is pain. And the treatments for sprains and strains are, for the most part, the same.

STEP AHEAD OF ANKLE PAIN

An injured ankle will usually feel better after a few days of TLC. But serious damage, like the tear that put Lou to bed, requires an x-ray or other tests to determine how bad the injury is, and possibly surgery to repair it. It's always a good idea to have a doctor check out ankle injuries that cause a lot of swelling or don't get better within a few days. You need to know what you're dealing with as soon as possible. (I once thought I had a sprained ankle, but an x-ray showed I'd broken a bone.)

In most cases, though, you can treat a sprain or strain your-

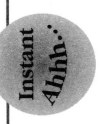

Instant Ahhh...

Pump Out the Fluid

A lot of the pain of a sprained ankle comes from the buildup of fluids in the area. A quick way to reduce swelling is to gently move your ankle through its full range of motion now and then. Just sit in a chair and gently raise and lower your foot, then rotate it, moving as much as the pain allows. Keep going for a minute or two, but don't push yourself to the point of severe pain. Try it a few times a day while your ankle is recovering. "It helps pump fluids out of the area," explains physical therapist Chris Miller.

self. Here's what doctors advise to get you on the road to recovery.

RICE is right. Emergency room doctors see a lot of sprained ankles. Their advice is almost always to take the following four steps.

R.I.C.E.

- *Rest it.* As soon as you feel pain, quit doing whatever it was you were doing and get some rest. Even gentle walking on a sprained ankle will probably make the swelling and inflammation worse.

- *Ice it.* Immediately apply an ice pack to the place it hurts most. It's fine to wrap some ice cubes in a small towel or washcloth and hold them on your ankle for about 20 minutes. Remove the ice, wait 2 hours, then ice it again. Applying cold for the first day or two after an injury makes blood vessels constrict, which reduces tissue-damaging inflammation, explains John Nowicki, N.D., a naturopathic physician in Issaquah, Washington.

- *Compress it.* Wrap the ankle with an elastic bandage. Make it snug, but not so tight that you can't slip a finger underneath.

- *Elevate it.* Raising your leg helps fluids drain out of the ankle, explains Chris Miller, a physical therapist near Riverside, Connecticut. "You need to lie flat with your entire leg elevated at or above the level of your heart," he

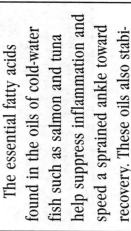

Fish for Relief

The essential fatty acids found in the oils of cold-water fish such as salmon and tuna help suppress inflammation and speed a sprained ankle toward recovery. These oils also stabilize cell membranes that may have been damaged by the injury. It's a good idea to eat fish three or four times a week until you're feeling better.

If you aren't a fish fan, you can get healing amounts of essential fatty acids by eating a tablespoon of ground flaxseed daily. Try sprinkling it on cereal or mixing it with a serving of yogurt.

says, "Just putting your leg on the coffee table while you sit on the couch doesn't count."

Continue these steps, known as RICE, for at least two days after the injury—longer if the pain and swelling don't subside.

Add herbs. Boost the benefits of cold by adding herbs. Instead of using ice cubes, fill a bowl with ice water and sprinkle in several drops of herbal oil. Camphor, eucalyptus, chamomile, and rosemary are all good healing choices that you can get at a health food store. Soak a washcloth in the herbal water, wring it out, and lay it on your sore ankle. Surround it with an ice pack for extra cooling power and leave it in place for about 20 minutes. Repeat the treatment once or twice a day until your ankle's healed.

Switch to heat. Once the swelling is gone, you can apply a heating pad set on low or a warm compress. The warmth will penetrate into the tissue and help improve the flow of nutrients into the area while promoting the outflow of pain-causing substances.

Keep up the pressure. If swelling persists for more than a few days, you may want to get a compression stocking from your doctor or a medical supply store (the ones sold in drugstores aren't measured as precisely). It won't come loose and

Wrap It Up!

A natural way to help your injured ankle back to health is with a comfrey wrap. Buy three or four whole leaves of this traditional trauma-treating herb from an herbalist or health food store. Blanch the leaves by dipping them briefly in boiling water. Let them cool a bit, then drape them over the injured area and cover with an elastic bandage. Replace the leaves daily until the sprain heals.

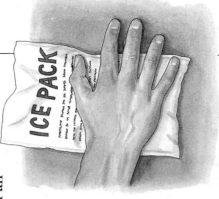

require rewrapping the way bandages do.

Compression stockings provide different amounts of pressure, Miller says. Get one labeled "25–35," which is about the same amount of pressure that you'd get with an elastic bandage.

Continue the cold. Even when your ankle's feeling better, it's a good idea to give it a dose of ice whenever you've been on your feet for a while. "Ice it after any sort of activity, even if you've just been out and about for a few hours," Miller says. Once you've sprained an ankle, it may be months before it's fully healed.

Ride herd on your calves. When your ankle can handle your weight again, you may want to take the time to stretch your calf muscles. Stretching will help strengthen your ankle and keep the nerves moving freely, Miller says. "We call it 'nerve flossing' because you're using your nerves like floss, moving them back and forth through the skeletal system."

Here's an easy exercise. Lie on your back with your legs extended and your toes pointed toward the ceiling. Gently bend your ankle so your toes are tilted toward your head. Hold for a moment, then relax. Repeat the stretch several times with both feet.

Work your toes. Toe raises can help stretch and strengthen a recovering ankle. First, stand in front of a wall or chair. Put your hands on the wall or chair for balance, then rise up on the toes of both feet. Hold the stretch for a moment, relax, then repeat several more times. Make toe raises a regular part of your workout routine.

STRETCHING

Bunions

Kick Away Foot Pain

Most of the men I know, myself included, have two or three pairs of shoes: a pair of sneakers for walking, working out, and lounging around the house, plus something a little fancier for dress-up. We're not really into shoes as fashion accessories, so we tend to buy what feels good.

Most of the women in my life, on the other hand, are very much into fashion footwear. They want shoes that look sharp—high heels, pointy toes, and all. So what if their feet hurt at the end of the day?

Unfortunately, buying shoes for style instead of comfort can literally change the ways your foot bones grow. Can you feel a knobby bump at the base of your big toe? If you can, that's a bunion, and it means your shoes are forcing your bones to grow in some pretty unnatural ways.

BAD TO THE BONE

A bunion is a bony protrusion that usually appears on the outside of your big toe, although smaller "bunionettes" can form on one or both of your little toes. If you went barefoot all the time, bunions wouldn't be painful. But once you have a bunion and squeeze it into a tight-fitting shoe, pressure and friction do the rest. Bunions really hurt—and they can make your feet feel tired and achy at the end of a long day.

FAVOR YOUR FEET

Short of surgery, there's no way to get rid of bunions once they form. Surgery is a reasonable choice when they hurt so much that you can't get around very well or when the pain doesn't go away even when you slip out of those sleek-looking pumps. Before you consider foot surgery, though—and the risk of complications that comes with it—you'll want to explore some gentler ways to reduce the pain and keep the bunions from getting worse. Here's a few that may help.

Try a doughnut. Made with spongy, synthetic materials, doughnut-shaped pads are perhaps the fastest solution to painful bunions. When you place a pad between the bunion and your shoe, the painful pressure is almost instantly reduced.

Slip in something comfortable. Drugstores stock a variety of over-the-counter orthotic inserts, comfortable pads that slip inside your shoe and reduce bunion

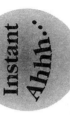

Instant Ahhh...

Comforting Comfrey

A comfrey footbath soothes painful bunions fast. Comfrey contains chemical compounds that reduce skin discomfort and help sore areas heal. To make a footbath, steep an ounce of dried comfrey leaves (available at health food stores) in a few cups of simmering water for 10 minutes. Add enough cool water to make the temperature comfortable, pour the water into a basin, and soak your feet for 20 minutes or so. If you can't find comfrey, it's okay to substitute Epsom salts, says Rowan Hamilton, Dip.Phyt., professor of botanical medicine at Bastyr University near Seattle.

pressure. If over-the-counter inserts don't help, you may want to try prescription orthotics made by an orthopedist. They're expensive—usually more than $250—but they're generally a better choice than going under the knife.

Beach your bunions. They may appreciate a trip to the seashore as much as you do. Walking barefoot in the sand is a great way to strengthen your feet and make them less sensitive to bunion pain.

Keep those socks snug. The more tightly your socks cling to your feet, the less likely they are to rub your bunions the wrong way.

Shake hands with rubber bands. They can be your best friends when you're fighting bunion pain, because they'll make your toes strong and flexible. Sit with your feet together and loop a thick rubber band around both big toes. Move your feet as far apart as they'll go, hold the stretch for 5 seconds, then relax. Repeat the exercise 10 times at least once a day.

Here's another good stretch. Place a rubber band around all

Healing Hands

Massage is an excellent way to rub out bunion pain, and you'll get even better results when you combine it with a soothing bath. The next time you're in the tub, lather your hands with soap. Slip your fingers between the toes of one foot and gently reach around to massage the bottom of your foot. Bend your wrist while you rub so your foot moves in every direction. Then do the same thing with your other foot. You may be a little sore the first few times you do it, but after that, your bunions should start feeling a lot better, says Mark Hoch, M.D., president of the American Holistic Medical Association.

of your toes on each foot. Spread your toes wide so they pull on the rubber band, hold for about 5 seconds, then relax.

Buy some new shoes. The main cause of bunion pain, and the one thing that always makes it worse, is wearing shoes that don't fit. Shoving your foot into a poorly fitting shoe literally changes the shape of your foot. "It takes on the shape of the shoe," says Cherise Dyal, M.D., an orthopedic surgeon in Wayne, New Jersey, and chair of the Public Education Committee of the American Orthopedic Foot and Ankle Society.

Always have your feet measured when you buy new shoes, she advises. Avoid narrow shoes with pointy toes. You want shoes that are wide enough for your feet to slip into comfortably, preferably with a flat or low heel.

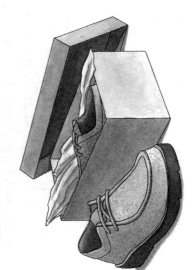

Soothing Salves

BUNION-BUSTING HERBS

The next time your bunions are barking, stop off at a health food store and get the ingredients for a soothing herbal rub. A time-tested formula consists of 6 parts oak bark, 3 parts marshmallow root, 3 parts mullein, 2 parts wormwood, 1 part lobelia, 1 part skullcap, 6 parts comfrey root, and 3 parts walnut bark. Put the herbs in a double boiler, add olive oil to cover, and cook for 1 to 2 hours. Strain out the herbs and throw them away. Add an equal amount of beeswax to the oil and store the mixture in an ointment jar with a tight-fitting lid. Apply it daily whenever your feet are hurting, advises Rowan Hamilton, Dip.Phyt. "You'll probably notice good results within a few days," he says.

Calf Pain

Muscle-Soothing Magic

There's not enough room here to explain how I ended up in a local Halloween parade dressed as a gorilla in a leisure suit. Suffice it to say that my position in the parade was between a woman in hot pink disco pants and a man with an Afro the size of Rhode Island.

While we were waiting to begin our long march down Main Street, I felt a sudden twinge of pain in my right calf. Honestly, it hurt like the dickens, and I wasn't at all sure I'd be able to keep up with my fellow revelers. But I remembered a conversation I'd had a few weeks earlier with Stephen Rice, M.D., Ph.D., director of Jersey Shore Sports Medicine Center in Neptune, New Jersey. He told me that calf pain is usually caused by a muscle cramp and that cramps feel better when they're stretched out.

Walk on tiptoes

This is a great way to reduce an existing cramp and strengthen your calf muscles to help prevent future ones. At first, walk on your tiptoes for about 10 seconds. As you get stronger, increase the time until you're tiptoeing for a minute or so. Do it at least once a day. (If anyone asks what you're up to, you can always say that you're trying out for the local ballet troupe.)

With that advice in mind, I limped to the curb and carefully pressed the ball of my foot against it. As my calf muscle stretched, the pain suddenly eased. So I marched, the cramps stayed away—and our marching group won third prize!

ROUTINELY OVERWORKED

The two major muscles in the calves—the gastrocnemius and the soleus—are big and heavy, but they have a short job description: All they do is lift your heel. That may not sound like much, but consider for a moment how many of your daily activities require this movement.

Walking is one of them. So are squatting, running, going up and down stairs, swimming, and stretching up to get a can of wax beans off a high shelf. If your calves aren't up to these tasks, they're going to cramp—and you'll be pretty much grounded until they feel better.

Calf pain is almost always caused by a temporary muscle spasm, probably brought on by fatigue or muscle strain. Also known as a charley horse (see page 290), this type of pain usually goes away in a few minutes, although in some cases, you may find yourself limping around for a day or two.

Of course, calf pain can also be caused by actual muscle damage—if you've been in an accident, for example, or you

▷ A Cup of Comfort

If calf pain is making it difficult to rest or sleep, try this herbal pain fighter. Get some dried passionflower, ginger, Jamaican dogwood, and meadowsweet at a health food store. Mix equal parts of the herbs, then steep a teaspoon of the mixture in a cup of hot water for about 10 minutes. Strain out the herbs and let the tea cool slightly. Sip two or three cups throughout the day and have an extra cup just before you go to bed to help ensure a good night's sleep.

really wrenched the muscle while playing sports or working around the house.

CALM A CALF CRISIS

There isn't a whole lot that doctors can do about run-of-the-mill calf pain. Even if you've torn a muscle, the injury will heal naturally within a few weeks. Cramps don't last anywhere near that long, but they can be terribly painful in the meantime. To get back on your feet, here are a few ways to coddle your calves.

Don't force it. I mentioned that I was able to defuse my calf pain just by stretching the muscle. While this works for cramps, it doesn't help if you've injured the muscle. In fact, if the pain gets worse when you stretch, that's probably what happened, and the best thing you can do is relax for a while. You certainly don't want to force the muscle to move when it doesn't want to, says Dr. Rice.

Healing Hands

A quick massage is almost sure to make your calf feel better. Just reach down with both hands and massage the muscle thoroughly, working across the muscle fibers rather than up and down. "This encourages new connective tissue to form," says Stephen Rice, M.D., Ph.D. Follow the massage with a spicy herbal salve made by mixing about a teaspoon of dried turmeric (the same powdered herb found in your spice rack) with enough water to make a paste. Spread the paste on the affected area and leave it on for about 20 minutes. Turmeric is a traditional remedy for reducing pain as well as inflammation.

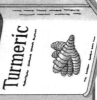

"A muscle that hurts wants to be left alone," he says. "Just try to keep the leg comfortable and let the muscle relax."

Listen to your body. Injured muscles can take a long time to heal, and the last thing you want to do is overuse them before the healing process is complete. As a general rule, calf pain that's only slightly irritating will probably take about 10 days to heal completely. Injuries that are slightly more serious may take 10 to 20 days, and really bad ones may take months. When you start to feel better, don't try to pick up right where you left off, or there's a good chance you'll get hurt all over again.

Soothe the swelling. It's normal for muscles to swell after injuries, but swelling is your worst enemy because it increases pain and increases the time it takes the damage to heal. The more you minimize swelling, the faster your calf will start feeling better.

Start by resting your injured leg. At the same time, apply an ice pack—or ice cubes wrapped in a washcloth or small towel—to the area, says Dr. Rice. Keep the ice in place for 20 minutes, remove it for at least 20 minutes, then repeat the treatment. Ice the area at least three times a day for a few days, or until the pain and swelling are gone.

It's also helpful to keep your leg elevated above the level of your heart, he adds. This allows fluids to drain away from the

Calf Calmer

A quick trip to the kitchen will probably yield everything you need for a soothing solution to your aching calf. Mix equal parts of water and vinegar in a saucepan, then heat the mixture until it's comfortably warm (it should feel hot on your skin, but not hot enough to burn). Soak a kitchen towel in the mixture, wring it out, and apply it to the painful part of your calf for 5 minutes.

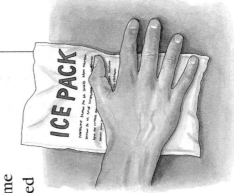

injured tissue. In addition, wrap your calf with an elastic bandage. It should be snug, but still loose enough that you can slip a finger underneath it.

Add some heat. If your calf is still hurting after a day or two, you may want to drape a heating pad over it. Set the heat control on low and warm your calf for about 20 minutes at a time. Heat increases circulation, which will flush pain-causing chemicals from the area while bringing in healing nutrients.

Raise your heel. At drugstores, you can buy little wedge-shaped pads that slip inside your shoe and elevate and stretch the calf muscle. "It shortens the distance your calf has to stretch on its own," Dr. Rice explains.

You should use a heel lift for only a few days. While it helps reduce pain, it also reduces the muscle's normal range of motion, which can actually slow your recovery time.

Stretch the muscle. Once the pain and swelling have receded, you can promote healing with a daily stretching routine. Here's an easy exercise you can do just about anywhere to strengthen the main muscle groups. It also helps relax painful cramps.

STRETCHING

• Stand a few feet away from a wall and extend your injured leg slightly behind you, with your other leg in front and slightly bent at the knee.

• Keeping both feet flat on the floor, brace your hands against the wall and lean forward. Lower yourself by bending your good leg while keeping your injured leg straight.

• Next, stand with your injured leg in front and repeat the stretch.

INSTANT HEAT
microwaveable

Trade in your sneaks. Good athletic shoes with slightly raised heels are a good investment if you're prone to calf injuries. They'll keep the muscles from overstretching.

If you can't remember the last time you bought new sneakers, do yourself a favor and get some new ones. Athletic shoes lose their cushioning ability over time, even when they look fine on the outside. You should replace them at least once a year, and more often if you do a lot of walking or hiking. If you're a runner, you'll need to trade in your shoes even more frequently—at least every 300 miles.

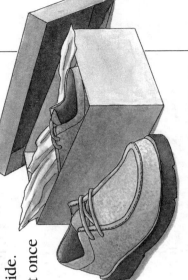

Charley Horse

So Long, Charley!

No one knows for sure where the expression *charley horse* came from. It may indicate that those awful calf cramps can make you feel as if you've been kicked by a horse. Another theory is that it's a reference to a little-known baseball player named Charlie, who apparently walked like a lame horse. Other experts suggest that the name came from night watchmen in London known as "Charleys," who walked so much that their legs were always sore.

Mysteries, mysteries! I never did find out where the term came from, and I guess it doesn't matter much. Doctors know very well what a charley horse is, and that's the first step toward getting rapid relief.

WHOA, CRAMPS!

All sorts of things can cause a charley horse. If you overwork a muscle, it will naturally shorten, or cramp; it's painful, but it's simply the muscle's way of protecting itself from further damage.

Muscle cramps can also be caused by nutritional shortfalls. If you don't get enough magnesium, potassium, or other minerals in your diet, the muscle won't function properly. The same thing can happen if you don't drink enough water.

CALM THE CRAMPS

Most muscle cramps go away on their own with rest and time, although there may be some lingering soreness. But if your charley horse keeps returning to the corral, you're going to have to do something to rein it in. Start by seeing your doctor. It's possible that you have a vascular condition called intermittent claudication, in which there isn't enough blood flow to the muscles (see page 311).

Chances are, however, that you're perfectly healthy, and a few simple steps will take away the pain—and more important, keep it from coming back. Here's what the experts advise.

Take a stand. The next time a charley horse takes hold, simply stand up, advises Chris Miller, a physical therapist near Riverside, Connecticut. "Putting weight on the muscle will stretch it out," he explains.

Raise your toes. The reason a charley horse is so painful is that the muscle is shortening more than it should. The obvious solution is to make the muscle longer by flexing your calf. It can be excruciating, though. You'll just have to try it to see if it makes things better or worse. While standing, lift your toes and the ball of your foot, keeping your heel on the ground. Hold the stretch for 10 to 15 seconds, then relax.

Stretch it out. Don't wait until you have a charley horse to

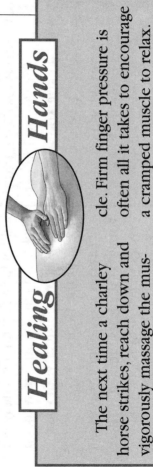

Healing Hands

The next time a charley horse strikes, reach down and vigorously massage the muscle. Firm finger pressure is often all it takes to encourage a cramped muscle to relax.

STRETCHING

stretch your calves; you should be doing it all the time. Regular stretching keeps muscles loose and limber and helps prevent cramps from getting started, says Stephen Rice, M.D., Ph.D., director of Jersey Shore Sports Medicine Center in Neptune, New Jersey. "It's especially important to stretch before and after exercising," he adds.

Here's another good stretch to prevent or treat calf cramps: Stand a few feet away from a wall, then extend your arms and brace your hands against it. Stretch your cramped leg straight behind you, with your other leg forward and bent at the knee. Keeping both heels on the floor, lean toward the wall until you feel a good stretch. Hold it for 10 to 15 seconds, then relax.

Strengthen the muscles. You're a lot less likely to get charley horses if you keep your calf muscles strong. One of the best workouts, known as plantar flexion, involves nothing more than sitting in a chair and flexing your ankles for a few minutes daily. For a slightly tougher workout, walk on the balls of your feet with your heels off the floor.

Take it easy. Once you've got your charley horse reined in, don't expect to get right back in the race. "If you try to keep going and

Loose Sheets, Better Sleep

A surprising number of people suffer from painful charley horses while they sleep. A lack of stretching undoubtedly contributes to the problem, but it's possible that the real culprit is your sheets. If they're tucked too tight, they restrict your leg movement, which can cause cramping. Before dozing off, pull the sheets loose so your legs have plenty of room. And if you do tend to get charley horses in bed, take the time to do some stretches before going to sleep.

use that leg immediately, you're likely to cramp again," says Dr. Rice. The best thing is to slow down and take it easy for a few days.

Mine for minerals. Sometimes, muscle cramps are signs that your body is lacking the minerals that help transmit electrical signals between the nerves and muscles. These minerals, known as electrolytes, include magnesium, potassium, and calcium. To ensure you get enough, eat plenty of whole grains, legumes, fruit, and vegetables. In addition, you may want to take a daily supplement that includes each of these muscle-protecting nutrients.

Drown your pain. Dehydration is a common cause of muscle cramps, including charley horses.

The reason the pain often occurs during exercise is that you may be using up more water than you're taking in.

The solution, of course, is to drink plenty of water throughout the day, not just when you're hot and sweaty. As a general rule, plan on drinking eight full glasses daily—more if you live in a hot climate or are perspiring heavily.

Soothing Salves

LOVELY LINIMENT

If you're prone to charley horses, here's a homemade liniment you can whip up in advance. In a small container with a lid, combine 1/2 ounce of powdered cramp bark (available at health food stores), 1 cup of apple cider vinegar, and a pinch of red pepper. Keep the mixture in a cool, dark place for a week, shaking it every day. When the week's up, transfer the solution to a clean glass bottle. Then, the next time a charley horse strikes, rub your affected calf with the liniment to stop the cramp.

Corns

Fight the Friction

Corns are a royal pain. The ugly little things usually appear on the outer part of your little toe or on the side of your foot, areas that are exposed to a lot of friction. Days of constant rubbing make the skin thicken and accumulate layer after layer of extra cells.

You'd think that all that extra padding would protect the skin, but often, the opposite is true: Pressure against the corn can cause the hardened area to exert painful pressure on the tender tissues underneath. Women are more likely than men to have corns because the fashionable shoes they like tend to be narrower than a straw.

CAN THE CORNS

If your corns hurt so much that you can barely hobble, you'll probably want to see a podiatrist, a foot doctor who can remove them surgically. But this is hardly ever necessary. For one thing, corns are easy to prevent—by wearing comfortable, well-fitting shoes, for example. And even if you already have corns, they're pretty easy to get rid of. So kick off your shoes, put your feet up, and learn how to shuck those corns forever.

The ol' soft shoe. Stiff leather shoes look great, but they don't feel so good when you have corns, says Pamela Taylor, N.D., a naturopathic physician in Moline, Illinois. The only way to get rid of corns is to get rid of friction. That means wearing shoes made from cloth or soft leather for a few weeks, she advises. Sandals are also a good choice as long as the straps don't rub against the tender areas.

File, don't fillet. Corns are just dead skin, so you'd think they'd be easy to cut away. But don't try it: There's a good chance that you'll damage healthy tissue and wind up with a painful sore—or even a nasty infection. "It's much safer to use a nail file or a pumice stone to file the corn down," says Dr. Taylor.

Don't file it all the way down at one time; instead, remove just a little bit of skin each day. Most of the corn will be gone in a week or two, and you'll be less likely to hurt yourself in the meantime.

Soften before scraping. Corns are a lot easier to remove if you soften the skin before using a file or pumice stone. First, soak your foot in warm water for 5 to 10 minutes. Once the skin is soft, gently abrade the corn to remove a few layers of skin, then leave it alone for the rest of the day. Repeat the soak-and-scrape routine once a day until the corn is gone.

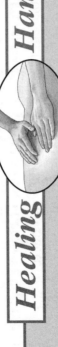

Healing Hands

A foot massage is a super soother when your corns are a-poppin'. But don't put a lot of pressure directly on the corns—it hurts! Instead, work around them. Massage your entire foot, starting at the tips of your toes and working backward to your heel. If your foot is particularly tender, you may want to use a massage technique called effleurage: long, stroking movements with just a little bit of pressure.

Go for a walk. It may be too painful if you already have corns, but taking regular walks is a great way to prevent them because it increases circulation to your feet and promotes healthier cell growth. "Increased blood flow brings more oxygen and nutrients to the tissues and removes waste products," says Dr. Taylor.

Forget about breaking them in. A lot of people buy shoes that don't fit because they're convinced that new shoes have to be "broken in" before they feel comfortable. It's not true. Shoes that are uncomfortable in the store won't get any comfier after you wear them for a while—and there's a good chance that the resulting pressure and irritation will trigger corns.

Insist on getting measured. Twenty years ago, clerks in shoe stores routinely measured your feet to ensure a good fit. These days, you're lucky if you can even find someone to help you find the size you *think* you need.

"Find a store where the clerks measure both of your feet," says Dr. Taylor. "They should check the fit at both the heel and the toe. After that, wear the shoes and walk around to make sure they're truly comfortable."

Instant Ahhh…

Oil Away Aches

Herbal oils are nearly perfect for corns. Any oil softens the skin, but herb-infused oil blends stimulate circulation and help keep your feet healthy and ache-free, says Pamela Taylor, N.D. She recommends a blend of the following oils, which you can find at health food stores. Add two drops each of peppermint oil and carrot seed oil to an ounce of calendula oil, then mix in five drops each of lavender oil and geranium oil. Store the mixture in a small bottle and massage it into your feet once a day—more often when your corns are aching.

Foot Soreness

Save Your Soles

The next time your feet are so tired that you can't even jump to conclusions, sit down and try to calculate just how many miles those tired tootsies have walked in your lifetime. You probably won't believe the number!

According to the American Orthopedic Foot and Ankle Society, the average person takes 10,000 steps a day. That adds up to more than 3 million steps a year, or more than 1,000 miles between birthdays.

That's pretty good mileage, especially when you consider that your feet never have to be rotated, retreaded, or replaced. So don't begrudge them a little much-needed rest from time to time, and do read on to find out how to keep them feeling better from one step to the next.

ENDLESS PRESSURE

It's a wonder that we walk upright at all, considering that the first ape who decided to walk on two legs instead of four probably spent the next day moaning about his aching feet.

Just consider the stress factors. You carry your weight with you everywhere you go. In fact, each step you take puts pressure equivalent to one and a half times your body weight on the weight-bearing foot. As you get older, your feet also become stiffer, which makes them less able to withstand the daily burden.

BE A SOLE SURVIVOR

You can almost always take care of sore feet yourself. Obviously, if you have diabetes, circulation problems, or other conditions that cause pain or fatigue in your feet, you'll have to work with your doctor to find the proper solutions. But for most people, a little TLC goes a long way. Here are a few tips you may want to try.

Insert an insert. Sometimes, sore feet just need a little cushioning to get back in gear. "As people get older, the padding on the bottoms of their feet decreases," says Pamela Taylor, N.D., a naturopathic physician in Moline, Illinois. Drugstores stock many different kinds of padded shoe inserts. Try a pair or two and see if they help. In many cases, that's all your feet will need to feel better.

Shear a sheep. Inserts made from sheepskin or wool are a good choice for padding your favorite shoes. You can buy a square foot or two of the material at a fabric or leather store, then cut it to fit your shoes.

"Wool has naturally springy fibers," says Dr. Taylor, "and it tends not to hold moisture. It will keep your feet warm in winter and cool in summer." Flannel is also a good material for homemade foot pads, she adds.

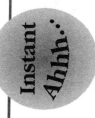

Instant Ahhh...

Pass the Salts and Oil

A great way to relax your kickers at the end of the day is to soak them in water spiked with Epsom salts and a few drops of lavender, chamomile, or peppermint essential oil, says Pamela Taylor, N.D. The oils, which are available in health food stores, reduce inflammation as well as muscle spasms, she explains. "They really help."

Step out of your rut. Have you been wearing the same type, or even the same brand, of shoes for years? It may be high time to switch to a style with more padding. "When I was younger, Birkenstocks felt great, but now they're not comfortable at all," says Dr. Taylor. "So I switched to sandals with cork padding. That made all the difference."

Soak your feet. A soothing footbath can make a real difference when your feet are beat at the end of the day. You can make it twice as effective by switching between hot and cold water, a technique called contrast hydrotherapy.

Put comfortably hot water in one basin and cold water in another. Soak your feet in the hot water for about a minute, then switch to the cold for 30 seconds. Repeat the cycle two or three times, ending with the cold water. Alternating hot and cold will stimulate circulation in your feet and make them feel better.

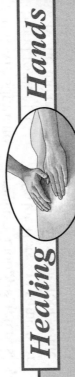

Healing Hands

Two great soothing moves for tired feet are "ankle wobbles" and "toe boogies." (I know, the names are ridiculous, but that's what the experts call them.)

To wobble your ankle, put your palms on either side of your foot, covering your ankle. Shake your palms while keeping them pressed against your ankle. If you do it right, you'll feel the vibration all the way up to your abdomen, says Pamela Taylor, N.D.

To do a toe boogie, put one finger on either side of a toe, right where it's connected to your foot. Vigorously vibrate it back and forth for a few seconds, then repeat the movement for the rest of your toes.

Stick 'em up. Your dad had the right idea when he came home and propped his feet on the coffee table while he read the paper (or your report card). Raising your feet not only gives them a chance to rest, it also allows gravity to drain away any swelling that's contributing to your discomfort. For this strategy to be really effective, though, you have raise your feet higher than your head, which usually means lying down and propping your feet up on a few pillows.

Stretch your steppers. You can wake up tired feet by giving them a good stretch. Regular stretching also helps keep your feet strong, flexible, and less prone to aching.

"The simplest thing is to do range-of-motion stretches," says Dr. Taylor. Here are some to try.

• Raise one foot while you're standing or sitting. Flex your ankle and move your foot in circles.

• Bend your foot at the ankle so your toes point toward the ceiling, then bend the other way, pointing your toes toward the floor.

• For a more challenging stretch, combine the two movements: Do ankle circles while keeping your toes pointed toward the floor.

Toe the line. If you tend to

Soothing Salves

CALMING CAMPHOR

"Anything that has menthol or camphor in it will stimulate the flow of blood to the feet and wash away the inflammation that causes soreness," says Pamela Taylor, N.D. "Creams that include the herbs arnica, comfrey, or hypericum (St. John's wort) also work well." You can buy a cream with one or more of these ingredients at a health food store, or add 6 to 12 drops of one of these herbal oils to an ounce of grapeseed, olive, or almond oil to make a soothing liniment.

STRETCHING

get cramps and aches in your toes or the balls of your feet, exercise them by gripping a small towel with your toes and pulling it toward you. Or you can pick up marbles with your toes.

Roll with it. To stretch your foot and leg muscles and get a foot massage at the same time, take off your shoes and roll a golf ball along the floor with the sole of your foot. Alternate with a tennis ball to get a slightly different stretch.

Check your shoes. It's pretty obvious that high heels can do a number on your feet, but even sensible shoes can leave your dogs barking if they're too worn out to give you any support. Check your shoes regularly for signs of wear and replace them as needed.

Shop for full service. Buy your shoes at a store where the clerk measures both feet. Shoe sizes vary by brand, so always try the shoes on, even if you already know your size.

It's also helpful to shop toward the end of the day, when your feet are naturally a little bit larger. Keep in mind also that shoes that fit properly should feel good right away. There's really no such thing as a "breaking in" period.

A Cup of Comfort

The next time your feet are aching, drink a cup of chamomile tea, suggests Pamela Taylor, N.D. It contains chemical compounds that reduce inflammation and have relaxing effects. Just steep a tea bag or a teaspoon of dried herb (available in health food stores) in a cup of hot water for at least 10 minutes. Strain the tea if using loose herbs, then sip and enjoy. Unless you're allergic to ragweed, drink a cup or two whenever you need quick relief.

Heel Pain

Tips to Heal Sore Heels

I was having dinner with my buddy Dave the other night, and he casually mentioned that he had plantar fasciitis. I nearly fell off my chair—not only because I'd been researching that very topic but also because he used such a high-falutin' medical term for this very common, very painful foot problem.

I thought at first that he'd gone to see a doctor. But, like many people (especially men) who are blessed with good health, Dave hates to go to the doctor, even when he's really sick—and this time, he'd been true to form. His heel had been bothering him for quite a while, so he checked the Internet, trying to figure out what was wrong. His attitude seems to be that it's silly to take his health problems to someone who actually graduated from medical school. (Sound familiar?)

In this case, it wasn't a bad

Instant Ahhh...

Heel, Sit, Stay

When heel pain strikes, sit down. Sitting with your foot comfortably elevated can reduce the pain in a hurry. In fact, get used to taking it easy for a few weeks. The less time you spend on your feet, the sooner the injury will heal.

choice, since there isn't a whole lot that doctors can usually do about plantar fasciitis that you can't do yourself.

TROUBLE AFOOT

If you bump your heel against something hard, the pain is predictable. But heel pain sometimes follows a peculiar pattern: After the initial trauma—which may or may not be especially painful—you may feel a burning sensation in your heel when you get up in the morning or at other times when you haven't been on your feet for a while.

Here's what happens: The plantar fascia, a band of connective tissue that stretches along the bottom of your foot from heel to toes, sometimes gets inflamed. This usually happens when the tissue has been irritated—from too much walking, for example, or simply because it's lost some of its natural stretch over time. The inflammation itself may not hurt very much. But when you stand up in the morning, the tissue is stiffer than usual, so the pain can flare up in full force.

HEEL THYSELF

The pain of plantar fasciitis usually goes away once the underlying inflammation clears up. The bad news is that it can take a really long time—up to six months in some cases—for that to happen.

A Cup of Comfort

Ginger tea will make you feel good from your head to your toes: It tastes great, and best of all, it can ease inflammation in your foot. You can buy ginger tea at most supermarkets and health food stores, or you can make your own. Cut some fresh ginger into several pieces and steep them in freshly boiled water for 10 to 15 minutes. Strain out the ginger and enjoy the delicious tea. Have a cup or two a day until your heel pain is just a memory.

Most people with plantar fasciitis start feeling better within a month or two. You don't want to ignore the pain in the meantime, though, because it will keep getting worse unless you take care of the inflammation. In severe cases, your doctor may need to inject steroids, powerful drugs that knock out inflammation. You may also need to wear shoe inserts to reduce the painful pressure. Most of the time, however, you can manage this problem with home care. Here's what doctors advise.

Pop a pill. As soon as you notice pain, a limp to the medicine cabinet can bring relief. Over-the-counter anti-inflammatory drugs, such as aspirin, ibuprofen, or naproxen, can be very effective, says Joseph Caporusso, D.P.M., a podiatrist in McAllen, Texas, and spokesperson for the American Podiatric Medical Association. "They block pain and reduce inflammation," he explains.

Give it the cold shoulder. Applying an ice pack, ice cubes wrapped in a washcloth, or even a bag of frozen peas can be just the thing to freeze the pain in its tracks. You can ice the area for up to 20 minutes every hour.

Stretch it out. Regular stretching exercises can relieve flare-ups and help the injured plantar fascia recover. First, hold one end of an old belt (or a tie or towel) in each hand and stand with your toes on the middle portion. Pull up on the belt while pressing down with your foot. Relax for a moment, then do it again. Repeat the exercise 10 to 15 times several times a day. It's particularly helpful to do this exercise just before bedtime to help keep the plantar fascia from tightening up overnight.

Put your mules out to pasture. Shoes without heels should stay in the closet when you're suffering from plantar fasciitis, says Dr. Caporusso. "You want firm, supportive shoes with good cushioning," he says. "An open-backed shoe doesn't support your heel, and it might allow your heel to move in a way that it shouldn't."

Shop like Cinderella. If your shoes don't fit, you won't live happily ever after. Ill-fitting footwear aggravates plantar fasciitis, and it may have triggered it in the first place. Make sure that the shoes you buy feel comfortable the first day you wear them; don't expect to "break them in."

Bike to the pool. You'll recover more quickly if you don't put too much strain on your feet. On the other hand, you don't want to stop exercising altogether. The answer is to switch from an activity that takes a toll on your feet, such as running or step aerobics, to one with less impact, such as swimming, bicycling, or walking.

My friend Dave, mentioned earlier, is a serious runner who couldn't bring himself to turn in his running shoes. He found, though, that cutting back on his mileage for a while eased his pain while he was recovering.

Healing Hands

Everyone loves a good foot massage, and if you happen to have plantar fasciitis, you're going to love it even more. Having someone firmly rub your foot will reduce pain, increase circulation, and help the area heal more quickly. If you have the time, follow the rub with a castor oil pack to really soothe the pain. First, rub castor oil onto the painful area, then cover with plastic wrap and wrap the whole thing in a towel soaked in warm water. Leave it in place for 20 to 30 minutes.

STRETCHING

Up against the wall! No, you're not under arrest. You're going to do a stretch that will loosen the muscles and tendons in your feet and calves.

Stand about an arm's length away from a wall. Put both palms against the wall and step forward with your right foot. Keep your weight on your right foot while straightening your left leg behind you, with the foot flat on the floor. You'll feel a stretch in your heel and the Achilles tendon at the back of your foot. Hold for 10 seconds, then relax. Repeat several times, then switch positions and stretch your other foot. Doing this several times a day will help plantar fasciitis heal more quickly. If you're lucky, it will even prevent it from coming back.

Wear shoes at home. If you pad around the house in slippers or socks in the evening, you're cheating your feet of hours of much-needed support. Wearing shoes right up until you go to bed will help keep the inflammation from getting worse.

Don't shop for soles. At least, not yet. Over-the-counter orthotic inserts can relieve pressure on your feet, but only if you get the right kind. "People often buy them and then find that they don't work," says Dr. Caporusso.

If your foot pain isn't getting better after a few weeks, visit a podiatrist. It may turn out that you do need some kind of shoe insert, but at least you'll know you're getting the right kind with the right fit.

Wake up your feet. If your pain makes it hard to get out of bed, try this morning stretch: Hang your feet over the side of the bed with your heels touching the floor, then slowly raise and lower the balls of your feet. After a few repetitions, your heel pain should ease.

Ingrown Toenail

Hammer Out Nail Pain

Back in the bad old days, when the criminal justice system was really designed to make a point, prisoners were sometimes tortured with relentless pressure from a hard, sharp object. The pain must have been agonizing, to say the least.

We don't do things like that anymore, but Mother Nature has her own form of medieval torture: the ingrown toenail. More than a few people have been reduced to tears by the sharp, searing pain of an errant nail growing into their flesh—and by the infection that all too often comes along for the ride.

NATURE'S NAILS

Humans don't have the dagger-like claws that cats do, but if you've ever had an ingrown toenail, you know that your nails are still plenty

---

Guided Growth

Here's a safe, painless way to "train" ingrown nails to head in the right direction before they cause real trouble. Take a small piece of cotton and roll it into a tight cylinder. Slip the cylinder under the nail right where it's touching (or almost touching) the skin. The cotton will relieve the pressure and may cause the nail to grow out rather than in.

sharp. An ingrown toenail starts out like any other nail, but sometimes its sharp edge curves into the side of your toe instead of growing out straight. The more the nail grows, the deeper it digs into your skin.

Some people are simply prone to ingrown toenails. Others get them when they wear too-tight shoes or trim their nails in the wrong direction.

THE SHARPEST PAIN

You should never ignore an ingrown toenail for very long. Apart from the fact that it can be excruciatingly painful, there's a very high risk that the area around it will get dangerously infected.

If one of your toenails has started to penetrate the skin, get to a doctor right away—and make the appointment even sooner if you see redness, swelling, or other signs of infection. At the very least, you'll need to have the dangerous part of the nail removed, and you may need antibiotics to knock out infection-causing germs.

If you can't get to a doctor right away, or if the nail hasn't penetrated too deeply, there are a few things you can do at

Healing Hands

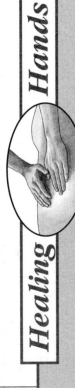

An herbal foot massage can soothe the pain of an ingrown nail and protect the area from a potentially serious infection. Start with a trip to the health food store for infused calendula oil and oregano, thyme, and lavender oils. Then combine 1 ounce of the calendula oil with 10 drops each of the others and apply the mixture all over your foot. The hands-on attention will make the area feel a lot better, and the oils will help reduce swelling and pressure around the sore nail.

home to keep the problem under control.

Soak it in salt. "An Epsom salts bath will help draw out pain and infection," says Pamela Taylor, N.D., a naturopathic physician in Moline, Illinois. Fill a basin with warm water, add a cup of Epsom salts, and soak your foot for 20 to 30 minutes.

Have feet of clay. A clay pack, available at health food stores, will help keep swelling and infection under control. "I'd use French green clay," says Dr. Taylor. "Or ask a pharmacist for pharmaceutical-grade kaolin clay."

Apply the clay to the affected toe and leave it on until it dries, usually 30 minutes to an hour. Then rinse away the clay and dry your foot thoroughly. Repeat the treatment once or twice a day.

Sock the germs. To reduce the risk of infection, change your socks two or three times a day. For additional protection, add a few drops of lavender, oregano, or thyme essential oil (available at health food stores) to a basin of water and soak your socks in the solution overnight. The germ-killing action of the oils will help ensure that your socks don't allow infection-causing bacteria to thrive.

Bare your troubles. Germs are never happier than when they're in

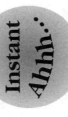

Instant Ahhh...

Tea for Toes

Here's a tea treatment that's taken by foot, not by mouth. Put a quart of water in a saucepan, then add 1 cup of dried calendula flowers, 1 tablespoon of dried thyme, and 1/2 cup of dried lavender flowers (all available at health food stores). Simmer the mixture for 5 minutes, then let it cool to room temperature. Put it in a basin and soak your foot for about 5 minutes. "It will reduce infection and painful swelling," says Pamela Taylor, N.D.

a dark, tight space. To keep them under control, expose the toe with the ingrown nail to the air as frequently as possible. "Going barefoot is always the best," says Dr. Taylor. At the very least, take off your shoes and socks when you're lounging around the house.

Dress like a gladiator. Sandals are a wonderful option for airing out an ingrown toenail. Footwear made of natural materials, such as leather and cork, will probably be the most comfortable and least aggravating to your toe.

Take a multi. A daily multivitamin will help ensure that your body has the right nutrition for proper nail growth. Healthy nails are less likely to become ingrown or infected.

Keep it in line. If you know that one of your nails is prone to becoming ingrown, check it every week so you can cut it before it gets too long. "Trim straight across the top of the nail," says Dr. Taylor. Don't try to round the edges so the nail follows the shape of your toe; this just makes it more likely to curve into the flesh.

Find footwear that fits. Shoes that don't leave enough room for toenails to grow naturally can force them to grow into your tender toes. Take the time to try on a lot of shoes until you find the ones that fit well and feel good.

Don't dig in. It's fine to snip away a toenail that has just started to grow in the wrong direction, but you don't want to mess with a nail that's already embedded in the skin. Trying to trim them at that point is likely to damage the tissue and increase the risk of infection. To play it safe, see your doctor.

MAXIMUM
Daily Pack

MULTIVITAMIN
& MINERAL SUPPLEMENT

Intermittent Claudication

Go for Better Blood Flow

I suspect that the patients of Peter T. Beatty, M.D., are in good hands. When I talked to him about intermittent claudication, a circulatory problem that can cause nagging leg pain, he didn't mince words about the fact that it's our own unhealthy habits that are often to blame.

"When I look around and see people eating fast food and fatty snacks, I worry about them," he told me. "They're at great risk."

But Dr. Beatty, an interventional radiologist at Legacy Meridian Park Hospital in Tualatin, Oregon, and national co-chair of the Legs for Life Program, is also unflinchingly positive. Nearly everyone with intermittent claudication can dramatically improve, he says. "There's no question about it."

LEG ATTACKS

We all know about heart attacks. Well, the same things that cause them—buildups of cholesterol and other fatty substances that restrict blood flow, for example—can also occur in the legs.

If a blood vessel in your leg is narrowed by fatty buildups, the muscle that depends on that blood vessel won't get enough blood or oxygen. This may not be a problem when you're just sitting around, because the muscle isn't demanding very much blood. When you're active, though, the muscle calls for more fuel than it's able to get.

The result: a painful cramp that forces you to stop moving and rest the muscle. The condition is called *intermittent* claudication because it comes and goes.

STEPS TO HEALTHIER LEGS

Intermittent claudication usually follows a distinct pattern. The pain comes on when you walk or are otherwise active, and it goes away when you relax. Another telltale sign is the regularity of the attacks. You may feel pain whenever you're 100 feet into your daily walk, for example, or 20 minutes into your weekly bike ride.

If you think you may have intermittent claudication, you need to see a doctor. You may need medications to improve blood flow or reduce deposits in your arteries. You also need to be checked out to be sure you don't have a more serious circula-

▲ A Cup of Comfort

If you have intermittent claudication, make your tea the green kind. It's a great source of bioflavonoids, natural chemical compounds that make blood vessels stronger and less vulnerable to blockages and pain. You can buy green tea bags in most stores where tea is sold; just steep a tea bag in a cup of hot water for 10 minutes, then enjoy. Try to have a cup or two every day.

tory problem, such as coronary artery disease.

Think of intermittent claudication as something of a wake-up call: If something's wrong with your circulation, you have to take care of it—the sooner, the better. Fortunately, there's a lot you can do. Here's what doctors recommend.

Get going. Exercise is good for your heart, and it's just as good for improving circulation in beleaguered leg muscles. "Get 20 minutes of exercise every day," says Dr. Beatty. "It's the most important thing you can do."

The type of exercise is up to you; swimming, cycling, and walking are all great choices. "The goal is to get your heart rate up and to break a sweat," he says.

If you haven't been exercising regularly up to now, talk to your doctor before starting a new regimen. Then do it!

Become an activist. People with intermittent claudication sometimes become isolated and afraid to go out or even to do things around the house. "They just don't move because they're afraid of hurting," Dr. Beatty says. It's much healthier to be as active as your symptoms allow. The fitter you get, the less pain you're going to have. "Don't just sit on the sofa and watch TV," he advises.

Eat heart smart. The same type of diet that's recommended for preventing heart disease will also go a long way toward protecting your legs.

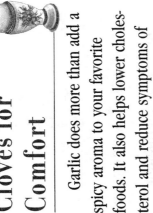

Cloves for Comfort

Garlic does more than add a spicy aroma to your favorite foods. It also helps lower cholesterol and reduce symptoms of intermittent claudication, says Erica LePore, N.D. She recommends eating at least a few cloves a day. Cooked garlic is acceptable, but raw garlic has the most cholesterol-lowering and pain-relieving power.

The basics are simple enough: Quit eating fatty foods, eat five servings of fruit and vegetables a day, use olive oil in place of butter, and load up on legumes and whole grains. Eating a healthier diet will keep all of your blood vessels, including those in your legs, a whole lot healthier.

Feed on fish. Salmon, tuna, mackerel, and other cold-water fish are loaded with omega-3 fatty acids. These healthful fats help prevent blood clots and may lower cholesterol. Have at least two or three servings of fish a week.

Eat fewer processed foods. "People with intermittent claudication should try to eliminate refined carbohydrates and processed foods from their diets," says Erica LePore, N.D., a naturopathic physician in Wakefield, Rhode Island. White flour, white sugar, white rice, and foods that contain partially or fully hydrogenated oil can all push cholesterol into the danger zone, she says.

Go for ginkgo. Some studies have shown that this healing herb can help open narrowed blood vessels and enhance circulation in the legs. Dr. LePore suggests taking the herb in capsule form. Look for a product that's standardized to

---

Instant Ahhh...

Stop and Recover

Attacks of intermittent claudication can be intensely painful because your leg muscles are literally starved for blood and oxygen. For almost instant relief, stop whatever it is you're doing. The pain will probably go away in a minute or two, but don't take that as an excuse to call it quits altogether. Once the pain is gone, start exercising again. "There's no harm in continuing once the pain goes away," says Peter T. Beatty, M.D.

contain 24 percent ginkgo heterosides and take 40 milligrams three times daily.

Other herbal helpers. "There are a number of herbs that can help with intermittent claudication because they increase circulation to the extremities," says Kimberly Beauchamp, N.D., a naturopathic physician in Wakefield, Rhode Island. Among the options are burdock, ginger, prickly ash bark, and gotu kola.

It's fine to take herbal supplements that you buy at a health food store (following the label directions, of course). But because intermittent claudication is a potentially serious health problem, talk to your doctor before launching into a full-fledged herbal treatment plan.

Max out on magnesium. Anyone with intermittent claudication should have the mineral magnesium in their medicine cabinet, says Dr. Beauchamp. "It relaxes smooth muscles in artery walls, and it's helpful in lowering blood pressure." Consider taking 300 to 600 milligrams daily, she advises.

Ease it with E. Like magnesium, vitamin E is a vasodilator, meaning that it opens narrowed blood vessels and allows more blood to flow through, says Dr. Beauchamp. "It can allow people to walk farther without pain," she says. The recommended dose is 400 to 800 IU daily, but check with your doctor before taking E.

A Cup of Comfort

Here's a triple-herb cocktail that can really improve sluggish leg circulation. Mix equal parts of dried hawthorn, lime blossom, and ginger, available at health food stores. Add a heaping teaspoon of the mixture to a cup of freshly boiled water, steep for 15 to 20 minutes, and strain out the herbs. Try drinking two or three cups of tea a day. Check with your doctor before using hawthorn.

Feed on fruit. If you blow right by the produce aisles when you do your food shopping, turn your cart around. Just about every kind of fruit is full of a natural fiber called pectin, which helps clear your arteries of cholesterol that's gumming up your leg works. Apples and grapes are particularly rich in pectin, so grab a bunch and munch.

Wrap and Raise

Herbalists use yarrow and peppermint to improve circulation, and after a visit to a health food store for the herbs, so can you. Steep 2 tablespoons of each herb in 2 cups of hot water for about 15 minutes. Strain out the leaves and put the teapot in the refrigerator to chill. Meanwhile, gather enough gauze, cheesecloth, or muslin to wrap your lower legs. Soak the cloths in the chilled liquid, wrap them around your legs, and rest with your legs elevated for about 20 minutes. If you do this once a day for several weeks, you'll notice quite a reduction in discomfort.

Knee Pain

Knock Out the Aches

When I was on the cross-country team back in high school, Coach McGarvey had one answer for just about every gripe. Cramp in your side? Run some hills. Tired? Run some hills. Anaconda wrapped around your neck? Run some hills!

As I recall, there was only one complaint that didn't result in a command to run up and down the nearest grassy knoll a couple of hundred times. Knee pain was always taken seriously, and for good reason: Once your knee is hurting, the underlying injury is almost sure to get worse if you overdo it. And the damage can last a lifetime.

BENT OUT OF SHAPE

Your knees endure a lot of wear and tear, even on ordinary days. They not only allow your legs to

---

Save Your Dough!

You've probably seen people wearing knee braces when they exercise. While these over-the-counter contraptions may reduce swelling somewhat after an injury, they aren't very helpful for treating or preventing knee pain, says Jerry Cochran, M.D. "They may help remind you to be careful about the joint, but they don't provide any extra stability at all."

bend, they also act as shock absorbers. The tendons and ligaments that hold your knee joint together are pretty good at managing life's hard knocks. But if you move in a way they don't like (twisting moves are especially bad), the stress can cause painful tears in the connective tissue.

Knee pain isn't always caused by sudden injuries, of course. The stress from repetitive motions—doing the same things again and again, such as jogging, kneeling in the garden, or hiking on steep trails—can also make tissues inflamed and sore.

ON MENDED KNEE

Most knee pain clears up on its own within a few days, or a few weeks at most. If the pain doesn't improve fairly soon, or if the joint is swollen and stays that way, there's a good chance that you've done some real damage. You're going to need x-rays or other tests to find out exactly what's going on.

While surgery may be necessary for serious knee injuries, most problems can be easily managed with a combination of medication and good home care. Here's what doctors advise.

Start with ice. Your first-line treatment for knee pain is as close as your freezer. Take out some ice cubes, wrap them in a washcloth or small towel, and hold them on your knee for about 20 minutes. Remove the ice for at least 20 minutes, then reapply it. Keep

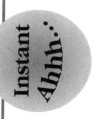

Instant Ahhh...

Unlock the Pain

When you're spending a lot of time on your feet and your knees are aching, you can get quick relief just by shifting position a bit. The best thing you can do is relax your legs so they're not locked at the knees. Standing in this slightly squatted position puts much less pressure on your joints.

doing this for about two days, advises Jerry Cochran, M.D., president of the Midland Orthopedic Clinic in Texas and spokesman for the American Academy of Sports Medicine. Ice causes blood vessels to constrict, which will dramatically reduce swelling and pain, he explains.

Follow up with heat. After two or three days, stop using the ice treatment and switch to heat. You can drape a heating pad set on low over your knee for about 20 minutes at a time. Unlike cold, heat causes blood vessels to expand. This increases the flow of blood and healing nutrients to the joint while also speeding the removal of pain-causing waste products.

Wrap and raise. As soon as your knee starts hurting, wrap it with an elastic bandage. In addition, keep your leg elevated as much as possible for the first few days after the pain starts.

"I can't emphasize enough the importance of elevation," says Dr. Cochran. "You want your foot to be higher than your knee, and your knee should be higher than the bottom of your breastbone." Wrapping your knee and keeping it elevated will help reduce painful swelling, he explains.

Soothing Salves

REACH FOR THE WITCH

Witch hazel is a traditional herbal remedy that's been used by Native Americans for centuries to ease sore muscles and joints. When your knees are hurting, apply the liquid to a clean cloth or towel, then rub it onto your sore knee with a gentle massaging motion, reaching around to rub the back of your knee as well. If you do this twice a day during painful episodes, you'll notice a big difference right away.

Work your quads. Strengthening your knees is the best way to coax them back to health, and it will help prevent further injury. "You should stretch all of the main muscle," says John Nowicki, N.D., a naturopathic physician in Issaquah, Washington.

Here's an easy exercise to start with: Stand up straight, bend your right leg behind you, and grip your right foot with your right hand. Slowly pull your foot toward your buttocks, keeping your lower back straight. Hold the stretch for 15 to 20 seconds, then relax and repeat with the other leg. (If this causes pain, give your knee a few more days of healing time before trying it again.)

Stretch your hams. To stretch your hamstring muscles, stand straight, then bend over and lower your hands as close to the floor as you can comfortably get. Hold the stretch for 15 to 20 seconds, then relax. Be sure to bend from your hips, not your lower back.

Build up your glutes. Strong gluteals (the muscles in your buttocks) reduce strain on your knees. To work your glutes, lie on your back with your knees bent and your feet flat on the floor. Place your right foot over your left knee, then wrap your hands around your left thigh and pull it toward your chest. Hold for 15 to 20 seconds, relax, then reverse positions and stretch your other leg.

Add some ab work. Strong abdominal muscles don't just look good, they also protect your knees by stabilizing your hips. Lie on your back with your knees bent and your feet flat on the floor. Using a twisting motion, slowly lower both legs to the right side of your body while keeping your lower back flat on the floor. Hold for 15 to 20 seconds, relax, then twist and lower your legs toward the left.

Take-it-easy exercise. It's a good idea to do non-weight-

STRETCHING

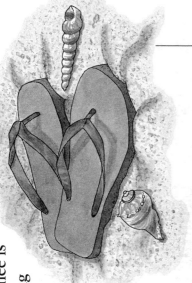

bearing exercises while your knee is recovering. "Swimming or riding an exercise bike works well," says Dr. Cochran. Walking isn't a true non-weight-bearing exercise, but it's fine as long as you take it easy and walk slowly until your knee is fully recovered.

Get up and about. If you spend most of your day at a desk or in a relatively sedentary position, your knees will experience a sudden jolt if you suddenly go into high gear after work. Doctors treat a lot of knee injuries in people who decide to go for a hard run after work or on weekends without adequately preparing their knees for action.

It's essential to keep your knees loose and limber throughout the day. If you have a desk job, for example, take a break at least once an hour to walk to the copy room or stroll around the building. Even standing up while you talk on the phone will help keep your joints limber.

Your sole support. Your beloved sneakers may come with a lifetime warranty, but that covers their lifetime, not yours. Don't wait until you can feel the sidewalk through the soles to get a new pair. Plan on getting new athletic shoes after using the old ones for about 300 miles—600 at the most. Worn-out shoes lose a lot of their cushioning ability, which will put unnecessary stress on your knees, Dr. Cochran explains.

Seek stability. Doctors usually advise staying active (in a gentle way) following joint injuries, but there's an important exception. If your knee feels unstable—it's wobbly or it won't hold your weight—you should stay off it for a while. Keep applying ice and elevating it for a day or two more.

Restless Legs Syndrome

Calming the Kicks

Imagine going to bed every night knowing that as soon as you begin to drift off, your legs will start feeling numb or tingly. You may feel as though irritating electricity is flowing through your muscles. Some people even report that their legs feel as if they're crawling with ants.

Welcome to the odd nighttime world of restless legs syndrome (RLS). This condition is unlikely to be a serious health threat, but people who have the attacks night after night can go months or even years without a good night's sleep. The resulting fatigue can make it nearly impossible for them to hold down a job or function at full alertness during the day.

FROM MILD TO MADDENING

People who have RLS often have a hard time describing the symptoms. Their doctors are equally baffled, because no one really knows what causes it. What they do know is that people with this mysterious condition experience their symptoms only when they're lying down or are otherwise immobile. As soon as they move their legs vigorously, the symptoms go away. When they stop moving, the irritating feelings return.

This perverse torture can last for minutes or even an hour or more, so you can see why people with RLS are so tired all the time. They're almost forced to keep moving, even when they'd much rather be asleep.

NO MORE RESTLESS LEGS

There aren't any definitive tests for RLS. Your doctor, probably a neurologist, will take a look at blood flow and nerve functions to make sure that your symptoms aren't caused by something else. Even if you appear to be perfectly fine—most people with RLS have no obvious health problems—the doctor may prescribe medications to relax the muscles and help you sleep. Most people, however, don't need drugs. "Almost all restless leg patients can get very good relief from their symptoms and live a normal life," says Mark Buchfuhrer, M.D., a sleep specialist in Downey, California, and medical director of the Southern California Support Group for RLS. Here are the best ways to keep your legs calm and get a better night's sleep.

Stand and stretch. When your legs start aching or tingling, sometimes just standing up will make the sensation go away. It's not uncommon, in fact, for people with RLS to get out of bed and read while standing.

Instant Ahhh...

Give In, Get Up

Trying to sleep when your legs are aching to move never helps. If anything, the frustration will make it harder to sleep. Rather than fight it, it's better to get up and move around for a while. The symptoms will go away almost instantly, and after 10 minutes or so, you (and your legs) may find that it's easier to rest.

Stretching your legs also seems to help, so you might try doing some deep knee bends, rising up on your toes, or flexing your thighs, calves, and ankles. Some people report that stretching before going to bed makes attacks less likely.

A soothing soak. Some people with RLS find that heading from the bed to the bathtub calms their restless legs. A soak in warm water will sometimes reduce symptoms enough so you can get to sleep.

Running hot and cold. While soaking in warm water is a common strategy for calming restless legs, some people do better when they alternate heat and cold. Soak a towel in warm water and drape it over your leg. After a minute, replace it with a towel soaked in cool water. Keep doing this for both legs until they feel better.

Cut back on alcohol and coffee. Both seem to cause an increase in RLS symptoms. As a general rule, limit yourself to one or two daily servings of either alcoholic or caffeinated beverages. If you still have trouble, you may want to give them up entirely to see if things improve.

Don't scream for ice cream. It pains me to knock one of my favorite treats, but many people with RLS find that ice cream makes their problem worse, and no one knows why. "For some reason, ice cream just tends to bother a very high per-

Healing Hands

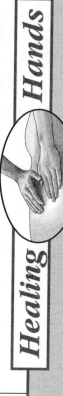

The next time you're tossing and turning because of restless legs, reach down and firmly massage the areas that are bothering you. While massage won't cure the condition, it does seem to ease symptoms for some people.

centage of people with RLS," says Dr. Buchfuhrer.

Make a menu memoir. Since there seems to be great variability in how food affects people with RLS, it may help to keep a record of everything you eat to see if there's a connection with your symptoms. After a few weeks, your diary may reveal that specific foods tend to make your RLS worse.

Iron it out. Even though the cause of RLS isn't known, there does seem to be a clear link between restless legs and low levels of iron in your body. "Every patient with RLS should have a serum ferritin level test," says Dr. Buchfuhrer. "It's a super-sensitive test for iron."

If your ferritin level is less than 45 micrograms per deciliter (45 mcg/dL) of blood, your doctor may advise you to take supplemental iron intravenously. Oral iron supplements help only about 20 to 30 percent of the time, says Dr. Buchfuhrer.

A busy mind is... A good approach for just about any kind of physical discomfort, and RLS is no exception. When you feel an attack coming on, get your mind in gear: Do a crossword puzzle. Play a computer game. Dig into a good novel. The less you think about your legs, the less bothersome the sensations will be.

Take a hike. People who exercise regularly often find that their RLS symptoms improve. Even a daily walk seems to

---

Watch Out!

Drugstore shelves are loaded with over-the-counter sleep aids, many of which contain antihistamines that promote sleepiness. Unfortunately, antihistamines tend to make restless legs worse, says Mark Buchfuhrer, M.D. "When people with RLS can't sleep, they sometimes take one of these drugs, and that only makes things worse," he says. It's best to consult a physician who's familiar with RLS before trying any sleep medication.

help. "It's best not to exercise right before going to sleep," adds Dr. Buchfuhrer. "You should do it at least a few hours before going to bed."

But take it easy. While moderate exercise can ease RLS symptoms, people who really exert themselves may find that their symptoms flare up. "Vigorous exercise can be a problem," says Dr. Buchfuhrer. "I have several younger patients who train to run marathons, and invariably, they get into trouble when they're really training hard."

Know your patterns. If there's any saving grace about RLS, it's that the symptoms tend to strike with predictable regularity. Once you know your patterns, you can take medication (assuming your doctor has prescribed it) to head off attacks. "Medications are much better at preventing the problem than at reducing symptoms once they get started," Dr. Buchfuhrer says.

Shift your schedule. Depending on when your symptoms tend to occur, you may be able to make schedule changes that will help you cope. You might take a later shift at work, for example, so you won't be going to bed until after the time your symptoms usually flare up. Or you might schedule an afternoon walk for the time when you often have trouble.

Shinsplints

Caring for Tender Tendons

I've never had shinsplints, and now I know why. The only people who tend to get them are athletes who are, well, more enthusiastic about their fitness endeavors than I could ever hope to be.

Even when I ran cross-country back in high school, I wasn't the type of runner who would impress the coach by doing an extra lap around the gym or showing up for practice even when I had the sniffles. But maybe you were (or are). If you get temporarily sidelined by shinsplints, consider them a badge of honor. They show that you're dedicated to your sport—and they won't hold you back for very long.

PUSHING TOO HARD

The doctors I talked to weren't sure where the term *shinsplints*

Change Your Rural Route

One of the quickest solutions for shinsplints is simply to run on level ground—a running trail, for example, or the track at a local high school or college. Runners who stay off rocky or uneven terrain often improve right away—and stay pain-free in the future.

comes from. It's not a medical term. It simply means that you're experiencing pain in the front of your lower leg—pain that's invariably aggravated by exercise.

What's probably happened is that you've strained or slightly torn one of the tendons in your lower leg. This usually happens at either end of the athletic spectrum: Elite athletes who push themselves really hard often get shinsplints; so do beginners who aren't quite as fit as they think they are.

A GENTLE WARNING

Shinsplints hurt, but usually not as much as a serious sprain or strain—and the pain almost always goes away once you get a little rest.

In fact, if the remedies I've included in this chapter don't make your leg feel as good as new, it could be a sign that the pain is due to something more serious, and you should see a doctor. In most cases, though, consider the pain of shinsplints to be a warning that it's time to take things a bit easier. In the meantime, try these tips to recover more quickly and prevent future problems.

Take a break. You're likely to get shinsplints only when you're dishing out more stress than your body is able to handle, says Thomas Ayers, D.C., team chiropractor for Sprint Capital USA, a training center for world-class athletes in Raleigh, North Carolina.

"We often see shinsplints in weekend warriors

who go out and push themselves too hard," he says.

The solution, obviously, is to rest. For most recreational runners (shinsplints are a problem mainly for runners), taking a week off is enough to eliminate the pain.

Cube 'em. Ice cubes are your best friends when you're coping with shinsplints. Putting cold on your lower leg will help reduce swelling as well as pain.

Apply a cold pack or ice cubes wrapped in a washcloth or small towel to the area that hurts. Keep it in place for about 20 minutes and repeat the treatment every hour or two until you're feeling better.

The pain of shinsplints often disappears within 5 to 10 minutes after you quit exercising. When that happens, a single application of ice is probably all you need.

Pop a pill. Most nonprescription pain relievers, including aspirin and ibuprofen, are very effective at easing the pain of shinsplints, says Dr. Ayers. Take them every 4 hours, following the directions on the label.

Hit the wall. If ice and pain pills don't make you feel better, you may want to try some gentle stretching. It helps the muscles relax and flushes away waste products that contribute to the pain.

Here's a stretch that will help: Stand in front of a wall with

Make Some Custom Slush

For a cold pack that fits the contours of your leg, fill a zipper-lock plastic bag with 4 parts water and 1 part rubbing alcohol, then toss it into the freezer until it's cold. (You may need to double-bag it to prevent leaks.) In a pinch, a bag of frozen vegetables makes a quick custom cold pack.

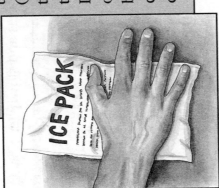

STRETCHING

your legs shoulder-width apart and one foot a step or two in front of the other. Bend the knee of your front leg while keeping your rear leg straight, then lean into the wall, keeping both heels flat on the floor. Hold the stretch for 5 to 10 seconds, then switch leg positions and repeat.

Sit and stretch. Here's an even easier stretch that will help ease shinsplint pain. Kneel with your legs together under you and the tops of your feet against the floor. Sit on your heels and slowly lean back. Hold the stretch for a few seconds, relax, and repeat.

Change the grade. A lot of runners who practice on treadmills adjust the machines so they're slanting upward. While running uphill provides a great workout, it can also lead to shinsplints if your legs aren't ready for the strain.

While you're training, you may want to reduce the pitch or even make it completely level. Once you build up more leg endurance and strength, you can return to uphill running.

Support your arches. If you have flat or fallen arches, you may be at risk for shinsplints. One of the easiest solutions is to drop by a drugstore and pick up some orthotic shoe inserts, which will support your feet and help keep your lower legs pain-free.

Shin Solutions

Moist heat is a great treatment for shin pain, and adding vinegar to the mix increases the anti-inflammatory power. Heat a mixture of equal parts vinegar and water, soak a small towel, wring it out, and apply it where you hurt. Leave it on for about 20 minutes. If you don't have any vinegar in the house, you can get similar results with castor oil. Rub the oil onto your sore shin, cover the oil with plastic wrap, then top that with a hot, moist towel. Leave it on for about 20 minutes, then wash off the oil with soap and water.

BURNETT'S CASTOR OIL

Tap your toes. The underlying cause of shinsplints is often muscle weakness—especially in the shin muscle, says Timothy Tyler, a physical therapist at the Nicholas Institute of Sports Medicine and Athletic Trauma at Lenox Hill Hospital in New York City.

"When you run, that muscle has to pull really hard," he explains. You can make the muscle stronger simply by tapping your toes. No kidding, it's as easy as it sounds. A few times a day, sit in a chair and tap your toes up and down, keeping your heels on the floor. Continue until you feel a slight burn in the muscle at the front of your shin. "That's how we prevent shinsplints," says Tyler. "It works."

Go back gradually. You may be eager to start running again, but after you've given your shins time to rest and recover, don't tear out of the starting gate at full speed. "It's best to gradually get back into the activity again," says Dr. Ayers.

This is especially important if you haven't exercised regularly in the past. It's great to change your life and take up regular exercise, but you want to do it slowly and give your body a chance to adjust.

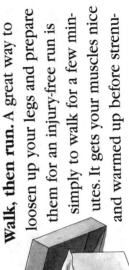

Walk, then run. A great way to loosen up your legs and prepare them for an injury-free run is simply to walk for a few minutes. It gets your muscles nice and warmed up before strenuous exertion.

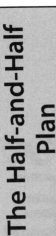

The Half-and-Half Plan

You're more likely to get shinsplints if you run every day. A better approach, especially if you're just beginning a workout program, is to run one day, take a day or two off, then run again. Giving your muscles a little recovery time means that you'll be less likely to limp home with shinsplints.

Stubbed Toe

Get Out of a Toe Jam

Oh, how I hate stubbing my $%^&# toe! It's not just the pain that gets me upset, it's also the fact that the pain is usually my own stupid fault.

I'm a big fan of walking barefoot. Unfortunately, I'm not the most organized person in the world. It's almost inevitable that at some point, one of my exposed toes is going to collide with some heavy object that I've left in an inconvenient place. I can't decide which is the better solution: Wearing shoes more often or straightening up the house a little more.

PAINFUL PIGGIES

Toe-stubbing is a fact of life. It's also nature's way of telling you to watch where you're going. When you stub your toe, you literally mash nerve endings as well as tiny blood vessels called capillaries. If you stub it hard enough, you'll bruise—which means that dozens of capillaries have burst. You could also cut through the skin or cause painful damage to the nail.

TLC FOR TOE TRAUMA

The pain of a stubbed toe usually doesn't last very long. Obviously, you'll have to exercise common sense. If the pain is severe or you have a bad cut, you'll want to see your doctor. This is especially true if you have diabetes or another condition that diminishes sensation in your feet, since even a slight injury could wind up being pretty serious.

Apart from these exceptional cases, it's easy enough to care for your traumatized tootsie yourself. Here are some things that can help.

Go for the cold. "Besides hopping up and down and screaming, which we all do, a cold cloth or some ice is probably your best first bet for a stubbed toe," says Karen Barnes, N.D., a naturopathic physician in Burlington, Ontario, Canada, and author of *Naturopathic First Aid.*

Wrap some ice cubes in a washcloth or small towel and hold them on the toe for about 20 minutes. Keep applying ice every few hours until the soreness is better.

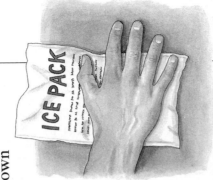

Put your foot up. Elevating the injured foot will help reduce swelling caused by inflammation. This, in turn, will help your toe heal faster and with less pain. Plan on staying off your foot for at least 10 to 15 minutes.

Bring on the heat. If your toe is still painful a day or two after it's been stubbed, you may want to warm it up with a heating pad. Use the low setting and keep the heat in place for about 20 minutes. This will help take the edge off any lingering aches.

Go homeo. The homeopathic remedies arnica and hypericum help reduce pain, swelling, and bruising, says Dr. Barnes. She advises taking a 30C dose of each as soon as you stub your toe. Keep taking them five times a day until you're feeling better. You can buy homeopathic products at many health food stores.

Try a tincture. Another

herbal remedy for toe pain is St. John's wort oil, available at health food stores. Soak some gauze with the oil, then wrap it around your toe. It may sting at first, but it will definitely help speed up the healing.

If you have an open cut, be sure to dilute the oil before applying it. Add 10 drops of oil to a cup of water, then dip the gauze in the solution.

Cream it with calendula. Did your stub break the skin? The herb calendula is a popular choice among herbalists for healing cuts and open wounds. Buy some calendula cream at a health food store and apply it to the area once or twice a day.

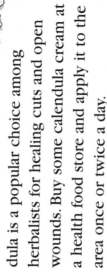

Reach for an analgesic. Aspirin, ibuprofen, and other over-the-counter painkillers are very effective at relieving stubbed-toe pain. Keep in mind, though, that aspirin and ibuprofen may make bruising worse. If your toe is the color of an eggplant, you may want to use acetaminophen instead. It has the same painkilling effects as aspirin without the bruise-promoting properties.

Change shoes. Your tenderized tootsie won't be happy if you cram it into one of your usual shoes. If you can't go barefoot (carefully!), switch to a sandal or other open-toed shoe until your toe feels better.

Pain-Pounding Produce

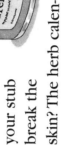

Bioflavonoids are natural chemicals found in most fruits and vegetables that help your body repair and replenish broken tissue. While you're recovering from a stubbed toe, load up on fresh produce—especially berries, which are absolutely jammed with these protective chemicals. Treat yourself to a bowl of cherries, blueberries, or raspberries every day. You can also take bioflavonoid supplements to make sure you're getting enough. "Take about 100 milligrams a day for a week or two," suggests Karen Barnes, N.D.

Take a C cruise. You need extra amounts of vitamin C when you've stubbed your toe. This all-purpose nutrient (which was probably voted "most likely to succeed" in high school) is essential for skin repair, says Dr. Barnes.

Unless you have stomach or kidney problems, take 500 milligrams four times a day for a few weeks, she suggests. Taking vitamin C with food will help prevent it from upsetting your stomach.

Get oil-E. Vitamin E oil will encourage healing without scarring. "Wait two or three days to let the healing process get started," says Dr. Barnes. After that, break open a vitamin E capsule and apply a little of the oil a few times a day.

Leave well enough alone. If you stubbed your toe so hard that the future of the toenail is in question, don't try to fix it yourself. Pulling a damaged nail can be excruciatingly painful, and it's also likely to result in infection. "Don't mess around with it," says Dr. Barnes. "You really should see a doctor."

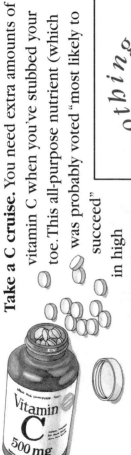

Soothing Salves

TRUST ST. JOHN'S

Herbal oils made from arnica and St. John's wort can make a real difference when you've stubbed your toe. They help relieve pain, promote healing, and reduce the risk of infection. Combine 6 to 12 drops of either oil with a few tablespoons of olive or almond oil, then apply the mixture to the sore area a couple of times a day.

Another easy option is to crumble dried arnica or St. John's wort, add enough water to make a paste, and apply it to the stubbed area. Leave it on for about 20 minutes, then rinse it off. You can find these herbal oils and dried herbs at health food stores.

Varicose Veins

Vanquish Vein Pain

Most people think of varicose veins as just a cosmetic problem. They're certainly unsightly, especially if they're large and discolored, but the main problem is that they can make your legs feel tired and sore.

Even though nearly everyone has some varicose veins, there's a lot of confusion about what they really are. As one doctor told me, they're nature's proof that gravity only pulls one way. Confused? Let me explain.

UPHILL BATTLE

A varicose vein is simply a blood vessel that doesn't have quite enough strength to push its cargo of blood uphill and back into circulation. When blood leaves your heart, it's traveling at tremendous velocity. The initial speed, combined

Chill the Ache

Cold witch hazel is a cool solution to aching veins. Chill a cup of witch hazel in the refrigerator for about an hour, then soak a washcloth in the liquid and apply it to the parts of your legs that hurt. Keep the compress in place for about 15 minutes while also elevating your legs. Witch hazel has astringent properties, which means that it improves blood flow and eases pain.

with gravity, means that blood doesn't have any trouble reaching the blood vessels in your legs.

But consider the return trip. This time, the blood has to go uphill, without the heart's pumping action to help it along. As it moves upward from veins in your legs—assisted by the pumping action of your leg muscles—the blood passes through tiny one-way valves, which snap shut behind it at intervals. Basically, it moves uphill in stages.

Sometimes, the valves aren't strong enough to support the weight of the blood, so it slips backward, forming pools inside one or more veins. After a while, the accumulated blood causes the vein to swell, resulting in a varicose vein.

KEEP THE BLOOD MOVING

As I mentioned earlier, varicose veins can make your legs feel tired and achy. That's the most common problem, but there's also a risk that the poor circulation that accompanies varicose veins can cause ulcers on your lower legs. Less often, the swollen veins can promote the formation of blood clots that are potentially serious.

So you see, you have to do something when you have vari-

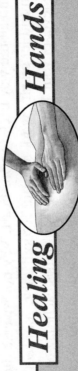

Healing Hands

There's nothing like a massage for soothing tired legs (or tired anything, for that matter). Besides making you feel good, massage can improve your circulation, which is a big plus if you have varicose veins. To help ease the ache even more, add a few drops of comfrey herbal oil to a few tablespoons of olive oil, then give yourself a soothing oil massage. Comfrey oil will boost circulation and help the discomfort fade a lot faster.

cose veins. If you really hate the way they look, or they're causing a lot of physical discomfort, surgery and other techniques can remove them. In most cases, however, you can bolster your veins with some simple home strategies. Here are a few things you ought to try.

Slip on some stockings. Snug-fitting hose, called compression stockings, are available from drugstores and medical supply stores. They provide extra support to the walls of blood vessels in the legs, which helps keep blood moving upward, says Peter Beatty, M.D., an interventional radiologist at Legacy Meridian Park Hospital in Tualatin, Oregon, and national co-chair of the Legs for Life Program. (You can visit www.legsforlife.org for information about free screening for leg circulation problems.) Your doctor should write a prescription for the kind you need. Over-the-counter compression stockings work well, but they may not provide the exact amount of pressure that you need.

Get a leg up. The blood in your legs has to fight gravity to climb all the way back to your heart. Why not reverse the situation and let gravity work for you? To do it, raise your feet above the level of your heart for a couple of hours each day, or sit with your legs propped up on pillows. About 10 minutes after you elevate your legs, the ache will go away.

Sleep on a slant. Sleeping with your feet raised a few inches will give your veins a boost all night. You can prop your feet on a flat pillow or put some boards under the foot of your bed. Check with your doctor first, though, since this sleeping position may aggravate some health problems.

Take a break. If you spend most of your day on your feet, your varicose veins may feel as if they're going to pop out of your legs by the time the day's over. Don't wait until you get home from work to give your legs a breather. Take breaks as often as possible. If you stand a lot, take some time to relax in a comfortable chair. Put your feet up on a desk if you can.

Dress for success. Compression stockings are designed to give your veins the kind of pressure they need, but other garments that put pressure on your legs can interfere with circulation. Avoid tight panty hose, girdles, and other kinds of restrictive clothing.

Beef up with bioflavonoids. Strong, healthy veins are less likely to become varicose. One way to strengthen yours is to get more bioflavonoids in your diet. These natural plant chemicals, found in most fruits and vegetables, make the vein walls stronger and better able to push blood uphill. Most researchers recommend at least five servings of fresh fruit and vegetables a day.

Load up on C. Your body uses vitamin C to strengthen blood vessels, says Erica LePore, N.D., a naturopathic physician in Wakefield, Rhode Island. Unless you have stomach or kidney problems, she suggests taking 500 to 1,000 grams of vitamin C two or three times daily. Since taking this much vitamin C may cause diarrhea, it's a good idea to start with the lower dose and gradually work up from there.

Stay active. Having varicose veins isn't an excuse not to exercise. In fact, it's all the more reason to be active. "Exercise is helpful in managing varicose veins," says Kimberly Beauchamp, N.D., a naturopathic physician in Wakefield, Rhode Island. The more fit you are, the better your circulatory system will be able to cope with the diminished capacity of your leg veins.

"It's best to do exercise like yoga, swimming, or walking, which don't put excessive pressure on the lower extremities," Dr. Beauchamp adds.

Keep cool. You don't want your legs to get too hot when you have varicose veins, because it could result in tissue-damaging inflammation, says Dr. LePore. You should avoid long, hot baths and other activities that make your legs hotter than usual.

Stimulate the veins. You can improve the pumping action of leg veins with a technique called contrast hydrotherapy, in which you alternate between hot and cold treatments.

Soak a cloth in hot water, wring it out, and place it over the area where you have varicose veins. Leave it in place for 3 minutes, then replace it with a cold cloth for 30 seconds. Repeat the cycle two or three times, always ending with the cold cloth. "It's helpful for strengthening blood vessels and promoting healthy circulation," says Dr. Beauchamp. And it makes your legs feel good!

Pain in Your Skin

- Abrasions
- Bites and Stings
- Blisters
- Boils
- Bruises
- Burns
- Chafing
- Cuts
- Dry Skin
- Folliculitis
- Frostbite
- Ingrown Hair
- Pressure Ulcers
- Rash
- Shingles
- Splinters
- Sunburn

Abrasions

Patches for Scratches

I used to work at a company that was full of fitness enthusiasts—"health nuts," as I liked to call them. Often, at lunchtime, I'd pass a bunch of them in the halls, carrying their helmets and water bottles on their way out to ride their mountain bikes (there was a wooded trail near the building). One day, I noticed that one of them, a tall guy named Dan, had a huge scrape across the side of his leg. It looked as if someone had gone at him with a cheese grater.

"Doesn't that hurt?" I asked him.

"A little," he told me. "But you should see the rattlesnake I fell on."

He was probably kidding, but it was at that moment that I decided to do all of my cycling on paved roads.

A TOUGH SCRAPE

Abrasion is just a fancy word for a scrape. Most abrasions are more painful than serious, except when they cover a wide area. The more extensive the scrape, the more likely it is to damage sensitive nerves under the skin. But even big scrapes usually heal fairly quickly. The main risk is infection, because until the skin heals, it's easy for germs to get inside. That's precisely what you want to prevent.

HEAL, BOY!

There's no shame in taking your abrasion to a doctor just to be sure nothing's seriously wrong. In most cases, of course, you can probably handle it yourself with common sense and a little TLC. Here's how.

Clean and cover. The first step in healing any wound is to get it really clean, says Laura Pimentel, M.D., chair of emergency medicine at Mercy Medical Center in Baltimore. You have to flush out all the bacteria that get into any open wound, as well as any dirt, gravel, or whatever else your skin came in contact with.

Flush the area thoroughly with running water. Keep flushing it until all the dirt or other foreign matter is gone. Then carefully wash the abrasion and the surrounding skin with soap and water. Don't bother with antibacterial soap; regular soap will work just fine.

After the area is clean, cover it with a bandage that's tight enough to keep the wound clean, but not so tight that it's uncomfortable. Change it once a day.

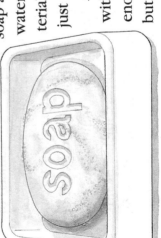

It's an Emergency!

Even minor abrasions sometimes become infected. When you change the bandage, look for redness, swelling, pus, or increased tenderness. These are all signs that bacteria are winning the battle, and you may need antibiotics to turn the tide.

Another risk to be wary of is tetanus, says Laura Pimentel, M.D. This is especially true if you got wood or rusted metal in your skin. Tetanus is a life-threatening condition, so be sure you're protected. If you haven't had a tetanus vaccination in the past 10 years, go to your doctor and get the shot. It stings for only a moment, but it provides long-lasting protection.

Instant Ahhh…

Wipe Out Pain

One of the quickest ways to ease the pain of abrasions is to apply a thick coat of triple antibiotic ointment, available at drugstores. The cool cream feels good going on, it protects the wound from infection, and it can even help prevent scars.

Sanitize with a saintly solution. If you want to be absolutely, positively sure that the abrasion won't get infected, paint on a little St. John's wort tincture. Available in health food stores, this herb kills just about all of the bacteria it encounters.

Try a little witchcraft. Distilled witch hazel, once a staple of medicine cabinets everywhere, is helpful when an abrasion continues to bleed, says Priscilla Natanson, N.D., a naturopathic physician in Plantation, Florida. "It's a styptic that slows blood flow," she explains. It stings a little, she adds, but only for a few seconds.

Start a healthy habit. If you're not taking a daily multivitamin already, this is a good time to start. The extra nutrients will ensure that your body has all the raw materials it needs to repair skin damage.

Heal with vitamin C. It helps your body repair blood vessels that were damaged. While the abrasion is healing, take about 2,000 milligrams a day, divided into two or three doses to prevent stomach upset or diarrhea. People with stomach or kidney disease should avoid large doses of vitamin C.

Cream it with calendula. It's a traditional remedy for abrasions and cuts, and there's good evidence that it works. "It's a great herb for wounds," says Dr. Natanson. Buy calendula cream at a health food store, then apply it to the abrasion every time you wash it and change the bandage.

Bites and Stings

Relief from Itchy Things

On a warm summer day more years ago than I care to admit, I was playing outside with my cousin and my sister, Suzanne. I was having a good old time on the swings, when I suddenly felt a sharp pain in my finger. I looked down and saw the business end of a bee sticking out of it.

I ran home, screaming for my mother. It wasn't my proudest moment, I admit, but that act of panic probably saved me from a lot more trouble. As it turned out, my cousin had inadvertently stirred up a beehive (or maybe a nest of yellow jackets; there have been a lot of family arguments about which it was), and the sky soon filled with buzzing avenging angels.

While I was at home with ice on my one little sting, Suzanne and

Soothing Sage

A sage poultice is sage advice if you're nursing an insect sting, because it reduces pain and swelling. Crush fresh sage leaves between your fingers, then simmer them in a saucepan with a little vinegar. When the leaves soften and cool, put them on the bite and cover the area with a warm, moist washcloth. Leave it in place for about 15 minutes.

my cousin were stung repeatedly. In fact, it was so bad that a little later, my mom put Suzanne in the shower to flush the remaining bees out of her hair.

PAINFUL VENOM

Now that I know something about bees, I can't really blame them for doing their best to defend their hives and honey. Most stings and bites are forms of self-defense, although some critters, such as mosquitoes and ticks, go for human blood as a delectable source of nourishment. Regardless of the reason, however, the discomfort we experience is caused by roughly the same thing: Insects inject chemicals that may make the skin swell and hurt.

TAKING THE BITE OUT OF STINGS

It's rare for insect bites or stings to cause serious health problems, but obviously, there are some notable exceptions. A bite from a black widow spider, for example, can make you seriously ill. And some people have a dangerous allergic reaction, called anaphylaxis, to insect bites.

That's why you should see a doctor if you have any unusual symptoms—such as serious swelling, hives, nausea, or breathing problems—after a close encounter with the insect kind. And the symptoms don't always occur right away; some people have reactions up to an hour or more after the bite or sting.

For people with insect allergies, an injection of epinephrine

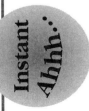

Instant Ahhh...

Nature's Venom Vacuum

The next time you get a bite or sting, mix a little baking soda with water and smear on a generous layer of the paste. It helps pull venom out of the skin, explains Heidi Weinhold, N.D. Don't have baking soda? Apply a dab of mud. Soil almost always contains a little clay, which also helps draw out the venom and reduces pain and swelling.

can be lifesaving. If you know that you're allergic, your doctor will probably give you a self-injector so you can take fast action if you're bitten or stung. But for most of us, the treatments are a lot simpler. All you'll really need is some home remedies to take away the pain and help the bite or sting heal more quickly.

Cool it with ice. As with other types of inflammation, some well-applied ice can freeze a painful insect sting in its tracks. Ice also soothes the itchiness of mosquito bites.

Wrap some ice cubes in a washcloth or small towel to make a cold pack, then hold it against the affected area for about 20 minutes. Remove the ice for at least 20 minutes, then reapply it until you're feeling better.

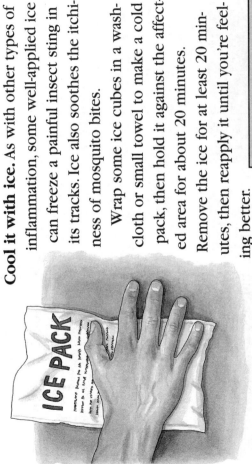

Even if you don't have any ice available, you can cool an insect bite to take away the ouch. Soak a cloth in cool water, wring it out, and drape it over the bite, suggests Laura Pimentel, M.D., chair of emergency medicine at Mercy Medical Center in Baltimore. "A cool compress is soothing and will help reduce itching," she says.

Tease with tweezers. If the insect left a stinger embedded in your skin, your best bet is to pull it out. Otherwise, it will continue to irritate the skin; a bee stinger continues to release venom even when the insect is long gone. Sterilize

Soak the Sting

Some insect bites really itch while they're healing, but an oatmeal bath provides quick relief. First, fill an old sock with about a cup of plain, dry oatmeal. Attach the open end of the sock to the bathtub faucet with a rubber band, then run warm water through it until the tub is filled. Settle in for a soothing, itchbusting soak.

An Anti-Insect Wardrobe

Mosquitoes and other insects tend to be attracted to bright, contrasting colors. One way to keep them away is to tone down your wardrobe when you're in the yard or hiking in the woods. Wear light-colored clothing during the day and darker clothing at night. Definitely avoid eye-popping shades as well as vivid floral patterns.

tweezers with some rubbing alcohol, gently grip the stinger, and pull it out.

Prepare to repair. To help your skin repair itself, be sure to get plenty of vitamins C and E, two nutrients that are critical for skin health. You'll get enough of both—along with other important vitamins and minerals—just by taking a daily multivitamin.

Grab some grapeseed. Available in capsule form at health food stores, grapeseed extract is rich in bioflavonoids, chemical compounds that will help your injured skin put itself back together. Follow the label directions.

Vitamin
C
500 mg

Blisters

Bubbles of Trouble

A few summers ago, I signed up for a week-long cycling tour through parts of Wyoming and Montana. I normally spend hours a week on my bike, but for a trip like this, I had to do some pretty serious training. I started taking long rides, confident that I'd be able to keep up with the group by the time my vacation arrived.

I had no trouble whipping my legs and lungs into shape, but there was one problem I hadn't anticipated. After the first few weeks of training, I had major blisters on my hands from leaning on the handlebars. They hurt so much that I thought I'd have to quit riding while they healed, which would have thrown off my entire training schedule.

Fortunately, that's when I happened to glance at the hands of some other cyclists going by. I saw their padded gloves—an obvious solution. I picked up some gloves of my own, and that was the end of my blister problem. I had a great time on my trip, and I haven't gotten any blisters since.

PROTECTIVE PADDING

This experience made me realize, once again, that our bodies are often smarter than we are. When we put ourselves (and our skin) in harm's way—by spending all day on our knees scrubbing floors, for example, or wearing tight shoes without socks—our skin responds to potentially damaging friction by forming a blister, which is nothing more than a protective, fluid-filled pad that works like those cycling gloves.

DON'T POP 'EM!

Most blisters don't hurt very much. As long as you don't tear them open, they protect damaged areas of skin and go away on their own, usually within a few days to a week.

The only time blisters are really dangerous is when they get infected. If the pain is getting worse, or if you notice the area is swelling or turning red, it's worth taking the time to apply an over-the-counter triple antibiotic ointment a few times a day. If that doesn't help, you're going to have to see a doctor to be sure the infection doesn't continue to spread.

Blisters that stay intact, however, are unlikely to get infected. That's why doctors say you should leave them alone; there's usually no reason to pop blisters to drain out the fluid, says Lisa Arnold, N.D., a naturopathic physician in Orleans, Massachusetts. "They usually heal on their own," she says. "The only time to pop them is if they get infected—and that's something a doctor should do."

Instant Ahhh...

Savory Infection Fighters

You probably have two of the strongest antiseptic herbs in your kitchen right now. "Rosemary and thyme can really help if you're worried about infection," says Lisa Arnold, N.D. Add a tablespoon of each herb to a cup of hot water and steep for about 10 minutes. Let the liquid cool to room temperature, pour some on a cloth, and hold it against your blister for about 20 minutes. You can repeat the treatment once or twice a day until the blister is gone.

This doesn't mean you should ignore blisters entirely, though. There are a number of steps you can take to prevent infection and help them heal more quickly. Here's what the experts have to say.

Keep 'em clean. The best way to keep infection-causing germs out of blisters is to clean them (and the surrounding skin) once or twice a day. Wash the area well with soap and water, then dry it thoroughly when you're done. Too much moisture will soften the blister and make it more likely to break open before it's ready.

St. John's to the rescue. The herb hypericum, better known as St. John's wort, is great for killing germs and easing pain. Use an alcohol-based tincture of the herb, available at health food stores, to moisten a square of gauze, then apply the oil to the blister after you've washed it.

Cure it with calendula. To reduce blister tenderness and help speed healing, apply a salve that contains the herb calendula along with skin-protecting vitamins A and E. "Calendula is really helpful for skin problems," says Dr. Arnold.

You can apply the salve, available in health food stores, once a day. Or buy dried calendula, crumble it between your fingers, and add enough water to make a paste. Cover the blister with the paste, leave it on for about 20 minutes, then rinse it off.

Give 'em some air. Even though it's good to protect blisters with a bandage, you want to expose them to the air for at least 20 minutes a day. A little air circulation will help protect the area from infection-causing bacteria, which thrive in dark, moist places.

Watch for hot spots. Before a blister appears, you'll usual-

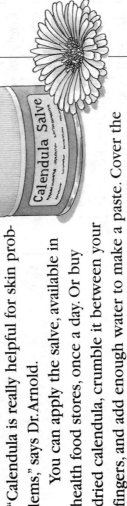

ly notice a hot spot—a red, tender area on your skin. Acting quickly at this stage may prevent a blister from forming.

If you've had a burn, for example, quickly apply ice to the area and keep it there for about 20 minutes. If the hot spot is caused by friction, cushion the area with moleskin, gauze, or another type of padding.

Go for clover. Red clover oil is a great choice for healing blisters. You can put the oil directly on the sore, then cover it with a bandage to promote healing. Repeat the treatment once a day until the blister's gone.

The oil is available in most health food stores, but be sure the product you buy is made for topical use. What you don't want is an essential oil, which is too concentrated to apply directly to your skin.

Forgo the friction. Blisters have an unfortunate tendency to occur in areas that get the most friction. The obvious solution is to quit whatever it is you're doing—hiking, scrubbing floors, hopping on one foot, or whatever—before the blister actually erupts.

By the same token, you should definitely avoid friction once a blister has formed. "A blister forms as a protective measure," says Dr. Arnold. "If you keep irritating the area, it isn't going to go away."

Soothing Salves

YEA FOR YARROW!

Big blisters sometimes take a long time to heal. You can speed things along by applying yarrow, an herb that naturally (and safely) draws out the fluid. "It's an astringent herb that will help dry it out," says Lisa Arnold, N.D.

If you're using fresh or dried yarrow (available at health food stores), chop or crumble it as finely as you can, then add enough water to make a paste. Apply the paste to the blister and cover it with an adhesive or gauze bandage. Replace the dressing once a day until the blister is gone.

Boils

Stop Infections from Simmering

A few months ago, I got hooked on a public television program about two great medieval emperors who struggled for control of what would one day become Korea.

Plots were hatched, armies clashed, schemes were thwarted, and victories passed back and forth between the two powers. What finally brought the saga to an end was the death of one of the emperors. He didn't fall in battle, nor was he assassinated. No, what brought him down was an ailment that confounded all of the court physicians: A boil on his backside. Hard to believe that such a humble problem led to the fall of an entire empire!

A BACTERIAL BREW

Boils are similar to pimples in some ways. They appear as red or pinkish, pus-filled bumps on the skin, sometimes with a white or yellow spot in the center. They're unsightly, but that's not why they're worrisome. When bacteria colonize a hair follicle (a tiny chamber from which a single hair grows), they have the potential to multiply to harmful levels. The immune system tries to keep them in check, but if it fails, the organisms can trigger a potentially serious infection. At the very least, they can cause boils, along with a lot of inflammation and pain.

BOIL OVER

If you're generally healthy, a boil is unlikely to be a serious problem. The pus will usually drain on its own, and the boil should disappear within one to two weeks. But if your immune system isn't able to combat the infection efficiently, the bacteria may spread to other parts of your body, and you'll probably need antibiotics to get things under control.

Large or painful boils should always be treated by a doctor, especially if you have other signs of infection, such as a fever, chills, or fatigue. Minor boils, however, are relatively easy to treat at home. It's mainly a matter of helping them drain, while at the same time boosting your body's immune response. Here's what you need to do.

Don't pop it. Opening a boil to remove the pus will certainly reduce pressure and pain, but it will vastly increase your risk of infection, warns Lisa Arnold, N.D., a naturopathic physician in Orleans, Massachusetts.

Most of the time, you should just leave the boil alone, she says. If it's too painful, ask your doctor to lance it. "Definitely

---

Soothing Salves

PASTE IT TOGETHER

Why buy fancy herbal creams to help boils drain, when a homemade salve may work just as well? Buy some dried yarrow, an astringent herb, from your local herbalist or health food store. Crumble the leaves, add a little water to make a paste, and apply it to the boil. Leave it on for about 20 minutes, then wash the area well, suggests Lisa Arnold, N.D.

A paste made with slippery elm is also effective, she adds. "You can buy slippery elm powder that you mix with water to make a paste," she says. Put a dab on your finger, then gently apply it to the boil and the surrounding area. Just be sure to wash your hands first to reduce the possibility of infection.

don't try it yourself," says Dr. Arnold.

Keep it clean. Boils can literally overflow with bacteria, and the last thing you need is for stray germs to cause an infection elsewhere. The most important home treatment is to keep the boil and the surrounding skin clean and dry. Wash the area with soap and water a few times a day. If you touch the boil, wash your hands immediately afterward, and don't let anyone else in the family use towels or washcloths that came into contact with the infected area.

Do the mashed potato. White potatoes contain natural chemicals that seem to help boils drain. Grate a potato and apply it directly to the boil, Dr. Arnold suggests. Leave it on for 10 to 20 minutes, then wash the area well. You can repeat the treatment once or twice a day

Lavender is lovely. Along with tea tree, lavender is one of the most powerful herbal oils for killing bacteria. Add a few drops of either oil, which you can buy at a health food store, to a cup of warm water. Moisten a washcloth with the water and hold it on the boil for about 10 minutes several times a day.

Cream 'em with herbs. A good choice is a cream that contains St. John's wort. If you apply it several times a day, it will help keep the infection from spreading, and it may reduce pain as well.

Another useful herbal cream is calendula, which reduces discomfort and helps the area heal more quickly. Look for a cream that also contains vitamins A and E, skin-friendly nutrients that promote faster healing.

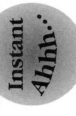

Instant Ahhh...

Bag It with Tea

One of the most effective remedies for a boil is to cover it with a tea bag. Black tea contains tannins, chemical compounds that help boils drain, says Lisa Arnold, N.D. Soak the tea bag in hot water just long enough to soften it. Let it cool slightly, then hold it on the boil for 10 minutes or so.

Bruises

Beat the Black-and-Blue Blues

There's nothing like a bruise to remind you—and everyone around you—of your own clumsiness. A friend of mine once showed up at work with an ugly bruise on his forearm. Each time he rolled up his sleeve, he had to explain to curious observers what happened. At first, he told the truth: how he'd slipped on some wet grass and slammed his arm against a railing. But he got tired of telling the same story. A few days later, I heard him telling someone that he got the bruise during a rugby match, when he knocked his arm against someone's head while making a critical interception. I have to say, this was far more entertaining, and better for his ego, than simply admitting that he was a klutz.

WHY AM I BLACK AND BLUE?

It's easy to understand what happens when you get a bruise. Any hard impact can damage tiny blood vessels, called capillaries, beneath your skin. Broken capillaries bleed, but you don't see blood because it's under the surface. What you do see is the dark "stain," which can range in color from slightly yellow to eggplant purple. Apart from the unsightly mess, bruises hurt because the same impact that damages blood vessels also injures skin and muscle. Most bruises are inflamed and tender for at least a few days, and sometimes a few weeks.

BRUISE CONTROL

Most bruises aren't a big deal. Each day, your body slowly cleans up the damage by removing fluids and damaged cells. The bruise gradually changes color as different chemicals are broken down and removed from the area. While you're healing, of course, the pain and tenderness can be a real nuisance—and you'll also have to answer those endless questions about how you got that ugly blotch. There's no secret strategy for making bruises disappear like magic, but there are ways to help them heal more quickly. Here's how to do it.

Make nice with RICE. The oldest treatment for bruises, and still the most effective, goes by the initials RICE: rest, ice, compression, and elevation. Doing these steps in sequence will minimize discomfort and help bruises heal much more quickly.

R.I.C.E.

• Rest means just what it says. When you've bruised an

Soothing Salves

THE CASTOR CURE

A traditional and powerful way to treat bruises is to apply a castor oil pack. "Castor oil has excellent anti-inflammatory properties, and it penetrates the skin very well," says Sean Sapunar, N.D. Spread castor oil over the bruise, then wrap the area with plastic wrap. Place a heating pad (set on low) or a washcloth soaked in hot water on top of the wrap. Leave it in place for about 20 minutes, then wash off the oil. You can repeat the treatment several times a day until the bruise is gone.

BURNETT'S
CASTOR
OIL

area, give it some downtime in order to let the damaged tissues start healing.

- Ice the area immediately after the injury. Apply an ice pack for about 20 minutes every few hours for the first day or two. Cold reduces the bleeding under the skin that causes pain and discoloration.

- Compress the area by wrapping it with an elastic bandage. You want the wrapping to be snug, but not so tight that it cuts off circulation. You'll know you're stretching it tight enough if you can see light through the bandage while you're applying it. The pressure restricts blood flow and helps prevent swelling.

- Elevate the bruised area above the level of your heart as often as you can. This allows excess fluid to drain away from the bruise and back into circulation.

In with the good, out with the bad. After a few days of RICE, switch to a technique called contrast hydrotherapy, in which you alternate between hot and cold compresses. "This creates an artificial pumping action that brings more nutrients to the area and pumps out waste products," explains Sean Sapunar, N.D., a naturopathic physician and clinical faculty member at the Bastyr Center for Natural Health near Seattle.

Blueberry Rescue

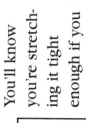

Remember the girl who turned into a giant blueberry in the film *Willy Wonka and the Chocolate Factory?* It wasn't a pretty sight, but the good news is that she probably never bruised again. Blueberries are loaded with vitamin C and chemical compounds called bioflavonoids, which are essential for blood vessel repair. "I advise people to eat a half-cup of blueberries a day," says Sean Sapunar, N.D. The nutrients in the berries will help bruises heal and make your blood vessels stronger and better able to resist future damage.

Here's how it works: Soak some washcloths in hot tap water and others in cold. Apply a warm compress to the area for 3 minutes, then switch to cold for 30 seconds. Several times a day, repeat the cycle three times, always ending with the cold compress. Alternating heat with cold causes blood vessels to expand and contract, Dr. Sapunar explains.

Pass the salts. Here's a chance to use that box of Epsom salts that's been sitting in the back of your bathroom cabinet all these years. Add a cup or two of the salts to a warm bath (or a smaller amount to a basin), then soak the area for about 20 minutes. "The magnesium in the salts is very soothing for bumps and bruises," says Dr. Sapunar.

Catch some fish oil. It sounds like something your grandmother would recommend—and, as usual, she'd be right on the money. Fish oil is rich in omega-3 fatty acids, natural substances that make your body less prone to inflammation. Take a tablespoon or two of fish oil daily until the bruise is gone, says Dr. Sapunar. "You can get similar benefits by eating fish and flaxseed, but it takes a little longer," he adds.

▲ Cup of Comfort

Ginger tea is an effective treatment for bruises. It reduces inflammation and dilates, or widens, blood vessels. Wider blood vessels allow more blood to circulate, which removes pain-causing compounds and brings in more healing nutrients. You can make ginger tea by steeping 1 tablespoon of powdered ginger in a cup of boiling water for 5 to 10 minutes. Drink the tea at least three times a day until the bruise is gone.

EPSOM SALTS

EPSOM SALTS

MAGNESIUM SULFATE

NET WT. 1 LB. 4 OZ.

"C" is for capillary. Your body uses vitamin C to repair damaged capillaries. When you have a bruise, you've injured dozens or even hundreds of them, so you need as much of this important nutrient as you can get. While the bruise is healing, eat plenty of fruit (especially citrus fruits) and vegetables, which are loaded with vitamin C. As long as you don't have kidney or tummy troubles, it's also helpful to take 2,000 to 3,000 milligrams of vitamin C supplements for a day or two. Since large amounts of vitamin C can cause diarrhea or upset stomach, it's a good idea to take smaller amounts several times a day. Taking it with food also helps.

Add a multi. Your body's need for nutrients increases dramatically when you have a bruise. Important bruise-beating nutrients include zinc, vitamin A, and selenium. You'll get plenty of these and other healing vitamins and minerals by taking a multivitamin every day until the bruise is gone.

Munch on nuts. Brazil nuts are loaded with selenium, the nutrient that's essential for skin health. Eat about a cup daily while the bruise is healing.

Ask for arnica. A major bruise buster, arnica gel is available at health food stores. If you'd rather not use a gel, you can take arnica in homeopathic form, following the package directions.

Beat it with bromelain. A natural substance found in pineapple, bromelain helps your body break down and remove the chemical spill that causes bruises. Fresh pineapple doesn't contain enough bromelain to be helpful, so it's better to take it in supplement form. The recommended dose is 400 milligrams two or three times a day on an empty stomach. If you take it with food, your digestive juices will make it inactive.

Burns

Easy Solutions for Seared Skin

When I was at a dinner party a little more than a year ago, one of the guests knocked over a full bowl of matzoh ball soup. That by itself would be enough to throw the most congenial gathering into disarray, but things quickly got worse because the scalding broth splashed another guest's arm. Startled as well as burned, she let out a loud yell.

Our host, Zella, was speechless—horrified that her favorite family recipe, the jewel in her culinary crown, could cause so much pain. But her daughter, Wendy, kept her cool. She immediately shouted, "Toothpaste, toothpaste!"

At first, I couldn't figure out what she was talking about. Then she explained that a welder once told her that toothpaste will stop the pain of any burn. I was intrigued, but

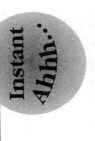

Instant Ahhh...

Minty Relief

I never would have believed this tip if I hadn't witnessed it myself. Applying toothpaste will quickly ease burns. Most toothpastes contain menthol, which has a cooling effect on the skin, explains Lisa Arnold, N.D.

doubtful. I'd heard about a lot of home remedies for burns, but never a word about toothpaste.

It just goes to show that there's a lot of good information out there that never makes it into the medical books. When Zella came downstairs with the toothpaste, Wendy applied a little to the burned woman's arm, and the pain almost instantly got better.

INSTANT PAIN

Burns are among the most painful injuries you're ever likely to get. Even a small burn damages nerves as well as the surface layers of skin. The exposed raw tissue can take a long time to heal. Worse, it's extremely vulnerable to infection.

The darned thing about burns is that they happen so fast. Unlike other types of injuries—a knife cut, for example—with burns, there's virtually no time to react and save yourself from danger. By the time sensations of heat have traveled from your skin to your brain, the damage has been done.

FIGHT THE FIRE

Doctors divide burns into three increasingly serious categories. A first-degree burn, the kind we all get from time to

---

Soothing Salves

SAINTLY RELIEF

The herb St. John's wort is almost custom-made for burns. It provides excellent pain relief, and it has mild antibacterial action. Daily applications will help reduce the risk of infection and may help burns heal more quickly. Your best bet is to get St. John's wort cream at a health food store, or you can buy an herbal oil. Add several drops of the oil to a tablespoon or two of olive or grapeseed oil. Apply the cream or oil mixture to the burn with a cotton swab, then cover it with gauze or an adhesive bandage. Reapply the cream or oil and change the dressing once a day until the burn is healed.

time, is merely red and painful. You may or may not get a blister, and the burn usually heals just fine with proper home care. A second-degree burn, which results in blisters and swelling, can be intensely painful. The worst is a third-degree burn, which involves much more than the upper layers of skin. Paradoxically, it may not be painful at all, because nerve endings may have been destroyed.

You need immediate medical attention for second- or third-degree burns or for any burn that's bigger than 2 or 3 inches around. Minor burns, however, are easy enough to treat at home. Here are some suggestions for cooling the pain and helping them heal more quickly.

Douse it with water. It's almost instinctive to throw water on something that's burning, and that's the perfect response when you've touched something that's too hot to handle, says Lisa Arnold, N.D., a naturopathic physician in Orleans, Massachusetts. "Cold water is the best thing," she says.

As soon as possible, flood the area with cold running water for about 10 minutes. This will stop the pain and help prevent swelling. If the pain persists, repeat the cold water treatment for 15 minutes each hour. "The cold water constricts the blood vessels, and taking it away opens them up again," she explains. This creates a pumping action that improves circulation and helps the burn heal more quickly.

Always improvise. If the closest cool liquid happens to be milk or even a soft drink, well, any port in a storm. "You have to work with what you've got," Dr. Arnold says. The more quickly you cool the injury, the sooner you'll stop the damage.

Don't reach for ice. Even though you want to cool a burn as quickly as possible, ice will probably make things worse. It will make the area too cold, and sometimes it sticks to the skin.

Quick Relief from Windburn

The frigid temperatures of winter, combined with dry skin, can make your entire face feel raw and irritated. To take the sting out of windburn, try these tips.

Warm up slowly. It's natural to rub your skin when you're cold, but the friction will make it more vulnerable to irritation. The next time you come in out of the cold, don't rub your face warm; just let it warm up naturally.

Clean it well. You know that gritty feeling you notice when you come in out of the wind? It's from windborne particles of sand and dust that can rub and abrade your skin, making the irritation worse. Gently wash your face, arms, and other exposed areas as soon as you come indoors. You may also want to apply a moisturizing cream to replenish all the moisture that the wind sucked out.

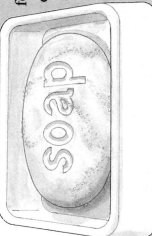

Keep it up. "Elevating the burned area, if it's on a part of the body that can be elevated, is definitely good," Dr. Arnold says. You want the area to be higher than the level of your heart so fluids that accumulate there will drain back toward the body as the normal flow of blood and other fluids mops up the damage.

If you can, keep the area elevated for about 20 minutes, Dr. Arnold advises. For larger burns, repeat the elevation several times a day during the first 24 hours.

Follow "Ow!" with aloe. The herb aloe vera is an all-around skin healer that takes away the pain of burns and helps them heal more quickly. If you have one of these low-maintenance plants in the house, you can grab one of the spiky leaves, snap it open, and rub the juice right on the burn. You can also get aloe gel at a health food store, then rub it on the burn a few times a day.

Soothe it with calendula.

Available as a cream in health food stores, the herb calendula helps fight infection and speed healing. You can also make your own calendula soother. Chop or crumble fresh or dried calendula leaves, then add water to make a paste. Dab the paste over the burn and leave it there for about 20 minutes, then gently rinse it off. You can repeat this treatment once or twice a day until the burn is healed.

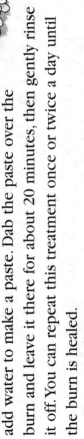

Mix and match. Even the best herbs for burns can be made a little better by using them in combination. Dr. Arnold advises picking up a cream or ointment that contains several skin-friendly herbs, such as comfrey, calendula, and goldenseal, at a health food store.

Keep the scene clean. One reason that burns are so dangerous is that they strip away the protective outer layers of skin—and there are plenty of germs that will jump right in. To prevent infection, wash the area with soap and water a few times a day. Cover it with a bandage if you think it's likely to get dirty, and be sure to change the bandage at least twice a day. Just remember to wash gently: Overzealous scrubbing can easily damage burned skin.

Spread on extra protection. To prevent infection, apply a thin layer of triple antibiotic ointment every time you wash the burn and change the bandage.

Leave blisters alone. Those ugly blisters that pop up after burns should be left alone, says Dr. Arnold. "They're part of the skin's healing mechanism, and they'll take care of themselves," she says. (For more tips on helping blisters heal, see page 349.)

Drink lots of water. When you're recovering from a burn, you want to drink as much water as you can hold—at least eight full glasses daily. Burns can result in dehydration because they break through your body's natural moisture barrier. Drinking a lot of water will hydrate cells in your skin and help the area heal more quickly.

Oil it up.

Forget the traditional advice about applying butter to a burn: It will trap the heat, cut off healing airflow, and generally make things worse. But vitamin E oil is another story. When it's applied after the initial pain is gone, the oil will soothe the area and help the skin heal more quickly. Just break open a vitamin E capsule, squeeze out the oil, and apply it to the entire area.

Shun the sun. Don't spend a lot of time in the sun while a burn is healing. Without its surface layer of protection, the skin will be vulnerable to the sun's burning rays. Stay covered up or stay inside until the burn is completely healed.

A Plant That Spurns the Burn

If you live in the northeastern or midwestern United States, you may have plantain growing in your yard right now. Consider yourself lucky, because fresh plantain—which is also sold in health food stores everywhere—is a traditional burn remedy. Simply squeeze or cut open a leaf and apply the juice directly to the burn. "You can even chew it up and then apply it," says Lisa Arnold, N.D.

Chafing

When You're Rubbed the Wrong Way

The last time I went camping, one of my friends, Lester, was sporting a new pair of hiking boots. Unfortunately, he failed to bring extra socks, and the socks he was wearing were a little shorter than the tops of the boots. By the time we'd trekked a few miles, his beautiful boots had etched a red, irritated line across the fronts of his shins.

It was obvious that another day of chafing would turn those red lines into painful, open sores, so we all got together and pondered what to do. We settled on The Great Sock Swap. That evening, we rummaged through our camping wardrobes to find socks that were long enough to protect Lester from his boots. The longer socks, plus a wrapping of gauze from the first-aid kit, kept Lester and his boots on the hiking trail for the rest of the weekend.

Soothing Salves

E IS EXCELLENT

The next time your skin gets rubbed the wrong way, break open a vitamin E capsule and apply the oil to sore spots. Your body uses vitamin E to repair damaged skin, and the oil will soothe and lubricate the area until it has a chance to heal.

PAINFUL RUBS

Chafing is basically what happens when something rubs against your skin long enough and hard enough to damage it. Prolonged friction wears away the surface layers of skin cells. Unless the pressure is relieved, the damaged area of skin will get inflamed, itchy, and sore. You'll eventually wind up with a painfully raw patch of skin, and when that happens, infection is a very real threat.

PADDING AND PROTECTION

Mild chafing sometimes resembles a rash, but if you look closely, you'll see that the skin is actually worn away. While severe chafing can result in infection, chafing is usually more of a nuisance than anything else. It can be mighty painful, however, and raw patches of skin typically take a long time to heal. It's definitely worth preventing if you can. If it's too late for that, here are a few ways to get the damage under control.

Lose the friction. The first step in dealing with a chafing problem is to eliminate whatever's rubbing you the wrong way, says Lisa Arnold, N.D., a naturopathic physician in Orleans, Massachusetts. The culprit is usually obvious, but sometimes you'll have to look around to figure out where the pressure is coming from. For example, you may have chafing on your thighs from a snug pair of pants or problems on your wrist from a too-tight watchband.

Instant Ahhh...

Jiffy Lube

A quick way to reduce painful friction in places where skin rubs against skin is to apply a little lubrication. A dusting of baby powder or cornstarch will let the skin surfaces glide smoothly past each other. Use a cotton ball to apply enough powder to lightly cover the chafed area; the best time is after bathing and before dressing. Reapply it as you need to, or check the area a few times a day and use more powder if it looks red or irritated.

Pain in Your Skin

Cover up. Once you've lost a few layers of your skin's protective cells, you'll need to cover the area to protect it from further damage. For small chafed areas, an adhesive bandage works well; for larger areas, use a square of gauze.

Keep it clean. When skin is chafed, it's more vulnerable to infection, so it's essential to keep the area clean. Wash it gently (you don't want to rub off more skin) with soap and warm water a few times a day. After washing and drying the area, replace the bandage. Keep doing this until the skin is completely healed.

Take extra vitamin C. Most multivitamins provide about 60 milligrams of vitamin C, the recommended daily amount. But that's not enough when your skin is damaged. You'll need more, probably 2,000 to 3,000 milligrams a day, to help your body repair damaged skin as well as blood vessels.

Taking that much vitamin C at once may cause stomach upset or diarrhea. To minimize any side effects, divide the total amount into smaller doses throughout the day and take them with food. Keep taking extra vitamin C until your skin is back to normal. If you have kidney or stomach problems, don't take any supplements without talking to your doctor first.

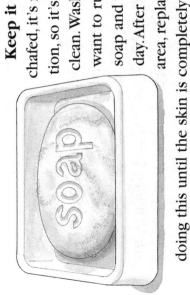

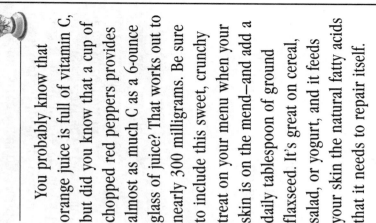

Pepper Power

You probably know that orange juice is full of vitamin C, but did you know that a cup of chopped red peppers provides almost as much C as a 6-ounce glass of juice? That works out to nearly 300 milligrams. Be sure to include this sweet, crunchy treat on your menu when your skin is on the mend—and add a daily tablespoon of ground flaxseed. It's great on cereal, salad, or yogurt, and it feeds your skin the natural fatty acids that it needs to repair itself.

Be a smooth dresser. If you keep getting chafed in the same place, there's a good chance that the problem is due to something you're wearing. Tight-fitting clothes are common offenders. You may want to switch to looser equivalents to see if that helps. It's also a good idea to wear clothing made from cotton or other soft weaves rather than coarse or synthetic fibers.

Wash and wear. Chafing is usually caused by the friction of hard things against skin, but sometimes, the problem is more subtle. Accumulations of dirt, sweat, or chemicals in your clothes can aggravate your skin as much as simple friction. If chafing is a persistent problem, take the time to wash clothes that get extra dirty, such as bike shorts, gardening gloves, or swimsuits, after every use.

Heed the signs. Most times, your chafed skin will heal without any problems, but it's important to keep an eye out for infection, since the damaged area is vulnerable to invasion by bacterial troublemakers.

Signs of infection include redness, pus, swelling, or increased pain. It's fine to apply a triple antibiotic cream once or twice a day for a few days, but if the infection doesn't seem to be getting better, see your doctor. You may need oral antibiotics to get the problem under control.

Cream It with Calendula

A traditional herbal remedy for skin injuries, calendula has antimicrobial properties that can reduce the risk of infection. You can buy calendula cream at a health food store, or you can make your own soother by adding a few drops of calendula oil to a tablespoon or two of olive oil. After washing and drying the area, apply a layer of cream or oil and cover it with a bandage. Leave it in place for at least 20 minutes, and reapply it once a day until all the chafing is gone.

Cuts

Save Your Skin

My cousin Jan is a big fan of Band-Aid–style bandages. She collects them the way other people collect stamps or coins. (Her favorites, from Japan, are decorated with strange, bug-eyed creatures.) She started collecting unusual bandages because she wanted something interesting to cover the small cuts that she's always getting on her hands and fingers.

Why so many cuts? Jan is a very hands-on kind of person. She loves carpentry, gardening, playing with cats, and other simple pleasures that are always putting her hands in harm's way.

SLICE OF LIFE

Your skin is your first line of defense against the often-harsh

---

Soothing Salves

CALENDULA CREAMS CUTS

Calendula is a traditional herbal treatment for cuts, and it does seem to help them heal more quickly. You can buy calendula ointment at health food stores. After washing and drying your cut, apply a generous dollop of ointment, then cover the cut with a bandage. Reapply the ointment each time you change the bandage.

The Perils of Paper

Have you ever wondered why paper cuts hurt so much? Doctors have wondered, too. It turns out that paper edges aren't as sharp as you may think. They're sharp enough to cause a cut, but not sharp enough to make a "clean" cut. "Paper tears the cells, and the cuts tend to be more painful than knife cuts," explains Sean Sapunar, N.D. The other reason that paper cuts cause so much pain is that your fingertips—where most paper cuts occur—are thick with sensitive nerve endings.

Paper cuts need to be treated like any other wound—flooded with water, washed with soap, and safely wrapped with an adhesive bandage. Before you do that, though, you can stop the sting almost instantly by firmly rubbing your finger near, but not on, the cut. "The sensation of pressure travels much faster than the pain," says Dr. Sapunar. "The pressure signals get to the brain first and block out the painful ones."

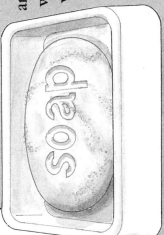

outside world. Nature made your skin a very effective barrier—so effective, in fact, that it can repair minor cuts with great efficiency. When you cut yourself, your body almost immediately mobilizes specialized cells in your skin and blood vessels. They secrete a host of chemical compounds, including gluelike substances that stop bleeding and seal the cut. The problem is, though, that some parts of your body, especially your fingertips, are jammed with pain-sensitive nerves. This is why even shallow cuts on your hands or fingers can deliver a surprising amount of pain.

REPAIRING THE DAMAGE

Cuts that bleed a lot or continue bleeding for more than a few minutes may be too much for you to handle. If you can see deep inside the cut—if it extends, say, more than 1/4 inch into the tissue—you should see a doctor right away. You may need stitches, and large cuts are much more likely to get infected than small ones. It's not worth taking chances.

Even a small cut can harbor untold numbers of bacteria, and the resulting infection can be painful as well as dangerous. Warning signs that an infection is brewing include redness, swelling, weeping, or increased tenderness. If you notice any of these symptoms, and they don't clear up within a day or two, call your doctor. You may need antibiotics to eliminate the infection.

Fortunately, most cuts aren't this serious. As long as you stop the bleeding and keep the area clean, you'll probably heal just fine. Here are the steps you need to take.

Clean thoroughly. The biggest risk from even small cuts is that harmful germs will get inside and trigger a painful, potentially serious infection. As soon as possible, flush the cut with cool running water to wash away debris and germs and help slow the bleeding. After flooding the area, wash it well with regular soap, which will kill any germs that remain.

Cover it up. Once the cut is clean, cover it with an adhesive bandage. "It should be snug enough to keep out dirt, but not so tight that it prevents circulation," says Sean Sapunar, N.D., a naturopathic physician and clinical faculty member at the Bastyr Center for Natural Health near Seattle.

Match the cover to the cut. You want the padded part of the bandage to cover the cut completely, and you should make sure that the adhesive part isn't touching the wound. Plain adhesive strips are fine for minor wounds, but deeper or more extensive cuts will heal better if you use a butterfly-style bandage to pull the edges of the skin together. The advantage of these bandages is that they don't need to be changed every day; they're designed to hold cuts together and give them a chance to heal.

Re-clean and re-cover. Even if you washed and covered a cut promptly, bacteria can get inside while it's healing. To prevent infection, it's important to change an adhesive bandage every day. Wash the wound with soap and running water, dry the area with a clean towel, and apply a fresh bandage. Most cuts don't require any more attention than that. "I'd stay away from hydrogen peroxide," says Dr. Sapunar. "It can actually damage the tissue in some cases."

Forget the Super Glue. It's a common home remedy for minor cuts, and in some ways, it works pretty well because it seals cuts almost instantly. "We use a medical bonding agent for cuts that's much like Super Glue," says Dr. Sapunar. But the glue that you have at home isn't quite the same. It isn't sterile, for one thing, and it probably isn't safe to get into an open wound. "I wouldn't use Super Glue on my own cuts," he adds. In most cases, a plain bandage is a better choice.

Seek out St. John. Tincture of St. John's wort (available in health food stores) will help keep cuts infection-free while they're healing, says Priscilla Natanson, N.D., a naturopathic physician in Plantation, Florida. "It has wonderful antibacterial properties, though it may sting a bit since it's an alcohol-based formulation," she says.

Feed your skin. There's never a better time to eat oranges than when you're nursing a cut. They're rich in vitamin C and bioflavonoids, natural chemical compounds that help skin and blood vessels heal more quickly.

Dry Skin

Time to Change the Oil

I don't live in a particularly dry part of the country, but it seems to me that I'm always hearing people complain about dry skin. Just the other day, the mom of a friend of mine was giving her daughter a good-bye hug and said to her, "Does my skin hurt you? It's so dry!" Another friend has five different moisturizers lined up by his bathroom sink. You'd think we were all in danger of drying up and blowing away!

When I talked to Christa Hinchcliffe, N.D., a naturopathic physician in the Seattle area, I found out two things. One is that dry skin is in fact very common. The second is that we bring much of this dryness upon ourselves.

LOW ON OIL

What does it really mean to have dry skin? Basically, it means that the tiny oil glands that pack your skin aren't churning out enough oil to hold in precious moisture. A few things can cause this to happen. If the glands don't get all the nutrients they need, they underproduce, and skin is stripped of its essential oils. Even if the glands work at full capacity, the air sometimes gets so dry that you lose moisture no matter what.

Dry skin, as you know, can feel itchy and irritated. If it gets dry enough, it may start cracking or flaking. Some people have to endure dry skin all their lives, and everyone tends to have drier skin as they get older. But don't make the mistake of assuming that dry skin is something you have to live with; usually, it's not.

MORE OIL, MORE MOISTURE

If dry skin is your only problem, there's no reason to worry about it. Dryness is sometimes a symptom of skin diseases or underlying health problems, but more often it's just what it appears to be: dry and uncomfortable.

One point to remember is that a parched pelt isn't merely uncomfortable. It also makes your skin more vulnerable to infection, so it's worth taking the time to stay moisturized, especially during the arid winter months. Here are a few strategies that will make all the difference.

Chew the right fat. Dry skin sometimes means that your body's not getting enough essential fatty acids, particularly the omega-3s found in fish and flaxseed.

Most Americans have low levels of omega-3s. The solution is

Soothing Salves

HOMEMADE MOISTURIZERS

The next time you're at a health food store, look for moisturizing creams that contain calendula, comfrey, chamomile, or yarrow. Herbalists call them vulnery herbs, which means that they're very soothing for dry skin. Another option is to whip up moisturizing oil treatments at home. You can buy oils of any of these herbs at a health food store, then add 6 to 12 drops to about an ounce of olive or almond oil. Rub the oil directly on your skin or add about 15 drops to a bath for a soothing soak.

to eat fish (some of the best choices are tuna, salmon, and sardines) two or three times a week. If you're not a fish eater, have 1 or 2 tablespoons of ground flaxseed a day. Try sprinkling it on your cereal, salad, or yogurt.

Drink lots of water. Dry skin is often nothing more than a consequence of not drinking enough water. Everyone's ideal H_2O quota is different, but eight glasses of water a day is a good place to start. You'll get the most benefit when you sip water throughout the day, rather than gulping it all down at once.

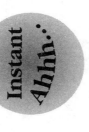

Ax the antacids. Sometimes, it's not poor nutrition but poor digestion that dries the skin. Millions of Americans depend on antacids, and overuse of these medications lowers levels of stomach acid and interferes with proper digestion and the absorption of skin-healthy nutrients, says Dr. Hinchcliffe.

For digestion-friendly ways to control heartburn, see page 159. If you take prescription drugs for heartburn, don't stop without checking with your doctor.

Make the moist of it. Using a moisturizer is the easiest way to help you feel more comfortable in your

Instant Ahhh...

Soothe Your Skin with Oatmeal

"Oatmeal is a really soothing herb for the skin," says Christa Hinchcliffe, N.D. You can buy colloidal oatmeal in drugstores, but it's just as easy (as well as cheaper) to use regular kitchen oatmeal. Add a scoop of oatmeal to an old sock, then use a rubber band to attach the open end to the faucet. Let the water run through the sock as the tub fills, then lie back and relax in the soothing, oatmeal-spiked water.

own skin. All moisturizers do pretty much the same thing: They add moisture to your skin while preventing existing moisture from escaping.

Look for a product that contains the mineral zinc, along with vitamins A, D, and E. These skin-healthy nutrients help improve moisture and reduce dryness from the inside out.

Moisturize when wet. Moisturizers are most effective when they're applied right after a bath or shower. That allows them to trap all that new moisture right next to your skin.

Don't be a killer. Antibiotic soaps and moisturizers may sound like a good idea. The truth is, though, that killing the bacteria living on healthy skin is never a good idea, because it makes it more likely that harmful germs will move in, Dr. Hinchcliffe says. "You need these organisms on your skin, so stay away from any type of bacteria-killing cream or soap."

Wash gently. Soaps are certainly good for cleaning your skin, but they often strip away the natural oils that protect it. Do a little label checking when you buy soaps. You want to use products that don't contain chemicals and do contain natural oils.

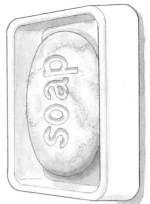

Patch the Cracks

If your skin is so dry that it's starting to crack, here are some tips to help it mend more quickly.

Cleanse gently. Use mild soap to wash the area once or twice a day. You have to keep it clean to prevent infection.

Don't bandage. "It's better to let the skin breathe and heal in the open air," says Christa Hinchcliffe, N.D.

Apply aloe. Squeeze the juice from an aloe plant and dab it on the cracked skin. Or use aloe cream, available at health food stores. "It's good for the skin and the immune system," says Dr. Hinchcliffe.

"A lot of good soaps are made with olive oil. Or try soaps made with safflower oil or castor oil," says Dr. Hinchcliffe. You can also find products that contain soothing herbs or nutrients, such as calendula, aloe, or vitamin E.

Try an herbal steamer. Skin naturally gets drier when you live in an arid climate or when the inside air is drier than usual. One way to add moisture to the air is to keep a kettle of water simmering on the stove. (Of course, this only works when you're home to keep an eye on it.) Add 10 to 12 drops of herbal oil to the water; any of the herbs mentioned in this chapter are good choices, including calendula, comfrey, and chamomile. They're all available at health food stores.

Soak without soap. The quickest way to pump soothing moisture into dried-out skin is to take a long, soothing bath. "The water gets absorbed into the skin," explains Dr. Hinchcliffe. But don't use soap when you bathe, and keep the water warm rather than hot. Hot water and soap are simply too drying when you're trying to moisturize your skin.

Hands of Milk and Honey

You can make your own moisturizer without leaving the kitchen by mixing equal parts of honey and milk. Use this homemade combo as a head-to-toe body lotion, then rinse off the excess. If you're feeling ambitious, toss the mix into a blender and add some apricots, avocado, or coconut oil. The blend feels wonderful, and you can keep it in the refrigerator and massage it into your skin whenever you want.

Folliculitis

Banish the Bumps

For a long time, I worked at a health magazine. I spent my days reading medical journals chock-full of photos and illustrations that were definitely not for the squeamish. Photographs of surgery or horrible injuries didn't usually bother me, but for some reason, pictures of skin conditions made *my* skin crawl.

The one that really gave me the creeps showed some poor soul covered from neck to waist with tiny yellow-white bumps. Much to my surprise, this wasn't some rare tropical disease. It was folliculitis, a skin problem that can affect just about anyone—though thankfully, in most cases, it's not so extreme.

A HAIRY TALE

No matter how often you wash, your skin is covered with bacteria. This makes sense because that's one of the main purposes of your skin: To act as a Great Wall that keeps out the bacterial barbarians.

Like any wall, however, skin sometimes cracks or breaks down. When that happens, bacteria that normally live harmlessly on the skin's surface get underneath. If these vagabond germs find their way into a hair follicle (a tiny chamber that produces a single hair), they can quickly cause infection. The infected follicles turn into small, yellow, fluid-filled bumps.

FAULTLESS FOLLICLES

Folliculitis is usually no big deal. As long as only a small area of skin is affected, you can take care of it at home, and it usually clears up in about five days. If it doesn't, your doctor will probably give you a topical steroid to control inflammation and an antibiotic to knock out the underlying infection.

Some people, unfortunately, are more prone to folliculitis than others, possibly because their immune systems aren't working quite as well as they should. Folliculitis is always ugly, but it isn't particularly painful. Once you know what's going on, you won't have any trouble keeping it under control. Here's what to do.

Start a soap opera. If you know you're prone to folliculitis, soap and water should be two of your new best friends. Frequent washing is the best way to minimize the number of infection-causing germs.

Ordinary soap is fine, but antibacterial soap has a little extra oomph, says Valerie Callendar, M.D., clinical assistant professor of dermatology at Howard University

---

Soothing Salves

BACTERIA BLASTERS

The healing herbs echinacea and goldenseal spell double trouble for the bacteria that cause folliculitis, says Heidi Weinhold, N.D. They kill some germs on contact, and they create an unfavorable environment for future populations.

The easiest approach is to buy an ointment that contains both herbs at a health food store or drugstore, then apply it several times a day until the outbreak is over.

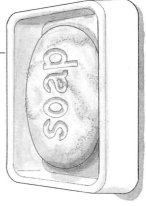

College of Medicine in Washington, D.C. During outbreaks, wash the area once or twice a day.

Create a custom combo cream. "I have some patients mix a hydrocortisone cream with an antibiotic cream," says Dr. Callendar. Hydrocortisone controls inflammation, itching, and swelling, and antibiotics kill the germs. You can buy the creams over the counter. Squeeze equal amounts of each into the palm of your hand, mix them together with your finger, and apply them wherever the bumps are making their unwelcome appearance.

Stay warm, not hot. People often think that bathing or showering in very hot water will kill aggravating bacteria. It doesn't work that way. In fact, hot water makes skin irritation even worse. You'll be a lot more comfortable if you bathe or shower in warm—or even cool—water until the outbreak is over.

Cut back on cosmetics. Makeup and skin-care products may irritate and aggravate skin that's trying to cope with a folliculitis outbreak. For faster healing, stop using them until your skin is back to normal.

Cover up with clay. Natural clay packs, available at many health food stores, are useful for fighting folliculitis, says Heidi Weinhold, N.D., a naturopathic physician in the Pittsburgh area. "They help dry out the skin and pull

Hot-Tub Folliculitis

There's nothing more relaxing and invigorating than soaking in a hot tub. Unfortunately, it's also a good way to come down with folliculitis. "Bacteria can live in the hot-tub jets," says Valerie Callendar, M.D. To keep the little critters from making the journey from the water to your skin, you need to disinfect the tub and the water frequently, following the manufacturer's directions. "It takes some work, but it's worth it," says Dr. Callendar.

out toxins produced by the infection," she says.

Most clays are left on the skin until they dry, she adds. Don't substitute hobby or modeling clay, though. Natural clay packs contain special ingredients that you need for really effective relief.

Don't oversoak your hose. If you take the time to read the directions on the detergents used to clean hosiery, you'll see that stockings should be left in the water for only a few minutes, "but some people leave them soaking overnight," says Dr. Callendar. The excess levels of detergent act almost like folliculitis factories by changing the bacterial balance on the skin. To be safe, soak your delicate items no longer than necessary to get them clean, she advises.

Switch razors often. During a folliculitis outbreak, it's easy for a razor's edge to be contaminated with bacteria. Each time you shave, you can push hordes of bacteria under your skin. To prevent this, buy some disposable razors and use each one only once during outbreaks.

Soak in cereal. If the itching of folliculitis is making you crazy, a colloidal oatmeal bath can put you at ease. "Oatmeal baths work very well," says Dr. Callendar. Most drugstores carry brands that are easy to use; you just add the mix to a warm bath. If the outbreak is on a small area of skin, such as on your arm, you can soak that area in the sink or a basin.

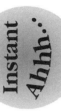

Instant *Ahhh...*

Compress for Success

Applying a warm compress will almost instantly ease itching and other folliculitis symptoms. As a bonus, moist warmth helps draw out infection so you heal more quickly, says Heidi Weinhold, N.D. "It also loosens up the oil glands that are blocked by the infection," she says. Just soak a clean washcloth in warm water, wring it out, and hold it against the affected area for 15 to 20 minutes.

Frostbite

Hot Tips for C-c-cold Skin

A friend of a friend of mine once spent a vacation mountain climbing in the Himalayas. As so often happens to intrepid souls who venture into those frigid climes, he wound up with a case of frostbite. The main reason that he was able to recover with all of his toes was that he not only knew what to do, he also knew what not to do.

That's an important distinction. The things that we instinctively do when we're cold—warm our toes by the fire, rub our frozen noses, or take a medicinal nip of whiskey—are absolutely the worst things to do when you have frostbite.

Incidentally, you don't have to be in extreme climates to get frostbite. If you're not properly garbed, you can get it while walking in the park on a chilly day in March. "A lot of frostbite occurs when people don't wear

---

Nuts to You!

While you're hibernating to heal frostbite, plan on eating like a squirrel. That means nuts—lots of them. They're a great source of vitamin E, the nutrient that you need most for repairing damaged skin. Sunflower seeds and almonds have the most E. Eat 1/4 cup a day until your skin's completely healed.

enough layers or fail to protect their faces from cold wind," says Christa Hinchcliffe, N.D., a naturopathic physician in the Seattle area.

BITTEN BY OLD MAN WINTER

The strange thing about frostbite is that it doesn't hurt right away. That's a good way to know if you're simply cold or if something worse is going on. The pinch of frost stings a bit, but frostbite doesn't feel like much of anything. Your skin may be a little numb or have a pins-and-needles sensation, but you won't be aware that anything's really wrong. At least, not at first.

Suppose that a part of your body—it's usually your nose or a finger, toe, or earlobe—is frostbitten. If you check your skin when you experience the tingling and numbness, you may notice that it's pale and very cold to the touch. No pain, just numbness. But later, when it's warmed up, it starts hurting like the dickens.

When you have frostbite, you have to warm the skin to prevent permanent damage, but it's important that you warm it in precisely the right way.

A Cup of Comfort

After any kind of injury, you want to maximize blood flow because it carts off harmful waste products and brings in healing nutrients.

"Ginkgo tea is very helpful for increasing circulation," says Christa Hinchcliffe, N.D. Plan on drinking a cup or two a day until you're fully recovered. Make tea the old-fashioned way by adding a tablespoon of dried herbs to a cup of freshly boiled water. Steep for 10 to 20 minutes, then strain out the herbs and sip.

THAW'S WELL THAT ENDS WELL

The mildest cases of frostbite, sometimes called frostnip, affect only a small area of skin. When frostbite is really severe, there may be damage to the underlying muscles or even the bones. Your skin may turn white or even black, and there's a good chance blisters will form.

Frostbite is always an emergency. If you notice any of these symptoms, get to an emergency room immediately if you can.

It's the only way you can hope to prevent damage to nerves, blood vessels, or other tissues. In the meantime, you'll have to take steps on your own to minimize—or even prevent—serious damage. Here's how to start your personal warming trend.

Warm up all over. The only antidote to frostbite is warmth. The sooner you can get yourself in a warm place, the less damage frostbite will do.

It's not enough just to warm the affected areas, though. The goal is to warm your whole body, says Dr. Hinchcliffe. Go inside if you can, or at least get out of the wind. And let yourself warm up slowly; you don't want to stand right next to a stove and heat up too quickly. That can make the skin damage even worse.

Apply moist warmth. Once you're inside, soak a cloth in warm (not hot) water and drape it over the affected area. "Stop the treatments when the affected area becomes red, not when sensation returns," Dr. Hinchcliffe says. The process may be painful, but that's normal.

Keep it up. It's advisable to keep the affected body part

Soothing Salves

HEAL WITH ALOE

Aloe vera is among the most potent herbs for skin problems. It will help frostbite heal more quickly, and it inhibits germs that can cause infection.

If you have an aloe plant, cut a leaf, squeeze out some of the gel, and slather it on the affected area once or twice a day. You can also buy aloe gel at health food stores. Buy the brand that has the fewest added ingredients (including artificial colors; natural aloe gel is clear, not green) and the highest concentration of aloe— at least 5 percent.

elevated during and after the warming process. This helps your body drain toxins away from damaged tissues.

Forget the libations. You may be tempted to take a shot of brandy or whatever happens to be sitting around the ski lodge, but it's best to pass on the booze. Alcohol can inhibit normal circulation, which is the last thing you need when you have frostbite.

Don't smoke. And ask people around you to refrain. Like alcohol, cigarette smoke inhibits the flow of blood and can potentially increase damage in the injured area, or at least slow the time it takes to heal.

Hands off. "Try not to jostle the body part or put a lot of pressure on it," says Dr. Hinchcliffe. When you have frostbite, your skin is very fragile. Rubbing or massaging it will make the problem worse. So will stamping your feet if your toes are frostbitten. And definitely forget the so-called Eskimo trick of rubbing frostbite with snow; you'll only make it worse.

Come clean. Once the area has thawed out, clean it gently with soap and water. The damaged skin is very susceptible to infection, so you'll want to clean it at least a few times a day. Don't scrub it, though; just wash the area thoroughly to eliminate any infection-causing germs that happen to be nearby.

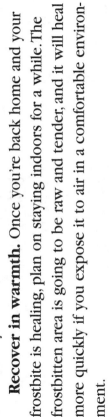

Recover in warmth. Once you're back home and your frostbite is healing, plan on staying indoors for a while. The frostbitten area is going to be raw and tender, and it will heal more quickly if you expose it to air in a comfortable environment.

Get moving. After your skin has had a day or two to start the healing process, get active. The idea is to exercise not only the injured area, but also your whole body. Moving around will improve circulation throughout your skin, which will help the injury heal more quickly.

"Start at a slow pace," Dr. Hinchcliffe advises. Walk for 10 to 20 minutes a day. Stretch your arms, legs, and back. As you start feeling stronger, you can increase the intensity of your exercise.

Relax in a whirlpool. Once the frostbitten area has started to heal, one of the most helpful (not to mention delightful) things you can do is lounge in a whirlpool. The flow of water will stimulate blood flow and improve your recovery.

"You want the water to be just below body temperature," says Dr. Hinchcliffe. She advises staying in the water for 15 to 20 minutes twice a day until the area is healed.

Give up the sweets. Taking a break from sugar is a good idea when you've been bitten by frostbite. The sweet stuff suppresses your immune system and will increase the risk of infection.

Take your vitamins. You never want to overdo it with nutritional supplements, but taking a daily multivitamin will ensure that you get all the key nutrients that your skin needs to recover.

Bundle Up

Even though it's best to stay indoors and warm until frostbite is completely healed, that isn't always possible. If you have to go outside, bundle up well to keep the cold away, says Christa Hinchcliffe, N.D. "The area will be sensitive to cold, and you'll want to keep it warm for at least three weeks after the injury," she says.

MAXIMUM Daily Pack

MULTIVITAMIN & MINERAL SUPPLEMENT

Ingrown Hair

Hair-Raising Strategies

An ingrown hair doesn't sound like much, right? Well, a good friend of mine, Sam, once told me a story that almost curled my hair.

Soon after graduating from college, he noticed that a small red bump had popped up on his back. He ignored it for a few days, but then he noticed that it was getting bigger and more tender. Naturally, he ignored it some more. A few days later, he was nearly overcome by dizziness and fever. That's when he got smart and called his doctor's office. He described his symptoms to the nurse on duty, and she told him to go straight to the closest emergency room. She even told him how to get there.

It's a good thing she did. The tiny bump on Sam's back was infected. Bacteria had slipped into his bloodstream, causing a whole-body infection that could have killed him if he hadn't gotten treatment within hours.

All from a little ingrown hair…imagine that!

THE RAZOR'S EDGE

You can get an ingrown hair anywhere that hair grows, but it's usually men who shave their beards who get them. When they shave, the razor cuts sharp points on the ends of the hair shafts. Beard hair tends to be curly, which means there's a chance that one of the newly sharpened hairs will curl downward and grow into the skin. It's like being stabbed with a sharp needle, except that it happens over days or weeks, instead of all at once.

SAFER SHAVES

Ingrown hairs aren't all that painful by themselves. Problems occur mainly when bacteria take advantage of the tiny wound, wiggle under the skin, and cause an infection.

Of course, anything that penetrates your skin is going to be somewhat uncomfortable. Even when ingrown hairs don't cause much of an infection, they can raise tiny bumps that don't make your morning routine any easier.

To prevent hairs from growing where they shouldn't—and to relieve the pain if they do grow there—here are a few things you may want to try.

The 10-minute solution. To ease painful or infected ingrown hairs, alternate hot and cold compresses. Soak a washcloth in hot water,

---

Soothing Salves

HERBAL SKIN SAVER

A quick way to take the sting out of irritated skin is to apply a cream that contains the herb calendula, says Heidi Weinhold, N.D., a naturopathic physician in the Pittsburgh area. Ready-made creams are available in health food stores, or you can make your own version. Just add 6 to 12 drops of calendula oil to an ounce of almond or olive oil. Rub it on the irritated area once a day until the problem is gone.

For ingrown hairs, Dr. Weinhold particularly recommends using calendula in the form of a succus, which is the watered-down juice of the herb. It's available at most health food stores. Apply it to the sore spots once or twice a day, using a cotton swab or a clean cloth.

wring it out, and drape it on the sore area. Keep it there for 3 minutes, then replace it with a cold cloth for 30 seconds. Repeat the cycle two more times, ending with the cold compress.

This technique, called contrast hydrotherapy, improves skin circulation and speeds healing, says Darrell Misak, N.D., a naturopathic physician in Mt. Lebanon, Pennsylvania.

Keep it clean. Trying to pull an ingrown hair out of your skin isn't necessary; your body will eventually expel it. But you should gently clean the affected area twice a day with soap and water, and definitely keep an eye out for infection. Warning signs include increasing redness, swelling, pain, or pus. If an infection doesn't clear up on its own in a day or two, see your doctor.

Go with the flow. "I recommend that people shave in the shower," says Dr. Misak. That keeps your skin clean and the pores open. It also reduces the chances that your skin will be irritated, and it allows for a closer shave, which can keep hairs from growing inward.

Wash well. It's important to wash your skin with soap and water before as well as after shaving. Thorough cleaning reduces the risk that bacteria will survive long enough to colo-

The Soap Dish

Many soaps dry and tighten your skin, leaving it vulnerable to irritation and infection. A nondrying soap or cleanser made with natural oils is a good alternative. Many premium soaps contain olive, safflower, or castor oil.

"I sometimes recommend a facial cleansing cream containing coenzyme Q_{10}," says Darrell Misak, N.D. It's a natural substance that helps skin stay strong and elastic. Most health food stores, as well as spas and hair salons, offer several choices. Buy the brand that contains the least alcohol and the fewest artificial colors or other ingredients.

nize tiny cuts that often occur when you shave.

Be anti-antibiotic. A lot of people insist on using antibiotic soaps and creams, but they shouldn't. These products tend to irritate your skin, including areas where hairs may be growing inward. So don't use them.

Lose the 'lectricity. Electric shavers may allow you to shave without using lather or water, but they're more likely than razors to irritate your skin, Dr. Misak says. "If you're having problems, go back to blades," he suggests.

Drink water—lots of water. When your skin's properly hydrated, it's better able to heal from injuries, including ingrown hairs. Eight glasses of water a day is about right for most people, but more is even better.

Shave, but don't save. You're less likely to get ingrown hairs if you shave once with a disposable razor, then throw it out, says Valerie Callender, M.D., clinical assistant professor of dermatology at Howard University College of Medicine in Washington, D.C. Reusing a razor makes it easier for yesterday's bacteria to get into today's shaving cut or ingrown hair follicle.

Give it up. For some men with extremely curly facial hair, not shaving may be the only solution to persistent ingrown hairs. Give it a try and see how well the bearded look suits you—or at least go a few days between shaves to give your skin a much-needed break.

Acidify. If you frequently get ingrown hairs or irritated bumps, you may want to use a soothing skin cleanser that contains alpha hydroxy acids or benzoperoxide to keep them at bay, says Dr. Callender. "They tend to be very effective."

Pressure Ulcers

Help for Painful Sores

The fact that there's an entire organization (the National Pressure Ulcer Advisory Panel) dedicated to these painful, slow-to-heal, and sometimes dangerous sores suggests just how serious—and common—they really are.

Adding insult to injury, pressure ulcers tend to strike people who are already facing significant health problems, either at home or in the hospital. Be warned: There's nothing minor about pressure ulcers. In fact, they're among the most serious issues that hospital patients face.

The good news is that most pressure ulcers can be prevented. There are also a number of ways to help them heal more quickly than they normally would.

THE PAIN OF TOO MUCH PRESSURE

Also known as bedsores or pressure sores, pressure ulcers tend to occur when people spend long periods of time sitting or lying without moving. When you stay in one position for a long time, the constant pressure can cut off circulation in small blood vessels near the surface of your skin. Without blood, oxygen, and nutrients, the area starts to break down.

The severity of pressure ulcers largely depends on how

long the pressure lasts. There may be just a red, irritated area or a shallow sore. In more extreme cases, there could even be a deep wound.

ALL THE RIGHT MOVES

Pressure ulcers occur mainly in people who are confined to bed or a wheelchair. Since the sores can potentially form within 2 hours, even a temporary loss of mobility can increase the odds that you'll get them.

Besides being painful, pressure ulcers frequently get infected. That can pose a very serious risk to someone who's already weakened by other health problems.

Prevention is obviously the best approach. It's essential to call your doctor at the first sign of pressure ulcers. If you already have them, you'll want to take immediate steps to prevent them from getting worse. Here's what you or your caregivers need to do.

Spot the spots. If you know what to look for, you can catch a pressure ulcer in the making, says Courtney H. Lyder, N.D., a naturopathic physician in New Haven, Connecticut, and president of the board of directors of the National Pressure Ulcer Advisory Panel.

The first sign is persistent redness, usually over a bony area such as the hip, says Dr. Lyder. If you have dark skin, look for a bluish color. As soon as you notice a sore spot, you need to

Movement Is Everything

The best way to prevent pressure ulcers is to move as frequently as you can, says Courtney H. Lyder, N.D. If you're spending a long time in bed, you need to move—or be moved—at least every 2 hours. If you're sitting, change positions about every 15 minutes.

"Frequent movement is ideal," says Dr. Lyder. Shifting position reduces the amount of pressure on different areas of skin, which is the best way to keep sores from starting.

shift position in order to reduce pressure on that part of your body.

Check early, check often. You or a caregiver should check for pressure ulcers at least once a day. If you're doing it yourself, use a small mirror to check thoroughly. Common trouble spots include the spine (especially below the waist), around the hipbones, or on the heels, knees, ankles, or shoulders. The sores can even form on the back of the head.

Mattress matters. Certain types of mattresses can help lower the risk of pressure ulcers. If you'll be in bed for a long time, replacing your mattress could

be a worthwhile investment. "Research has shown that solid foam and gel cushions can be quite effective at preventing pressure ulcers," says Dr. Lyder. Ask your doctor what type of mattress would be best for you.

Pad your seat. Padding is also important if you spend a lot of time sitting. Again, some pads work a lot better than others. Check with your doctor to see what kind of pad you should use.

The right slant on things. If your bed is adjustable, don't raise the head more than 30 degrees. Lying on too much of a slant can make you slide downward, creating additional pressure than can lead to skin damage. As a rule, it's best to keep your bed flat, only raising the head for short periods of time, such as when you're eating or drinking.

Place pillows strategically. Properly placed pillows can play an important role in preventing pressure ulcers. Use them to keep your knees and ankles from touching each other. It's also helpful to place them under your knees and calves to keep your heels off the bed.

Stay off your hip. When lying on your side, don't lie directly on your hipbone. It's among the main trouble spots for pressure ulcers, so the more you stay off it, the less likely you'll be to develop problems.

Bathe wisely. Regular bathing is important for cleanliness and comfort, but overdoing it may dry your skin and make you more vulnerable to pressure ulcers.

Doctors usually advise patients to bathe only as often as necessary for good hygiene. Warm water is less drying than hot. Be sure to use a mild soap; strong antibacterial soaps can be very drying. To pump extra moisture into your skin, use a soap that contains natural oil such as olive or safflower. Or use a water-based soap that contains a skin-friendly herb such as comfrey or calendula.

Clean and cover. Once a sore forms, it's important to keep

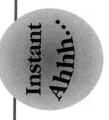

Instant Ahhh...

Witch Away Pain

For an ulcer that's still in the red, painful stage, a little witch hazel can help. This medicine-cabinet staple will cool inflammation and help the sore heal more quickly. Apply a little witch hazel to a cotton ball and dab the sore once or twice a day. You'll feel a moment of pleasant coolness while the witch hazel evaporates, and the pain will usually diminish right away.

it from getting infected. You don't want to add a widespread infection to the other health concerns that are on your mind. Be watchful for any sign that a pressure ulcer is becoming infected. Call your doctor if you notice any pus in or around the sore, if there's a foul odor, or if there's redness, swelling, or warmth around it. If you catch it soon enough, you'll probably be advised to gently wash the area twice a day with mild soap and water and to keep it bandaged.

Stay hydrated. Dry skin can greatly increase your risk of getting pressure ulcers, so it's important to drink plenty of fluids (at least eight full glasses, and maybe more) throughout the day, says Dr. Lyder. In addition, apply a skin moisturizer to ulcer-prone areas of your body.

Heat it up, cool it down. Alternating hot and cold compresses, a technique called contrast hydrotherapy, can help heal and soothe pressure ulcers, says Lisa Arnold, N.D., a naturopathic physician in Orleans, Massachusetts.

Soak a washcloth in hot water, wring it out, and drape it over the affected area. Leave it in place for 3 minutes, then replace it with a cold, damp cloth for 30 seconds. Repeat the cycle three times, ending with the cold. "It helps move blood through the area," Dr. Arnold explains.

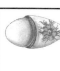

Fishy Skin Protector

Proper nutrition is the first step in building strong skin. Doctors often advise bedridden patients to eat fish at least once or twice a week. Cold-water fish, such as salmon and mackerel, are especially good because they contain the highest levels of omega-3 fatty acids, nutrients that go a long way toward keeping skin strong, supple, and better able to resist injuries. If you're not a fish lover, you can get plenty of omega-3s by having a tablespoon of ground flaxseed a few times a week. You can add it to hot or cold cereal, smoothies, yogurt, or salads.

Rash

Rush Away Redness

I don't use the word *hypochondriac* very often, because I really believe that everyone's opinions about their own health should be taken seriously. After all, who's in a better position to judge than the person who's suffering?

A friend of mine, however, whose name I'll withhold, comes close to making me use the H-word on occasion. He's always getting a strange rash on the top of his head, which he attributes to some obscure disease that he suspects he picked up as a child. I've often tried to persuade him that the rash is probably caused by stress, since it seems to erupt only when he's working late hours at his office. But he's not convinced.

That's not to imply that stress is the only cause of rashes, of course. There are probably hundreds of potential culprits—and the best treatments for you will depend on what's causing the rash in the first place.

Marigold Magic

Marigold blossoms are skin-friendly botanicals that are great for stopping a rash in its tracks. The next time a rash rears its ugly head, dab on some marigold oil with a cotton swab or clean cloth. Keep applying the oil, available at health food stores, until the rash is gone.

Know your ABCD's

You should always check with your doctor when you discover a new, unexplained blemish on your skin. It's probably a rash (or maybe a mole), but it could also be skin cancer. It doesn't pay to take chances.

Your suspicion level should be even higher if the "rash" displays any of the following characteristics, known as the ABCD's.

Asymmetry. In other words, the two halves aren't the same size.

Border irregularity. The blemish has a jagged, notched, or irregular edge.

Color variegation. It's not a solid color.

Diameter. It's more than 6 millimeters in diameter.

"Cancer is the biggest concern when these things happen, so don't wait," says Darrell Misak, N.D. "Get it checked."

TAKE RASH ACTION

Some rashes are just reddened skin. Others burn or sting. Still others are maddeningly itchy. It all depends on what's behind the rash and how your skin reacts to it.

If you keep getting rashes and you don't know why, you obviously need to see a doctor. Once you determine what's making you break out, you can take steps to avoid it. If that's not possible, your doctor may advise you to take antihistamines or use topical steroids to control the symptoms. In the meantime, here are a few ways to defend yourself.

Take notes. A recurring rash has so many possible causes that it may take careful observation to get to the root of it. "Almost every chronic condition or disease has some kind of rash associated with it," says Darrell Misak, N.D., a naturopathic physician in Mt. Lebanon, Pennsylvania.

Ask and answer as many questions about the rash as you

can. Has it been there a long time, or did it just appear? Is it a reaction to something that touched your skin? Were there any recent changes in your diet, clothing, or environment that preceded it?

"The answers to these kinds of questions determine the best way to respond," says Dr. Misak.

Keep a diet diary. "Food sensitivity is a big issue with rashes," says Dr. Misak. A recurring or chronic rash could be triggered by something in your diet—dairy foods, wheat, corn, or citrus fruits, for example. Keeping a record of everything you eat over the course of several weeks and noting when the rash occurs and subsides may flush out the cause—or at least narrow the pool of suspects.

"Remember, a rash can appear 24 to 72 hours after you eat the problem food," Dr. Misak adds.

Hydrotherapy helps. This is just a fancy way of saying that you may want to use warm or cool compresses to get relief. If you have a rash that feels warm to the touch, for example, you may want to soak a small towel in cool water, and drape it over the area to relieve the discomfort. If your rash feels dry and itchy, a warm compress may be more effective.

HOT
COLD

Instant Ahhh...

Soak in Oats

An almost-instant way to ease a dry, itchy rash is to treat it to an oatmeal bath. You can buy a colloidal oatmeal kit at most drugstores. Add the finely ground oatmeal to warm (not hot) water, then settle in for a soothing soak. You can also fill an old sock with plain dry oatmeal, then fasten the open end to the faucet with a rubber band. Fill the tub with warm water, letting the water run through the sock. (You can let the oatmeal bundle float in the bathtub when you're done filling it.) Oatmeal makes water soft and soothing—perfect for a painful rash.

The Solid-Gold Solution

Rashes often occur in areas where jewelry touches your skin—on your earlobes or wrist, for example. The reason is that the metal nickel is often used in jewelry, and it's a very common cause of rashy allergies.

The best (if not the cheapest) alternative to giving up jewelry is to avoid metal mixtures or alloys. Buy jewelry made from sterling silver or gold (18 karat or higher). These metals are unlikely to trigger skin reactions.

Lighten your load. Sometimes, a rash appears because your body's overloaded with stress or pain-causing waste products. One of the best things you can do is take some time to relax and get the stress out of your life. Start by taking an hour a day to just play. Go to the zoo, head for the pool, or dig in the dirt. That may be enough to make the rash go away.

Choose cosmetics carefully. Any type of makeup, perfume, lotion, or skin-care treatment that you smear on your skin is a possible rash-in-a-bottle. Choose products with no fillers, dyes, or added colors and those labeled hypoallergenic.

Beat the heat, lose the ooze. Prickly heat, a rash that pops up when hot, humid weather clogs up your sweat glands, responds well to the acidity in vinegar. For quick relief, add a teaspoon of apple cider vinegar to a cup of water and sponge the solution over the affected area.

If you have a wet, oozing rash, use this herbal combo: Mix equal parts of slippery elm and goldenseal powder (both available at health food stores). Wash and dry the affected skin, then dust it with the powder mixture to keep it dry and infection-free. If the rash doesn't clear up in two to three days or develops redness, heat, or yellow or green pus, contact your doctor right away.

Shingles

Flush Out the Hidden Virus

I'm grateful that I never got chickenpox when I was a kid. I never was very good at lounging around in bed, for one thing, and the idea of being covered with ugly, itchy red bumps for a few weeks makes me shudder even now. But mostly, I thank my lucky stars that I was spared because of what can happen after you have chickenpox: The virus that causes it doesn't necessarily disappear when you recover. It just goes into hiding. Sooner or later, it may reappear and cause a painful, blistering disease known as shingles.

BACK TO THE SCENE OF THE CRIME

If you've had chickenpox, there's about a 40 percent chance that you'll eventually have an attack of shingles. The virus that causes the original infection isn't completely destroyed by your immune system. Instead, it slips deep into

Pink Protection

It's been on drugstore shelves almost forever, and with good reason. Calamine lotion, best known for its vivid pink hue, can ease the itch of shingles and reduce pain as well. Apply the lotion after a shower or bath and several more times during the day.

the nerves and remains there in a dormant state. In some people, it stays dormant; in others, it wakes up, climbs up the nerves to the skin, and causes a painful, blistery outbreak. The sores usually appear in a band across the torso or buttocks and sometimes on the face.

When you first come down with shingles, you may have a fever or other flu-like symptoms. In most cases, you'll be completely recovered in a week or two, and you can consider yourself cured once all the blisters have healed. If you're over age 50, however, there's a good chance that nerve damage caused by the virus will cause lingering pain known as postherpetic neuralgia.

TAKE RASH ACTION

Shingles can be extremely painful, so it's worth getting in to see your doctor right away. You may need painkillers or other medications to tide you over. In addition, there are drugs that can shorten the duration of attacks if they're given within 24 hours of blistering.

The good news is that shin-

Soothing Salves

BATTLE BLISTERS WITH CALENDULA

Calendula is one of nature's most potent blister fighters, which is important when you've had a painful shingles outbreak, says Priscilla Natanson, N.D.

She advises applying calendula cream to the blisters. It's available ready-made in health food stores, or you can make your own healing remedy by crumbling dried calendula and adding enough water to form a thick paste. Apply it to the blisters and leave it on until the paste dries, then wash it off. You can repeat the treatment two or three times a day until you're better.

To make calendula even more healing, mix a few drops of St. John's wort oil into the paste or simply add 6 to 12 drops of the oil to an ounce of olive oil. Apply it to the blisters once or twice a day.

gles isn't dangerous in most cases, and it does clear up on its own. To reduce discomfort in the meantime, take the following tips to heart.

Suck down vitamin C. When you're battling the shingles virus, extra vitamin C is helpful as long as you don't have kidney or tummy troubles. "Vitamin C is a great immune booster," says Priscilla Natanson, N.D., a naturopathic physician in Plantation, Florida. Check with your doctor about the amount that's right for you.

Go ACE to Z. A potent nutritional combo that will strengthen your immune system and help the blisters heal more quickly includes vitamins A, C, and E, plus the mineral zinc. Look for a supplement that contains each of these important nutrients and follow the directions on the label.

Echinacea is excellent. It's one of the most powerful herbs for strengthening the immune system, and it will gear up your defenses to fend off the virus. Echinacea is more effective in the early stages, so start taking it as soon as you notice symptoms. It's available in capsule form at health food stores and drugstores; follow the directions on the label.

Ditch the itch. Don't let the name fool you: The herb chickweed is no mere weed. "It's a wonderful anti-itch herb," says Dr. Natanson. You

---

Immune-Boosting Veggies

Fresh vegetables, either raw or cooked in soups or other recipes, provide powerful protection when shingles strikes. All vegetables are rich in immune-boosting chemical compounds that can help your body fight back.

"Broths and juices are full of nutrients that are easy for your body to assimilate," adds Priscilla Natanson, N.D. Vegetable soup, minestrone, and chicken soup are good choices because of the variety of ingredients they include. Fresh, homemade soup is best, but canned or jarred soups are helpful, too. So eat up!

can buy creams or salves made with chickweed at health food stores.

Hit the showers. Alternating cold and hot water when you shower will strengthen your immune system by stimulating blood flow, improving the flow of healing nutrients, and flushing away harmful chemicals, says Dr. Natanson.

Start with your usual warm-to-hot shower. When you're almost finished, crank it up a little hotter than usual, then turn around a few times so your blisters get a good dousing. Then lower the temperature so the water is a little on the cool side. Let it run for a minute or so, then step out and towel off.

If you use this technique at the first sign of symptoms, there's a good chance that you'll get better a little more quickly, says Dr. Natanson.

Soak in cereal. A warm bath spiked with a cup of colloidal oatmeal can help keep itchy shingles from driving you crazy. You can buy colloidal oatmeal at most drugstores and supermarkets. Or fill a sock with regular dry oatmeal, fasten the sock to the faucet with a rubber band, and let the water run through it. If you don't have oatmeal, add a cup of baking soda to the water.

A Cup of Comfort

Hot tea made with rose hips not only tastes good, it's good for you when you have shingles. "It's high in vitamin C," explains Priscilla Natanson, N.D. Plus, taking the time to enjoy a cup of tea will help you relax and maintain optimal immunity. Drop a teaspoon of dried herb into a cup of freshly boiled water. Steep for about 15 minutes, then remove the bag or strain out the herbs and enjoy your tea.

Baby those blisters. Shingles blisters are a lot more painful than the kind you get from too much hiking or working in the yard. They can be so sensitive, in fact, that even the pressure from heavy clothes can be agonizing. Until they're gone, get in the habit of wearing loose, light clothing.

Keep friends and family safe. Shingles blisters are packed with live viruses that can potentially cause chickenpox in people who haven't had it. Don't let anyone touch the blisters, and take the time to clean them every day with soap and water.

St. John's wort works. As long as you're not taking antidepressants, the oral form of St. John's wort, available in health food stores and drugstores, is helpful for post-shingles pain. Take 300 milligrams three times daily. Be sure to tell your doctor you're taking it if you're thinking of using antidepressant medications. Taking both may be harmful.

Instant Ahhh...

Ease It with Ice

A fast way to reduce the itching and pain of shingles is to wrap a few ice cubes in a washcloth or small towel and hold them against the tender spots. Ice acts as a local anesthetic by temporarily numbing the skin, explains Priscilla Natanson, N.D.

If you have trouble keeping the ice pack in place, make a cold "slush pack" that conforms to the shape of your body. Mix 1 part rubbing alcohol with 4 parts water, fill a few plastic zipper-lock bags with the mixture, and put them in the freezer. After they're chilled, take one out to use on your shingles. When that bag warms up, put it back in the freezer and replace it with a cold one.

Splinters

Get Rid of Painful Skin Spikes

I dreaded getting splinters as a kid. The splinters themselves weren't so bad, but the whole torturous process of getting them out was agony. My mom had studied to be a nurse, so she treated a splinter as an occasion for major surgery.

First, she insisted on washing her hands, my hands, and the whole neighborhood's hands, if possible. Then she took a thin needle and held it over a match to sterilize it. That was a long 10 seconds as I watched that needle turn glowing red, knowing it was about to be used on my tender finger.

Finally, after giving the needle a quick wave to cool it off, she expertly slipped the offending sliver out of its hole. I can't say exactly how she did it, because I always looked away

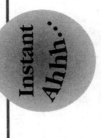

Instant Ahhh...

Soak Away Pain

The skin where a splinter was embedded hurts the most right after the sliver's been removed. For quick relief, soak the area in warm water for 10 to 15 minutes.. You can also use warm soaks to help propel difficult-to-remove splinters to the skin surface.

at that point. Then it was on with a bandage, and I was free to wander off to my next splinter encounter.

AN UNPLEASANT POINT

How can a tiny piece of wood be so dang painful? It's because your fingertips, the usual places that you get splinters, are filled with sensitive nerve endings. That's what makes your fingers so deft at knitting or putting puzzles together, but it's also what makes them sting like the dickens when a sliver of wood gets under your skin.

SPLIT, SPLINTER!

As moms have always known, splinters aren't exactly a medical emergency. Unless the area is badly infected or the splinter is lodged under a nail or somewhere else where you can't get at it, there's no reason to call a doctor.

The truth is, you can remove most splinters in the time it takes to read this chapter. But read it anyway, just to be sure that you get the nasty thing out—or not, in some cases—with a minimum of discomfort.

Leave it alone. If the splinter is lodged close to the surface of the skin, and the area isn't bleeding or painful, it's okay to

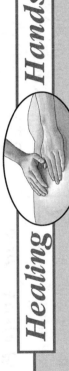

Healing Hands

If the pain of a splinter is driving you nuts, but you can't find a way to remove it right away, simply press or rub the skin close to the sliver, advises Sean Sapunar, N.D., a naturopathic physician and clinical faculty member at the Bastyr Center for Natural Health near Seattle. "The pressure signals travel faster than pain signals," he explains. "They get to the brain first and get all the attention, so you feel less pain."

ignore it, says Lisa Arnold, N.D., a naturopathic physician in Orleans, Massachusetts.

"Your body will generally work it out of there on its own," she says. Just keep an eye on it to be sure it isn't digging deeper into the skin or getting infected.

Tweeze it out. I described my childhood memories of splinter-ectomies to Dr. Arnold, hoping to get a little sympathy, but she simply said, "I do the pretty much same thing." Darn!

She recommends using tweez-ers rather than a needle to root out a splinter, though. Wash the area around the splinter with soap and water, sterilize the tweezers with rubbing alcohol, then grip and pull.

Here's a helpful piece of advice I didn't know: If you can, pull the splinter out of the hole at the same angle that it went in. This will reduce the chances that it will break off in the skin.

Pull it with plantain. If you don't feel up to splinter surgery, an herbal poultice can do all the work for you. Plantain is one of the best herbs to use. "It will actually draw the splinter out of the skin," says Dr. Arnold.

You can buy fresh or dried leaves at many health food stores. Chop or grind the herb and add enough water to make a paste, then slather it over the splinter. Cover it with a band-

$oothing $alves

SUPER SKIN HEALER

As soon as you say the word *skin*, herb experts start thinking "calendula." "It's a fan-tastic skin-healing herb, no mat-ter what the situation is," says Lisa Arnold, N.D.

You can buy calendula cream at health food stores. After washing the area, apply a little of the cream. Keep using it until the wound is completely healed. You can also whip up your own calendula cure by adding 6 to 12 drops of calen-dula oil to about an ounce of almond or olive oil. Apply it to the area, and cover with an adhesive or gauze bandage. Keep it in place for at least 20 minutes.

age and replace the poultice daily until the splinter comes out.

Wash and watch. Once the splinter's been removed, be sure to keep the skin around the injury clean. Wash gently with soap and water once or twice a day and cover the area with a bandage if it's likely to get dirty. Check the site of the injury for signs of infection—redness, pus, swelling, and so on. You can treat a minor infection with some triple antibiotic ointment, but see a doctor if it doesn't clear up in a day or two.

Bathe away the pain. To promote healing and ease the sting of splinters, try this triple herbal wash. Mix equal parts of the dried herbs calendula, echinacea, and comfrey, available at health food stores. Add a heaping tablespoon of the mixture to a pint of freshly boiled water and steep for 20 minutes. Strain the liquid, let it cool, and use it to wash the area thoroughly.

Consider a tetanus offensive. Had a tetanus shot lately? Probably not. Do you need one? Probably, says Laura Pimentel, M.D., chair of emergency medicine at Mercy Medical Center in Baltimore.

"Any sort of break in the skin could be an entrance for tetanus," she says. The tetanus germ can cause painful and potentially fatal muscle spasms, and it tends to live on wood or rusted metal. If you haven't had a tetanus shot in the past 10 years, you're probably due, she says.

Dab on St. John's wort. Available in health food stores as a cream or a tincture, this herb helps fight bacteria and eases the pain of splinters. Apply it to the area once or twice a day.

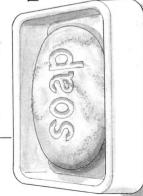

Sunburn

Terrific Tips to Cool Down

It happened on the last day of a three-day weekend at the shore. I must have slacked off on the sunscreen, and I paid dearly for it. In the few hours it took to drive home, what started as vague soreness on my reddened chest quickly escalated to painful stinging and horrible itching. I knew I had to do something fast, but I wasn't sure I would find an open drugstore if I got off the highway.

Then I remembered that there were a few bottles of water left in my cooler. I soaked my T-shirt in the cool water and pressed it against my chest. The sunburn still hurt, but at least I wasn't having fleeting thoughts of crashing into a bridge abutment just to end the pain.

When I got home, I went straight to a drugstore and bought some aloe lotion. It brought the pain down to a comfortable level, but I learned later that I really hadn't needed it. I had all

Antioxidant Rx

To help your skin heal, eat five or six servings of antioxidant-rich foods daily. Berries of any kind are tops, followed by citrus fruits, mango, papaya, dark leafy greens, broccoli, brussels sprouts, nuts and seeds, whole grains, and legumes.

the necessary remedies at home, and any one of them would have been the ticket to a pain-free night.

NOW YOU'RE COOKIN'

The source of sunburn is no big mystery. What you may not know is that it's not the rays you can see that do the damage, but the invisible ultraviolet rays. They pack so much energy that even brief exposure causes your skin to darken. The darkening is a handy mechanism to shield the delicate tissues underneath, but it provides only so much protection. With too much exposure to these rays, surface layers of your skin can burn painfully.

TURN DOWN THE HEAT

If you've been severely burned, you may need prescription ointments to minimize the damage and perhaps painkillers to help you cope. Most sunburns aren't this serious, of course, at least in the short run. The long-term story is a little different, because too much sun exposure and repeated burns greatly increase your risk of

skin cancer. But we all make mistakes now and then. If you happen to get burned despite your best efforts, here's what you need to do.

Crack the medicine chest. You'll probably find some

Soothing Salves

MARIGOLD MAGIC

Calendula is one of the best remedies for sunburn, but what if there isn't a health food store in your neighborhood? You can make your own calendula oil from marigolds, says Heidi Weinhold, N.D. Cut off the flowers and hang them to dry. Remove the dried petals, put them in a jar, and add enough olive oil to cover. Seal the jar and put it in a dark place, but take it out and shake it every day for two weeks. Then strain out the petals and store the oil in a tightly covered jar in the refrigerator. The next time you get a sunburn, you'll have a very cool remedy all ready to go.

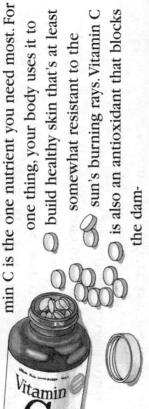

aspirin, ibuprofen, or other pain reliever. The drugs won't help the burn heal, but they're very effective at reducing pain while nature takes its course.

Play it cool. Cool water is a refreshing treat for sunburned skin. As soon as you can, soak a washcloth, wring it out, and apply it to the burned area, or simply lounge in a cool bath or shower. Apart from providing nearly instant relief, cool water helps hydrate the skin and prevents it from drying out.

Tank up on vitamin C. If you're a sun worshiper, vitamin C is the one nutrient you need most. For one thing, your body uses it to build healthy skin that's at least somewhat resistant to the sun's burning rays. Vitamin C is also an antioxidant that blocks the damaging effects of free radicals, harmful oxygen molecules that are produced in profusion when the sun's burning rays toast the skin. Finally, vitamin C helps repair sunburn damage.

As long as you don't have stomach or kidney problems, you should already be taking supplemental vitamin C every day. The Daily Value is 60 milligrams, which is enough under normal circumstances, but not if you've gotten burned. Then you'll need a lot more—your doctor can tell you exactly how much. If you want to avoid possible diarrhea or stomach upset, don't take it all at

It's an Emergency!

Most sunburns are only minor annoyances, but sometimes they're severe enough to require emergency care. If your skin blisters or develops open sores, or you feel dizzy or nauseated, go to a doctor immediately. Severe sunburn can also cause chills or fever, which are early signs that you may be going into shock.

Sunburn Savvy

Did you get burned even though you slathered on sunscreen? It's possible that you used the wrong product. Most sunscreens protect against UVA and UVB, the sun's two types of burning rays, but they don't necessarily give all the protection that you need, says Min-Wei Lee, M.D., a dermatologic surgeon and director of East Bay Laser and Skin Care Center in Walnut Creek, California. Here's what to look for when you buy sunscreen.

- Buy only products that contain zinc oxide or Parsol 1789 (also called avobenzone). They provide optimal protection against both types of rays.
  - Choose a sunscreen with a sun protection factor (SPF) of 30 or higher.
  - Use a waterproof brand if you'll be swimming or you perspire heavily.
  - Reapply sunscreen every 2 hours, no matter what it says on the label.

once. Divide the total amount into smaller doses and take them throughout the day (for example, 500 milligrams in the morning and another 500 milligrams later). It will also be less likely to upset your stomach if you take it with food.

Have a sun-E day. Another sun lover's nutrient is vitamin E. Like vitamin C, it's a protective antioxidant that helps prevent, or at least minimize, skin damage. Take 800 IU daily when you're nursing a sunburn. You can also use vitamin E cream or oil. When you apply it to the burned areas, they'll heal more quickly, and you'll be less likely to have permanent scars.

Make moisturizer magic. Moisturizers pump healing fluids back into the skin and create a temporary cooling sensation, says Richard Wagner, M.D., professor of dermatology at the University of Texas Medical Branch in Galveston. "Make sure it's fragrance-free, or your skin may be irritated by an allergic reaction," he says. "That would make the sunburn worse."

Shun soap. For the first day or two after getting burned, don't use soap on the painful areas. It dries the skin and can make the pain worse. Of course, you may have to use soap if the area is dirtier than usual. Better to have a little irritation than to risk infection.

Drink like a sponge. Sunburns remove part of your body's natural moisture barrier, so you'll need to drink plenty of water to compensate. "It helps to offset fluid loss," says Dr. Wagner. Drinking water also helps your body repair the burn and keeps your immune system in good shape to repel any bacteria that invade through the damaged skin. Drink as much water as you can hold—anywhere from four to eight glasses a day, depending on your size and how active you are.

Wallow in aloe. I suspect that the aloe plant was put on Earth just to help heal sunburned skin. Aloe thrives in any container, in any room, in any part of the country. If you get burned, break off a leaf, squeeze out the gel, and apply a generous amount. You can also slit a leaf lengthwise and tape the open area against your skin, says Heidi Weinhold, N.D., a naturopathic physician in the Pittsburgh area.

Cure it with calendula. Herbalists are quick to sing the praises of calendula when it comes to repairing damaged skin. "It's wonderful for sunburn," says Dr. Weinhold. At health food stores, look for it in succus form; it's the juice of the herb mixed with water. Apply it to the burn and cover it with a light bandage or gauze. "You can reapply it a few times a day," she says.

Pain **Anywhere**
(And Sometimes Everywhere!)

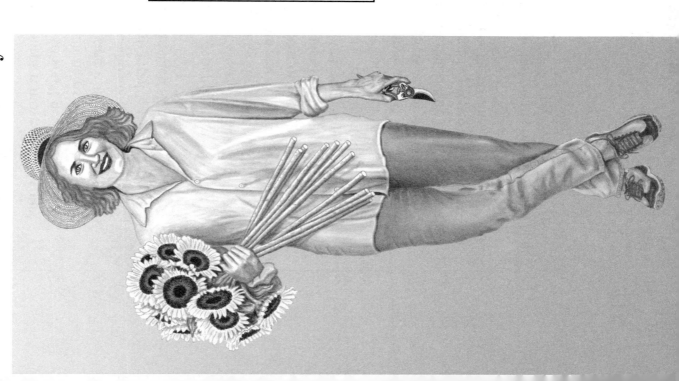

- Arthritis
- Bursitis and Tendinitis
- Cancer Pain
- Fibromyalgia
- Flu
- Lyme Disease
- Muscle Cramp
- Muscle Soreness
- Post-Amputation Pain
- Postoperative Pain
- Raynaud's Syndrome

Arthritis

Ease the Aches

Not long ago, a study from the Centers for Disease Control and Prevention reported that about one in three of us suffers from arthritis. One in three! I have to admit that I was shocked.

Yet there's plenty of good news on the arthritis front. For one thing, most people who get it will have a relatively minor form. In addition, doctors are discovering new treatments all the time—and I'm not necessarily talking about revolutionary new drugs or procedures. As it turns out, some of the most effective treatments for arthritis are the same ones used by your parents and grandparents.

INFLAMMATION AND PAIN

There are many, many kinds of arthritis, but the two you hear most about are osteoarthritis and rheumatoid arthritis. Osteoarthritis is by far the most common form. Also called

---

Soothing Salves

QUICK RELIEF

Boswellia oil can quickly relieve arthritis pain, says Grace Ornstein, M.D. "Massage it on painful areas," she says. You can find the oil at health food stores.

wear-and-tear arthritis, it's caused by the wearing down of the protective surfaces of the joints. Without the proper padding in the joint, moving it results in painful inflammation. Sometimes it hurts a lot, and sometimes it doesn't hurt at all, but the underlying problem never goes away entirely.

Rheumatoid arthritis is potentially much more serious. For reasons that still aren't clear, the body's immune system attacks and damages the joints. People who have rheumatoid arthritis may also experience occasional fever, fatigue, and other symptoms.

JOINT EFFORTS

Whether you have osteoarthritis, rheumatoid arthritis, or some other type, keep in mind that it's an ongoing problem that always requires a doctor's care. The sooner you get help (treatments range from prescription pain relievers to medicines that "tame" the immune system), the less likely you'll be to have long-term, potentially serious joint damage.

Incidentally, keep your doctor in the loop if you're using over-the-counter drugs to treat arthritis symptoms. Aspirin, ibuprofen, and other nonprescription products are pretty safe for most people, but they can cause all sorts of problems if you take large amounts every day.

Drugs are certainly an important part of a joint-protecting

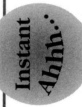

Instant Ahhh...

Pepper the Pain

A quick way to ease arthritis pain is to apply a topical cream that contains capsaicin, the hot chemical compound that's found in red pepper. "You get local numbing of nerve endings along with a warming effect," says Kevin R. Stone, M.D. Most drugstores carry the cream; brands include Zostrix and Dolorac. It comes in concentrations from 0.025 to 0.075; if you have sensitive skin, try a lower strength first. Follow the label directions for use.

strategy, but they're far from your only choice. As it turns out, there are many home treatments that are surprisingly effective. Here are the best ones that doctors recommend.

Cool a hot joint. When an arthritic joint is inflamed—it may be painful, swollen, or even feel hot—put some ice on the fire. "Ice is very good for inflammation and swelling," says James Herndon, M.D., chair of the department of orthopedic surgery at Brigham and Women's Hospital in Boston. He recommends putting an ice pack on the sore joint for about 20 minutes at a time. Repeat the treatment once an hour and continue for as long as it seems to help.

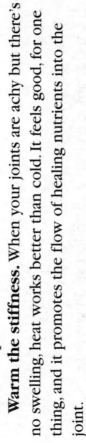

Warm the stiffness. When your joints are achy but there's no swelling, heat works better than cold. It feels good, for one thing, and it promotes the flow of healing nutrients into the joint.

Moist heat seems to work best, so you may want to use a warm compress instead of a heating pad. Soak a small towel in hot water, wring it out, and drape it over your painful joint. When the towel cools, soak it again and reapply it.

"I've found that patients with chronic arthritis like heat better than ice," Dr. Herndon says. Heat feels so good, in fact, that he routinely advises people who wake up stiff and achy to start the day with a soothing hot bath or shower.

Indian herbs help. Guggul, boswellia, gokshura, and madder are commonly used in India to relieve joint pain, and there's good evidence that they work, says Grace Ornstein, M.D., medical director and scientific advisor for Himalaya USA, a marketer of herbal formulas based in Houston. "They all have anti-inflammatory properties," she says.

These and other anti-inflammatory herbs are available in supplement form in health food stores. Follow the directions

Movement Matters

Exercise is a tricky issue if you have arthritis. You obviously don't want to push yourself too hard when you're hurting. On the other hand, regular exercise lubricates your joints and helps with weight loss. "I've had patients who lost as little as 10 pounds and experienced almost total relief from pain," says James Herndon, M.D.

If you're ready to start an exercise program—and you have the go-ahead from your doctor—keep the following points in mind.

• You'll get the most benefit by alternating high-impact forms of exercise, such as jogging, with low-impact workouts, such as yoga or cycling. Obviously this is true only if your arthritis is pretty mild.

• Walking is almost always a good choice. If you have too much knee or ankle pain to walk, ride a stationary bike. "Set the seat high so you don't have to bend your knees as much," Dr. Herndon says.

• Swimming is a very safe, very effective form of exercise. And because water supports your body weight, there's little or no painful pressure. The effect of gravity on the joints is eliminated.

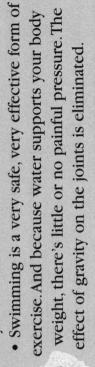

on the label, and be sure to let your doctor know you're taking them.

Lick it with licorice. The herb licorice root is a friend indeed when your arthritis flares up, because it can counteract the inflammation. "It's a wonderful herb," says Dr. Ornstein.

Licorice root is available in capsule form at health food stores. (Don't bother with licorice candy: which contains little or no real licorice.) Since a substance in licorice called glycyrrhizic acid can cause high blood pressure in some people, look for deglycyrrhizinated licorice (DGL) products, then follow the label directions.

To make licorice tea, mix about a teaspoon of dried licorice in a cup of hot water, steep for 5 to 10 minutes, let cool, and enjoy. If you have high blood pressure or other health problems, don't drink it every day without talking to your doctor first.

Spice up your menu. The herb turmeric is aromatic, spicy, and a great inflammation fighter, says Dr. Ornstein. You can add it to rice, stews, and meat dishes. Or you can take turmeric capsules, which are available in health food stores.

Rebuild with glucosamine. There's some evidence that supplements that contain glucosamine may help your body replenish joint cartilage that's been damaged by arthritis. Doctors usually recommend taking 1,500 milligrams daily, divided into two or three doses. Some people report significant improvement after just six weeks.

Try joint juice. The liquid form of glucosamine appears to work better than the pill form, says Kevin R. Stone, M.D., chair of the Stone Foundation for Sports Medicine and Arthritis Research in San Francisco. "With a pill, the absorption is vari-

A Cup of Comfort

It's unlikely that the Gingerbread Man ever had arthritis. I know, he was just a cookie, and a fictional one at that. But all of that ginger must have helped. Ginger is a powerful anti-inflammatory herb that can take the edge off arthritis pain, says Grace Ornstein, M.D. To make a healing tea, grate about an inch of fresh ginger and steep it in hot water for 10 minutes, then strain. Drink it once or twice a day.

able, but with the liquid form, you get all of the medication at once," he explains. So drink up!

Drink plenty of water. Like most people, you probably don't drink enough water, and that could be making your arthritis symptoms worse.

"If your joints are well hydrated, they tend to be less stiff in the morning, which is when the pain is usually the worst," says Dr. Stone.

He advises drinking at least eight full glasses of water every day—and don't wait until you're thirsty. By the time you feel thirsty, your body's water levels have already dropped too low.

Work out, heat up. If your joint pain tends to flare after you exercise, a heat treatment can help. Apply a heating pad set on low or a hot, moist towel to aching joints after your workouts. "I recommend it after exercise to cut down swelling and pain," Dr. Herndon says.

Experiment with drugs. What's the best pill to reach for when you need relief? There's no clear answer, Dr. Herndon says. "I have my favorites, starting with ibuprofen, then aspirin." Other people may do better with naproxen. You'll just have to try different painkillers until you find the one that works best for you. If you're going beyond the guidelines on the label or you have any chronic health problems besides arthritis, consult your doctor first.

Bursitis and Tendinitis

Join the Joint-Relief Team

Bursitis and tendinitis are completely different problems, but it makes sense to discuss them together because the symptoms—and the treatments—are almost always identical.

When it comes to pain, both can really put you out of commission for a while, but strangely, the pain isn't always due to obvious injuries. Even simple daily activity can trigger flare-ups.

A while ago, I talked to Phoebe Yin, N.D., a naturopathic physician and faculty member at Bastyr University near Seattle. She told me about a patient who regularly had flare-ups of bursitis, which she attributed to a bad fall years before. It turned out, though, that the pain was caused by washing dishes at the restaurant where she worked. "The sink was too high for her, so she was always holding her arms at a 45-degree angle," Dr. Yin told me. "That was putting pressure on her shoulder joints."

THE JOINT'S ON FIRE

Tendinitis and bursitis are both caused by inflammation in a joint that's been overworked. In the case of bursitis, the inflammation occurs in small, fluid-filled sacs called bursae that help your joints move smoothly. With tendinitis, what gets inflamed is a tendon, which connects muscles to bones. The pain is typically an aching, throbbing, or burning sensation around the joint. You'll probably notice swelling as well.

Although bursitis and tendinitis can affect just about any joint, it's usually the knees, elbows, shoulders, and hips that suffer the most.

PUT OUT THE FLAMES

Tendinitis and bursitis are rarely serious, and they invariably clear up on their own. Obviously, any joint pain that's severe or lasts more than a week has to be checked out by a doctor. It's always possible that there's damaged tissue or bone that won't get better without medical treatment. Nevertheless, it's fine to use home treatments for a few days to see if the problem goes away. Here are the main strategies that doctors recommend.

Turn down the heat. If your joint feels hot and swollen, the first thing you should do is get some ice on it. Applying cold constricts blood vessels and reduces the flow of fluid and inflammatory chemicals to the painful area.

Apply a cold pack or ice cubes

---

soothing Salves

COUNT ON CHICKWEED

The herbs chickweed and comfrey make a potent two-pronged attack against joint aches. If you have access to fresh herbs, get a handful of chickweed and a few large comfrey leaves, then blanch them by dipping them in boiling water for a few seconds. Layer the chickweed over your painful joint, then cover with the comfrey. You can also buy dried herbs at a health food store to make a paste. Chop the herbs, mix them in equal portions, and add enough water to form a paste. Use a bandage to hold the leaves or dried herbs in place if you need to, and leave them on for about 20 minutes. Repeat the treatment two or three times a day until you're feeling better.

---

wrapped in a small towel or a washcloth to the area for about 20 minutes. Repeat the treatment every hour or two until the pain goes away.

Elevate the area. You can't always do this, but whenever possible, raise the area that hurts higher than the level of your heart. Gravity will help pull out fluids and reduce swelling.

Wrap it up. Snugly wrapping the injured area with an elastic bandage will also reduce swelling. Don't make the bandage so tight that it cuts off circulation, though. If you can just barely slip a finger under the edge, it's tight enough.

Warm the ache. Pain that lingers after a day or two often responds well to a heat treatment. Soak a small towel in hot water, wring it out, and place it on the area that's hurting. Or you can use a heating pad set on low.

Run hot and cold. This traditional healing method uses alternating hot and cold treatments to improve circulation in an injured part of your body. It brings in more nutrients while flushing out toxins and waste products, says Dr. Yin.

First, soak a small towel in hot water, wring it out, and

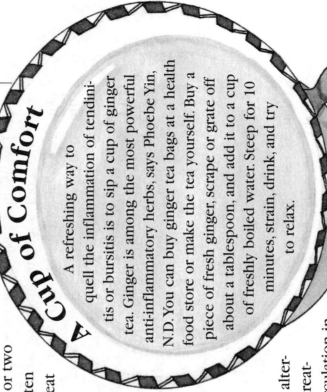

A Cup of Comfort

A refreshing way to quell the inflammation of tendinitis or bursitis is to sip a cup of ginger tea. Ginger is among the most powerful anti-inflammatory herbs, says Phoebe Yin, N.D. You can buy ginger tea bags at a health food store or make the tea yourself. Buy a piece of fresh ginger, scrape or grate off about a tablespoon, and add it to a cup of freshly boiled water. Steep for 10 minutes, strain, drink, and try to relax.

apply it to the sore spot for about 3 minutes. Then replace it with a towel that's been soaked in cold water. Repeat the cycle two or three times, always ending with the cold.

Call for castor. A castor oil pack is an old-time pain treatment that's never out of style. Smear some castor oil (available at drugstores, supermarkets, and health food stores) over the area that hurts. Put some plastic wrap on top of the oil, then cover the whole thing with a heating pad set on low.

The heat will push the oil's healing components into the aching joint. Since this is a heat-based treatment, don't use it if you have swelling or inflammation.

Turmeric is terrific. This pungent spice contains chemical compounds that can relieve an inflamed, irritated joint. If you're not a big fan of spicy foods, you can take supplements that contain curcumin, the active ingredient in turmeric. They're available at health food stores; follow the directions on the label.

A berry good cure. All dark berries, including cherries and blueberries, contain chemical compounds called bioflavonoids, which reduce inflammation. Eat about 1/2 cup of berries every day until you're feeling better.

Pop a morning multi. That multivitamin that you take every day with breakfast is especially important when you're coping with bursitis or tendinitis. "There are a lot of nutrients that are important for connective tissue health," says Dr. Yin. A multivitamin will provide them all.

Open the floodgates. "Your joints and bursae have a lot of water in them," says Dr. Yin, "so hydration is very important for joint health." Plan on drinking eight glasses of water throughout the day.

Oil your joints. The essential fatty acids found in fish are

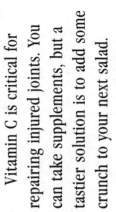

important for good health, especially when your body is coping with inflammation.

Until your joints are better, plan on eating two or three servings of fish a week. The oils will help tame inflammation and help you recover more quickly.

If you're not a fish fan, you can get healthy amounts of these fats by eating ground flaxseed. Every day, add a tablespoon or two of seeds to cereal, smoothies, yogurt, or salads.

Redesign your life. Sometimes, the best way to fight bursitis or tendinitis is to do some creative thinking. Pay close attention to what you do as you go about your daily life. Are repetitive motions putting your arms or legs in awkward or strained positions? Do you spend long periods of time with a knee or elbow pressed against the floor or a chair?

"Things that put pressure on a joint or tendon or restrict blood flow might cause problems down the road," says Dr. Yin. So try to eliminate them from your daily routine.

"C" Relief

Vitamin C is critical for repairing injured joints. You can take supplements, but a tastier solution is to add some crunch to your next salad.

"Green and red peppers are good sources of vitamin C," says Phoebe Yin, N.D. Not a pepper fan? Then load up on oranges—but don't peel them too carefully. "There's a lot of vitamin C in the white part next to the peel," says Dr. Yin.

Cancer Pain

Wipe It Out

This chapter brought back memories of someone I knew whose battle with cancer was inspirational. Marty had been many things in his life: A teacher, an actor, a tireless volunteer for charities and nonprofit groups. But in his heart, I'm convinced, he always wanted to be a comedian. The wit and good nature that he brought to his life's darkest moment were an inspiration to all of us who loved him.

I especially like the story he told after he returned home from cancer surgery. While he was being prepared for the operation, he asked, "What are you doing there?"

"We're shaving your head," a nurse told him.

Marty paused for a second, probably to make sure that the entire surgical staff was listening, then fired back, "But I'm having my gallbladder removed."

Marty never forgot the value of a good joke, despite the pain his illness caused him. The doctors I talked to told me that way too many people with cancer endure needless pain. As it turns out, it's almost always possible to keep the pain at minimal levels, or even eliminate it entirely. But you have to work with your doctors to make sure it happens.

THE ENEMY WITHIN

Entire textbooks have been written about cancer pain, but the causes are pretty basic. Often, it's due to a growing tumor that's pressing against surrounding tissue or nerves. Tumors can also damage tissue, block circulation, or irritate nearby nerves. In addition, cancer pain can be caused by the treatments themselves: surgery, radiation, chemotherapy, and so on.

As I mentioned, in many cases, cancer doesn't have to cause pain. For one thing, the drugs and other approaches to managing pain are getting better all the time. Some types of cancer don't cause pain, and even people who do have pain are unlikely to have it all the time.

COMFORT IS KEY

If you have cancer, don't hesitate to talk to your doctor about your pain. It's not uncommon for people to stay silent because they don't want to bother the doctors, or because they don't want to get addicted to powerful drugs.

Let me put that one to rest right now: Cancer patients who take painkilling drugs are very unlikely to become addicted. Furthermore, your doctors want you to be open and honest about what you're feeling. If you're in a lot of pain, you aren't going to recover as well. That's why most cancer-management teams include a specialist in treating pain.

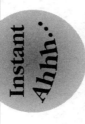

Instant Ahhh...

Busy Mind, Healthy Body

One of the quickest ways to reduce pain from cancer or other illnesses is to keep your mind busy. The more you focus on the pain, the more you're going to hurt, says Tim Birdsall, N.D. That's why aches and pains that you barely notice during the day become troublesome as soon as you try to fall asleep at night. "Having a conversation, playing a board game, going for a walk—any kind of distraction will help," he says.

The Alternative Route

A number of traditional healing herbs appear to be helpful for both treating and preventing cancer, says Tim Birdsall, N.D. You'll want to work with a naturopathic physician before using any herbs, of course, but the following herbs are believed to be particularly useful for coping with cancer. You can find all of them at health food stores.

Curcumin. This is the active chemical compound in the spice turmeric, and it's available in supplement form. "It's been shown to affect several stages of cancer formation and progression," says Dr. Birdsall.

Green tea. Antioxidants and other chemical compounds in green tea can help fight cancer. You'd have to drink about 10 cups of tea a day to get the healing effects, so it usually makes more sense to use green tea capsules, following the label directions.

Maitake, reishi, and coreolis. These gourmet mushrooms are sold at some supermarkets; they're also available in supplement form. "They contain components that stimulate the immune system," says Dr. Birdsall.

There are many different kinds of cancer, and everyone's situation is unique. I don't need to tell you how important it is to talk to your doctor before trying any of the remedies in this chapter, but don't be afraid to mention them. There's a good chance that a combination of these approaches will help you feel a lot better—and give you the strength to battle cancer on every front.

Tell the whole story. It's not enough to merely tell your doctor that you hurt. To get the best relief from pain, you have to be very specific about the kind of pain you have, and where and when you have it. Do you feel fine when you lie still, but have pain when you sit up? Do you have pain when you lie on your left side, but not on your right?

"These are the kinds of details that really help," says Tim Birdsall, N.D., director of naturopathic medicine at Midwestern Regional Medical Center in Zion, Illinois, and coauthor of *How to Prevent and Treat Cancer with Natural Medicine.*

Fight your fear. That's easier said than done, of course, but the fear of discomfort invariably makes actual pain even worse, says Dr. Birdsall. The best remedy for fear is to learn as much about your condition—and its treatments—as you possibly can.

"Once you understand that your doctors will do everything they can to help you get comfortable, you'll be less likely to worry about and anticipate pain," he explains.

Cool down or heat up. You wouldn't think that simple home remedies such as heat and ice would be helpful for cancer pain, but they're surprisingly effective. Each person responds differently to heat and cold, so you'll just have to try both to see which is most effective.

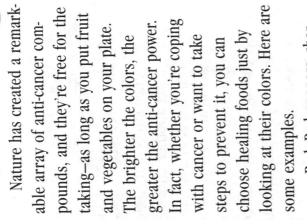

ICE PACK

Anti-Cancer Power

Nature has created a remarkable array of anti-cancer compounds, and they're free for the taking—as long as you put fruit and vegetables on your plate. The brighter the colors, the greater the anti-cancer power. In fact, whether you're coping with cancer or want to take steps to prevent it, you can choose healing foods just by looking at their colors. Here are some examples.

- Red: Red peppers, cherries, grapes, and raspberries.

- Purple: Beets, blackberries, and plums.

- Orange: Apricots, carrots, and squash.

- Dark green: Spinach and broccoli.

For cold treatments, apply an ice pack or ice cubes wrapped in a washcloth or small towel to the painful area. Hold it in place for 20 minutes, then let your skin warm up for 20 minutes. Repeating the treatment once an hour or so will numb nerve endings and help you feel better.

To use heat, cover the area with a heating pad set on low or a towel that's been soaked in hot water. Heat penetrates deeply into the muscles and improves circulation. It's also very soothing and can help reduce stress and anxiety.

Yet another choice is to combine heat and cold. Soak a small towel in hot water, wring it out, and place it on the painful area. Keep it there for 3 minutes, then replace it with a cold cloth for 30 seconds. Repeat the cycle two more times, ending with the cold compress.

Let your mind wander. A quick way to ease pain as well as stress is with a mental technique called visualization. Basically, it involves creating a soothing mental image in as much detail as you can.

Sit in a quiet place, breathe deeply for a few minutes, and fill your mind with an image that's relaxing and soothing: a beautiful garden, for example, or a lovely mountain pass. Put all your senses to work. Imagine the smells, sounds, sights, and so on. This form of meditation has been shown to decrease levels of stress chemicals in your body, which in turn goes a long way toward relieving pain.

Relax from head to toe. Another exercise that reduces pain is progressive relaxation. It involves making an effort to relax every part of your body, starting with your toes and traveling all the way up to the top of your head. "It can be really useful," says Dr. Birdsall.

Again, sit or lie in a quiet place. Close your eyes and focus on your toes. Tense them slightly, then mentally will them to relax completely. Enjoy the feeling of relaxation for a moment, then do the same thing with your ankles, your calves, your thighs, and so on up to your head. It takes only about 20 minutes to relax your entire body, and when you're done, you'll be surprised by how much better you feel.

Keep on moving. It's easy to give up exercise or even simple daily activities when you're sick. But regular exercise is essential for pain relief as well as recovery. Moving your body vigorously increases levels of pain-fighting chemicals called endorphins and reduces levels of chemicals that cause pain.

"Anything involving movement will be beneficial," says Dr. Birdsall. Your doctor will help you design an exercise plan that's right for you. The idea is to do as much as you're comfortable with, keeping in mind that the more you exercise, the more you'll be able to do.

Eat organic. When you're struggling with a major illness, the last thing you need is to weaken your body with pesticides or other chemicals found in conventional foods. Organic foods are best because they allow your body to use more of its energy to reduce levels of toxins produced by the disease or medical treatments, says Dr. Birdsall. "Reducing toxins from other sources makes the body more effective at dealing with the disease," he adds.

Fibromyalgia

Manage This Mysterious Malady

You wake up with so much pain in your body that it hurts to blink. When you call a friend to cancel an appointment, she's sympathetic, but you can tell by her voice that she thinks you're overreacting to some routine muscle soreness. She just doesn't understand how much you hurt!

I've talked to a few people with fibromyalgia, and they told me that the difficulty in getting others to understand what they're going through makes a difficult situation even worse. Even some doctors don't seem to get the picture. In fact, one friend told me that she went to a pain specialist, carefully described her symptoms, and explained what she knew about fibromyalgia. The doctor nodded thoughtfully and said, "Well, we'll do what we can, but personally I don't believe fibromyalgia is real." And this was just months after a major study about fibromyalgia was published in the *New England Journal of Medicine*! Needless to say, my friend found another doctor.

MYSTERY PAIN

Fibromyalgia is a baffling mystery to the experts who study it. What causes it? Your guess is almost as good as theirs. It's possible that fibromyalgia is somehow linked to brain chemicals such as serotonin (linked to depression) and substance P (linked to pain).

What doctors do know is that it can be incredibly painful. Most people with fibromyalgia experience an aching, burning sensation in their muscles. They're usually exhausted all the time, possibly because the pain makes it hard to get a good night's sleep.

BANISH THE HURT

Because fibromyalgia doesn't seem to cause changes in your body that can be detected by x-rays, blood tests, or other diagnostic techniques, the only way your doctor can tell if you have it is to rule out other causes for the pain. If no other problems are detected and you've had widespread aching that's lasted for at least three months—plus a minimum of 11 "tender points" that scream at the slightest pressure—there's a good chance that you have fibromyalgia.

As of now, there is no cure, and there isn't likely to be one until doctors figure out just what causes fibromyalgia. What they have found, however, is that most people can control symptoms with a variety of self-help techniques as well as with prescription medications for pain or sleep problems (in some cases). Just be prepared to be patient: What works for one per-

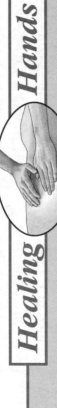

Healing Hands

Many people with fibromyalgia see their massage therapists at least as often as they see their doctors, because massage is an excellent way to reduce discomfort. Just be sure to get a light, gentle massage. Too-vigorous handwork often seems to make the pain worse, says Milton Hammerly, M.D.

STRETCHING

son with fibromyalgia won't work for everyone. You'll probably have to do some experimenting to find what's best for you. Here are a few strategies that experts recommend.

Stretch out. You know how much it hurts when you pull a muscle in your leg, back, or shoulder. The problem isn't so much the initial injury but rather how the muscle responds: It tightens to prevent further damage—and tight muscles are sore muscles. In people with fibromyalgia, their muscles are essentially stuck in a short, contracted position, says Jacob Teitelbaum, M.D., a fibromyalgia researcher in Annapolis, Maryland, and author of *From Fatigued to Fantastic*. One way to ease the pain is to get the muscles to relax by doing regular stretching exercises or simply by staying active.

The idea is to stretch the affected muscles slowly, says Dr. Teitelbaum. When you're going for a walk, for example, take long, slow strides at first. Try to feel a good stretch in all the muscles in your legs. Regular stretching will help "train" the muscles not to contract in painful ways. Just don't stretch too much at once. "If you try to stretch through the pain, the muscle will pull back and make the problem worse," Dr. Teitelbaum warns.

Get plenty of rest. Sleep does more than give you much-needed rest. It also gives your body a chance to repair tiny

A Cup of Comfort

Fibromyalgia is thought to cause painful muscle inflammation. The solution, of course, is to treat it, well, gingerly. A cup of ginger tea contains inflammation-fighting compounds called gingerols—and it tastes good, too! Just steep a few slices of fresh ginger in a cup of boiling water for about 10 minutes, strain, and sip the tea until it's gone.

muscle tears that occur during the day. It's essential to get at least 8 hours of sleep each night, says Dr. Teitelbaum, so set a reasonable sleep time and stick to it. Don't let late-night gatherings or classic movies on TV keep you up too late.

Consider 5-HTP. This amino acid, sold in health food stores, promotes the production of a feel-good brain chemical called serotonin, which helps promote good sleep. "Take 300 milligrams at night for 12 weeks," says Dr. Teitelbaum. "It will significantly improve pain and help you sleep." The supplement may interact with antidepressants and other drugs, he adds, so check with your doctor before trying 5-HTP, especially if you're taking any medications.

Soothe yourself to sleep. A lot of us get so wound up during the day that it's almost impossible to fall asleep. One thing that can help is to create a soothing nighttime ritual a few hours before going to bed. Turn the lights down. Turn off the TV and loud music. Light your favorite scented candles and make a conscious effort to wind down—by taking a long, relaxing bath, for example. If you do this every night, your body will get into the habit of unwinding as you prepare for sleep.

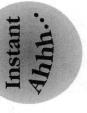

Get Your Signals Crossed

Here's a hot tip: Over-the-counter capsaicin creams contain the same spicy ingredient that's found in red pepper. When you apply the cream to your skin, it quickly blocks a chemical (substance P) that transmits fibromyalgia pain signals to your brain. The cream will sting a bit, so be careful to keep it away from your eyes or any areas of broken skin, and wash your hands thoroughly after using it.

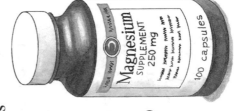

Dilute and doze. Over-the-counter sleep aids that contain the active ingredient diphenhydramine can be very helpful when you need extra sleep. The problem with these products is that they can leave you feeling hung-over the next day. To get the benefits without the problems, take a much lower dose than the amount listed on the label, says Milton Hammerly, M.D., medical director of complementary and alternative medicine at Centura Health in Denver and author of *Fibromyalgia: How to Combine the Best of Traditional and Alternative Therapies*. "Even a dose as low as 25 milligrams works for some people," he says.

Ice is nice and heat is neat. Both work for muscle pain flare-ups caused by fibromyalgia, but you'll have to experiment to decide which end of the thermometer works best for you. Apply either a heating pad set on low or a cold pack for about 20 minutes when your muscles are hurting. Take a break for a half-hour, then apply it again.

Sneak up on your workout. There's no question that regular exercise can reduce fibromyalgia flare-ups. Since exercising vigorously can make the pain worse, the trick is to warm up those muscles first, then exercise at a moderate pace. Walk slowly before jogging, for example, or swim slow laps before revving up the speed.

Mind your minerals. Two in particular, calcium and magnesium, are critical because they help ease muscle pain. As a bonus, taking these minerals at night can help you sleep. Check with your doctor to see how much will work for you. Some people report that taking 500 milligrams of calcium and 250 milligrams of magnesium an hour or two before going to bed is helpful. Magnesium may cause diarrhea in some people. If this occurs, reduce the dose.

Don't overdo the analgesics. Ibuprofen, aspirin, and other over-the-counter standbys for pain don't seem to help very much for fibromyalgia, says Dr. Teitelbaum. "Only about 10 percent of people with fibromyalgia benefit from them."

Pop some pulp pills. A supplement called MSM (methyl-sulfonylmethane), made from wood by-products, helps some people with fibromyalgia get through the day with less pain. Check with your doctor first, then start with 500 milligrams twice a day and gradually increase the dose to 1,000 to 2,000 milligrams twice daily, advises Dr. Hammerly. You should notice a difference within two weeks. If nothing happens within that time, the supplement probably won't work for you, he adds.

Favor fish. The oils found in cold-water fish help your body overcome painful inflammation. "Eat three servings of salmon, tuna, or sardines a week," says Dr. Teitelbaum. If you're not a fish eater, you can substitute fish oil or flaxseed oil, which contain the same beneficial oils. Follow the dosage directions on the label.

Get extra support. It's common for people with fibromyalgia to feel isolated and depressed because no one really understands what they're going through. Others who have the condition do understand, so getting together with people who are fighting the same battle is a great way to cope. To find a fibromyalgia support group in your area, visit the Arthritis Foundation Web site at www.arthritis.org.

Flu

Rally the Immunity Troops

I realize now just how hard my mom worked when my sister or I came down with the flu. Basically, it was her chance (which she would gladly have passed up) to roll up her sleeves and do some serious parenting.

Mom had a whole battery of procedures and products that she brought into play. Bed rest. Chicken broth. Tissues. Vicks. A humidifier. Lots of liquids. No sweets except sherbet to soothe our sore throats.

She certainly didn't mind using over-the-counter products to ease our aches and pains, but she knew that they didn't do all that much. I've since learned—and doctors agree—that Mom's anti-flu plan was about as good as it gets.

MUCH WORSE THAN A COLD

Flu is short for *influenza*, the name of the virus that causes the

A Cure to Cry Over

If flu has your nose stuffed to the rafters, harness the power of the humble onion. The same vapors that make cooks weep can help clear up your congestion, so start peeling and let them work their magic. Once you're breathing easier, chop the onion and toss some into a salad for lunch: Onions contain compounds that strengthen your immune system.

illness. Unlike viruses that cause the common cold, flu germs really hit with a vengeance.

Your symptoms may start with a mild cough, a headache, or a few sniffles, but it doesn't take long before you know that this is no ordinary cold. The flu virus can knock you right off your feet with fever, chills, aches, and a wracking cough, along with a sore throat and congestion.

Flu usually hits from late fall into the winter, although it can occur at any time of year. The virus is easily passed from one person to another, and it tends to last for a week or more.

FIGHT IT FROM WITHIN

If you're generally healthy, flu doesn't really require a trip to the doctor. The rules change, however, if you're over age 55 or you have an underlying health problem that could complicate your recovery.

Anyone with heart disease, immune-system problems, lung disease, or other serious health conditions should call their doctor at the first sign of symptoms. Even if you're in great shape, talk to your doctor if you don't start feeling better within about a week. It's not uncommon for a viral flu to lead to a secondary bacterial infection. You may need antibiotics in order to recover.

In the meantime, your best bet is to follow Mom's strategy: Get lots of rest and try to stay comfortable while your body takes care of the viral invader. Here are some super suggestions for reducing your discomfort and healing more quickly.

Know thy enemy. The earlier you start fighting back

Slick Soother

The herb slippery elm forms a slick coating that can soothe a sore throat faster than you can shout "Relief!" You can buy the powdered form at a health food store and make a slightly sticky tea by adding a teaspoon of the powder to a cup of hot water. Or take slippery elm lozenges, also sold at health food stores. Sucking on a lozenge will keep your throat coated and comfortable for hours.

against the flu, the more quickly you can recover from it. But in the early stages, it may be hard to distinguish flu from a cold. The key question to ask is, Where are my symptoms located? A cold is usually an above-the-neck affair, while the flu tends to involve your whole body with symptoms such as muscle aches or fever.

Stand the heat. Nobody enjoys having a fever, but that high temperature is doing you a favor. "An increase in temperature is one of the most potent defenses your body has against viruses," says Christian Dodge, N.D., a naturopathic physician and faculty member at Bastyr University near Seattle.

In other words, lowering fever with aspirin or other drugs may actually prolong your illness. Unless you're just too uncomfortable or the fever's very high (above 102°F), it's best to leave it alone.

Cool your skin. It won't affect the underlying fever, but applying a cold compress to your skin will make you feel a lot more comfortable. Soak a washcloth in cool water, wring it out, and put it on your forehead or neck. When it warms up, soak it again and repeat the process.

Take to the tub. If your whole body feels like it's burning up, soak in cool water to take the edge off the fever's fires.

Get cold feet. Put a pair of socks in the freezer until

A Cup of Comfort

Just about any herbal tea feels good when you have the flu. As long as you don't have high blood pressure, licorice tea is especially good because of its antiviral properties. Drink a cup or two a day until you feel better. Other good choices include chamomile and ginger. If you're using dried herbs, add a teaspoon of licorice or chamomile or a tablespoon of ginger to a cup of hot water, steep for 10 minutes, strain, and drink. Avoid chamomile if you are allergic to ragweed.

Garlic Is Great

As powerful as it is pungent, garlic is great for spurring your immune system to fight off a flu virus. Since raw garlic has the highest concentration of immune-boosting components, chop up a few cloves and toss them into your favorite hot soup. By the time the soup's cool enough to eat, the garlic will have softened and added its flavor to the meal.

---

they're good and cold. While they're chilling, take a long, warm bath, dry off, and bundle up in warm pajamas. Then put on the frozen socks.

"This draws a lot of circulation down to your feet, which can ease some of the inflammation in your upper respiratory tract and lungs," explains Dr. Dodge. The increased circulation also stimulates your immune system.

Since this treatment will make you sweat, keep clean pajamas next to the bed so you can change into them when you start feeling chilled. If you have circulation problems, heart disease, or other chronic health conditions, talk to your doctor before trying this remedy.

Be fluid. Lots of liquids are in order when you're battling the flu. When you're not adequately hydrated, your symptoms feel worse, and your immune system won't function as well as it should. Water is the best choice; try to drink at least eight glasses a day.

Eat light. Big, heavy meals aren't a good idea when you're sick, because your body will put more energy into digestion than into stomping the viral invaders. Nor do you want to go hungry, because your body needs nutrients in order to recover. A good compromise is to plan your menu around soups, vegetable juices, and other easy-to-digest foods.

Stop the sweets. I really appreciated the sherbet Mom gave me when I was sick, but it actually isn't such a good idea. It's best to keep sweet treats to a minimum because sugar reduces your immune system's ability to fight the infection.

Duck dairy. "Avoiding dairy foods is a good idea when you're sick," Dr. Dodge says. Milk, cheese, and other dairy products tend to make mucus thicker, which increases congestion and other symptoms.

Load up on vitamins. Some of the vitamins and minerals that you should be getting every day—including vitamins A, C, and E and the minerals zinc and selenium—are especially important when

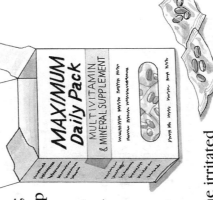

you're contending with the flu, because they strengthen your immune system.

You can't count on the amounts of vitamins in foods when you're sick; you need supplemental amounts. Drop by a drugstore and pick up a multivitamin/mineral supplement that provides 100 percent of the recommended daily amount of each of these important nutrients.

Steam away congestion. A mini-steam bath is a great way to open up your congested airways and soothe the irritated

---

Soothing Salves

MENTHOL MAGIC

Slathering a menthol rub over your chest is a traditional remedy for flu, and it seems to help with aches and pains as well as congestion, says Christian Dodge, N.D. "The active ingredient is eucalyptus, and it works very well." You can make your own herbal rub by adding 6 to 12 drops of oil of menthol, eucalyptus, or camphor (available at health food stores) to an ounce of olive or almond oil.

tissues. Just heat a pot of water on the stove, carefully move it to a table or counter, then lean over and inhale the steam. If you want, you can drape a towel around your head and shoulders to trap more of the steam.

To get even more relief, add a few drops of eucalyptus oil, available at health food stores, to the water. You'll benefit from the herb's germ-fighting properties.

Keep on resting. It's a prime requirement for defeating flu. Even once you start feeling better, ease back into your life slowly, suggests Dr. Dodge. "Doing this can help prevent a relapse," he says.

Get shot. If you're at high risk for getting the flu—you're elderly, work in a health care setting, or have chronic health problems—you should definitely get the flu vaccine annually, says Dr. Dodge.

The vaccine isn't 100 percent effective at preventing flu, but if you get the shot and practice good preventive measures—such as washing your hands frequently and supporting your immune system with a good diet—you'll dramatically improve your odds of getting through the flu season unscathed.

Instant Ahhh...

Pass the Salts

Flu is almost always accompanied by muscle aches and pains. A quick way to get relief is to soak in a bath spiked with Epsom salts. "They contain magnesium, which is good for relieving muscle tension," says Christian Dodge, N.D. Pour about a cup of the salts into the bathtub while the water's running.

Lyme Disease

Protection from Tick Infection

Lyme disease is simply a blood-borne infection, yet it's a bit more complicated than you might think. The basic facts are straightforward enough: A bite from a Lyme-infected tick fills your bloodstream with bacteria. You notice telltale symptoms and go to the doctor. You take antibiotics for a week or two. You're cured, and you get on with your life. At least, that's how it's supposed to go.

Sad to say, things are rarely that simple in real life. My friend John came down with Lyme disease, but almost nothing went the way it should have. First of all, he never knew he was bitten by a tick. He didn't have the classic bull's-eye rash that makes every doctor say "Aha, Lyme disease." When a sudden fever and intense leg pain prompt-

---

A Royal Treatment

To keep ticks from taking a liking to you, try tapping the power of pennyroyal. It's an herb that's a well-known flea and tick repellent. You can rub fresh leaves onto your skin and clothes, or put a few drops of pennyroyal oil (available at health food stores) on your shoes and socks. But don't get the oil on your skin—it's too strong for that!

---

ed him to make a Sunday afternoon trip to an urgent-care center, the physician did a blood test and said that he definitely did not have Lyme disease.

But John's a persistent guy, even when an infection has sapped almost all of his energy. When he still felt bad several days later, he insisted on a second blood test. Sure enough, it confirmed his suspicion that he had Lyme disease. He took antibiotics for a while, and fortunately, that was that.

SMALL BITE, BIG PROBLEM

If you're infected with Lyme disease, you'll probably have localized symptoms at first, such as pain and swelling at the site of the bite. As the infection spreads, you may experience more widespread symptoms, such as muscle and joint pain, fever, fatigue, and stiffness. Without prompt treatment, Lyme disease can cause arthritis-like aches and pains, along with muscle stiffness. Some people develop neurological problems, such as confusion and forgetfulness.

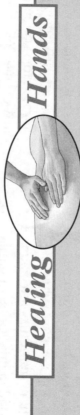

Healing Hands

One of the best home remedies for the aches and pains of Lyme disease is to thoroughly rub the affected areas. Better yet, have someone else do the massage for you. "Massaging painful muscle groups can help," says Sam Donta, M.D. Just be gentle, he adds. Your muscles and joints will be pretty sore, and an aggressive massage will hurt too much to enjoy.

To add an herbal soother to your rubdown, try St. John's wort, a traditional treatment for both nerve pain and muscle soreness. Buy some St. John's wort oil at a health food store and add 6 to 12 drops to an ounce of olive or almond oil, then rub it on.

But here's the tricky part. These lingering symptoms may occur soon after the bite, or they may take years to develop. And you may or may not experience localized pain.

That's why, if you're feeling achy and tired and you don't know why, you should ask yourself a few key questions, such as: Do you live an area inhabited by Lyme-causing ticks? Have you been spending a lot of time outdoors? Have you traipsed through grassy meadows (a favorite haunt of ticks)?

If you even suspect that you've been in tick territory, and you have some combination of Lyme symptoms—fatigue, fever, joint pain, and so on—don't take chances, says Sam Donta, M.D., an infectious disease specialist and professor of medicine at Boston University School of Medicine. Go to a doctor and request a Lyme test. It's the only way you'll know for sure what's happening.

THE ROAD TO RECOVERY

If you know you've been bitten by a tick and experience any symptoms at all, you have to see a doctor right away. The sooner you start treatment, the more likely you are to make a full recovery.

Once you've been diagnosed, the treatment almost always includes antibiotics, but sometimes that's not enough by itself. You'll also need to take steps to make yourself more comfortable while the drugs do their work. At the same time, you'll want to make sure you never get the disease again. Here's what you should do.

A Cup of Comfort

You may want to whip up some red clover tea if you're dealing with Lyme disease. The herb has been used traditionally as a blood purifier, for skin health, and for overall constitutional health. Steep 1/2 cup of fresh red clover flower heads in a quart of boiling water for 10 minutes, then strain. Let the tea cool, then sip it throughout the day.

Pick Off a Tick

It's easy enough to pull a feeding tick off your skin. With tweezers, grasp the head as close to your skin as possible and pull gently. The little bugger should pop right out.

Here's the good news: Ticks have to feed for about 24 hours to transmit Lyme bacteria. If you remove a tick within hours after it attaches, there's a good chance that you won't get infected.

If you do discover a tick merrily feeding away, don't panic! There's a good chance that it isn't even a deer tick, the kind that causes Lyme disease. Just remove the nasty little sucker, put it in a bottle, and ask your doctor to identify it.

That's what I did when I noticed a tick on my arm while I was on vacation. My doctor took one look and said it wasn't one of the species that causes Lyme disease. Boy, did I breathe a sigh of relief!

Don't drop everything. The pain and fatigue of Lyme disease can make it very hard to stay active; even walking across the room can seem like an insurmountable challenge. Don't give up. You have to do as much as your condition allows, says Dr. Donta. The more active you are, the more quickly you'll regain your energy. You'll even experience less pain.

Push yourself harder. Once you have some momentum going with your exercise, gradually increase the challenge. "Increase the activity week after week," Dr. Donta says. You don't have to push yourself to exhaustion. Just walk a little farther or stay on your feet a little longer. It will keep your muscles strong and make it easier to recover.

Get plenty of rest. You want your body to use as much of its energy as it can to fight the bacteria coursing through your blood. Do whatever you have to do to reduce the physical and emotional stress in your life.

This could mean taking a relaxing bath every day. It could mean taking naps, working fewer hours, or going to bed earlier at night. Your body has a big job ahead of it, and you want to make it easier for your natural resources to work in your favor.

Eye what you eat. Experts aren't sure why, but Lyme disease sometimes flares up when people eat certain foods. For example, coffee or sugar may cause a sudden increase in symptoms. The foods that can cause this vary widely, however, so there are no set rules about what you should or should not eat.

Dr. Donta advises keeping track of everything you eat, especially if you notice that you're feeling worse than you did before. The sooner you identify problem foods (if there are any), the sooner you can take steps to avoid them—at least until the infection is completely gone.

Heat up or cool down. Lyme is notorious for causing symptoms that wax and wane. You may feel fine one day and totally awful the next. When you're feeling achy or tired, you

Testing the Test

The blood tests for Lyme disease sometimes give false-negative results. In other words, they indicate that you're not infected, when you really are. You can increase your chances of getting a correct result by asking your doctor to perform a test called a Western Blot. It may catch Lyme disease infections that blood tests miss.

Keep in mind that tests won't reveal the presence of Lyme disease until you've been infected for about six weeks. That's why doctors sometimes go ahead and give antibiotics right away. Taking the drugs won't hurt if you don't have Lyme, but it can save you from a lot of trouble if it later turns out that you're infected.

may want to experiment with cold or heat treatments. Neither is best; different people respond in different ways.

For example, apply a cold pack or ice cubes wrapped in a small towel to an achy joint or muscle. Hold it in place for about 20 minutes, then repeat the treatment throughout the day. If that doesn't seem to help, use a heating pad set on low instead. Once you figure out which approach works for you, use it for soothing relief whenever symptoms are threatening to lay you low.

Avoid nutritional supplements. You may hear from friends or slick-looking advertisements that supplemental amounts of nutrients, especially B vitamins, are good for Lyme disease. Forget it, Dr. Donta says. For one thing, the bacterium that causes Lyme disease doesn't produce its own B vitamins; supplemental amounts could be just what it needs to keep going.

In fact, some scientists speculate that extra amounts of any nutrient could make Lyme disease worse, or at least increase recovery time. So until you're better, it's a good idea to stay away from supplements altogether.

Dress to protect. Preventing Lyme disease is the best way to spare yourself a world of hurt. When you're heading into tick territory, wear a hat, a long-sleeved shirt, and long pants. Use an insect repellent and thoroughly check your skin for ticks once you get home. In this case, an ounce of prevention is truly worth a pound of cure!

Muscle Cramp

Untie the Knots

I first met Dave, one of my lifelong friends, when we traded comic books in grade school. Since he's always been the more active of the two of us, I figured he'd be a good one to talk to about muscle cramps.

I expected him to tell me a story about how a cramp caused him to lose at a track meet, a karate competition, or something dramatic like that. Instead, he told me about what happened at a local pool. "I was swimming some easy laps one day, and my right leg totally locked up," he told me. "The pain was unbelievable, and I wasn't sure how I was going to get out of the water."

After a few seconds of panic, Dave regained his usual cool. He painfully made his way to the side of the pool and hoisted himself and his bum leg out of the water. The cramp went away after a few minutes, but the experience

---

It's an Emergency!

If you're taking cholesterol-lowering medication, report any muscle aches, pains, or cramps to your doctor immediately. They can indicate a rare life-threatening condition in which muscle—including heart muscle—is being destroyed as a side effect of your medication.

Pain Anywhere (And Sometimes Everywhere!)

stayed with him. "It was scary," he remembered. "The cramp came out of nowhere, and I still don't know what caused it—or what made it go away."

THE BIG SQUEEZE

Muscles don't contract and relax by themselves. They depend on electrical signals, which in turn are generated by electrolytes—minerals such as magnesium, calcium, and potassium. Your muscles work normally when levels of these minerals are properly balanced. If your body doesn't have the right mineral balance—because you're not getting enough of one or more electrolytes in your diet, your thyroid's out of whack, or the minerals have been depleted by hard exercise—the electrical signals to your muscles essentially get crossed. The result can be painful cramps.

LOOSEN UP

Muscle cramps rarely last more than a few seconds, but they're not something you want to put up with. For one thing, they're excruciatingly painful. More important, cramps that happen at the wrong time—when you're at the deep end of the pool, for example—can be dangerous. The next time you're clamped by a cramp, try one of these tips to get out of its grip.

Straighten up. A painful muscle cramp will eventually relax on its own, but the sooner you encourage it to do so, the sooner you'll get relief. Since the cramped muscle can't move

The Salad-Dressing Solution

Hot vinegar is great for relaxing cramped muscles. Mix equal parts of water and vinegar in a saucepan, heat until comfortably hot, and soak a small towel in the solution. Wring it out and hold it against the painful area for 5 minutes, then replace it with a towel that's been soaked in cold water. Repeat the cycle three times, keeping the hot towel in place for 5 minutes and the cold towel in place for 1 minute, always ending with the cold treatment. By the time you're done, the cramp should be gone, or at least feel a lot better.

itself, you'll need to use a free hand to straighten the affected leg, arm, or foot. Gently pull the muscle in the opposite direction of the cramp. Doing this a few times will usually relax the muscle.

Rub it out. Some firm finger-work will almost always ease a cramped muscle, says Ellen Potthoff, N.D., D.C., a naturopathic physician and chiropractor in Martinez, California. "During a cramp, muscle fibers stay contracted and forget how to relax," she explains. Massaging the cramped area will break up the contraction and loosen the muscle again.

Deposit some minerals. Your body needs healthful amounts of calcium and magnesium for proper

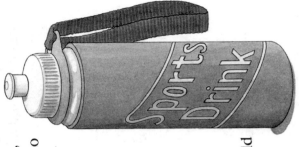

muscle function. If your stores of these electrolytes have been depleted by exercise or a poor diet, your muscles will become much more prone to cramping. You need between 500 and 800 milligrams of each mineral daily to prevent cramps. Your best bet is to take a daily multivitamin that contains these and other important minerals.

Slurp a sports drink. Drinks such as Gatorade contain minerals that your muscles need to function properly. If your cramps are caused by a lack of nutrients, a swig of an athletic beverage before and during exercise could prevent them from occurring (or recurring).

Instant Ahhh...

Stand Up for Yourself

The next time you get one of those awful foot or toe cramps in the middle of the night, relax: Relief is just a step away. All you have to do is stand up and put weight on your foot. This stretches the muscles and almost instantly stops the cramp.

Start with a stretch. Stretching your muscles before you exercise is essential if you want to prevent cramping. It's especially important to stretch if you haven't been active for a while.

Be well watered. Muscles that aren't properly hydrated are more prone to cramping. "People should drink at least six to eight glasses of water a day, more if they're going to be sweating heavily," says Dr. Potthoff. Don't wait until you're thirsty to drink, though; by the time you feel thirsty, you may already be dehydrated.

Reconsider your position. Some cramps happen because a muscle group becomes fatigued after being in the same position for long periods of time. If you can schedule your day so that you can break up long tasks with shorter ones, your muscles will appreciate the chance to switch gears. Get up from your desk a few times an hour. Rake leaves as a break from working on your knees in the garden. The more frequently you change position, the less likely you are to have cramps.

Roll away the pain. Here's a great way to instantly stop foot cramps that seem to come out of nowhere: Roll a golf ball across the floor under the bottom of your bare foot. Doing this for 30 to 60 seconds will almost always ease painful cramps.

Greens for Relief

The greener your midnight snack, the less likely you are to be rudely awakened by middle-of-the-night cramps. Leafy green vegetables, such as spinach, okra, and turnip and beet greens, are chock-full of cramp-stopping electrolytes—especially magnesium, potassium, and calcium. A daily salad or stir-fry that includes these ingredients should keep cramps at bay. (I like to use spinach leaves in place of lettuce in sandwiches and burgers.)

Muscle Soreness

Muscle Away the Pain

I was a cross-country runner in high school, and even though I loved the exhilaration of running, I always dreaded the first day of practice. Honestly, it was murder! I had to push my poor, out-of-shape muscles through stretches, calisthenics, sprints, hill runs, and LSD (long, slow distance) under a merciless August sun.

Actually, the toughest part was the day after practice. I'd wake up feeling as if my leg muscles had been replaced by wet cement—cement that was quickly drying. I'd haul myself out of bed and walk around as stiff-legged as Frankenstein. If I happened to drop a quarter during the day, well, it just had to lie there until I was able to bend down and pick it up.

ALL TORN UP

We've all had the experience of waking up sore after a day of exertion. Soreness means that you've pushed your muscles further than they were prepared to go, causing microscopic tears in the muscle fibers. Buildups of a chemical called lactic acid, a natural by-product of muscular exertion, also contribute to the overall ache.

Muscles have a tremendous capacity to repair themselves, however. In fact, they'll get a little bit stronger in anticipation of your next bout of hard work. In the meantime, of course, they'll hurt like the dickens!

DON'T BE A SORE LOSER

My solution for sore muscles was to lie around the house as long as possible, waiting for the pain to go away. Boy, was I ever wrong! Every doctor I talked to told me that's the worst way to coax muscles back to health. As you'll see, getting off the couch is an important step on the road to recovery.

Start with ice. As soon as muscle pain starts and for 24 to 48 hours afterward, put ice to work. Wrap some ice cubes in a washcloth or small towel, then put the cold right where it hurts for about 20 minutes. Cold numbs muscle pain and inhibits blood flow that can cause inflammation, says Ellen

---

Healing	Hands

Sure, it feels good, but massage does more than make you close your eyes in dreamy relaxation. It also stimulates blood flow, which can push pain-causing lactic acid out of your muscles and bring in healing nutrients. Whether you do it yourself or have someone else do it, it's best to use gentle pressure, always stroking toward the center of your body. (For example, you'd rub a sore upper arm by pushing up toward the shoulder, not down toward the elbow.)

To make massage even more soothing, use a little herbal oil. Add six to eight drops of St. John's wort, comfrey, or arnica oil (available in health food stores) to an ounce of olive or almond oil, then rub the mixture wherever you hurt.

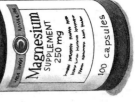

Potthoff, N.D., D.C., a naturopathic physician and chiropractor in Martinez, California.

Follow up with heat. A day or two after applying cold, switch to heat. It opens blood vessels and improves circulation, which helps remove pain-causing lactic acid from your muscles. Apply a heating pad set on low to the sore area and keep it in place for about 20 minutes.

Make the right moves. Sometimes, a sore muscle feels as if it never wants to move again—but gently stretching and moving it will speed recovery and keep it from getting tight, says Dr. Potthoff.

Try to move the affected muscle through its normal range of motion, stretching it slowly and carefully. This may mean flexing and extending your arm, arching your back, or taking a slow walk to stretch your legs. It's good if you feel the muscle pulling and stretching, but the pain shouldn't get worse. If it does, take it easy for a day before trying to stretch the muscle again.

Load up on minerals. Calcium and magnesium are critical for proper muscle function. To help your aching muscles recover, make sure that your body's stores of these nutrients are filled

---

Soothing Salves

EASE ACHES WITH ARNICA

A great way to take the kinks out of sore muscles is to apply arnica cream, which relaxes muscles and helps them recover more quickly. You can also make your own muscle soother. Chop or crumble fresh or dried arnica, add enough water to make a paste, and spread the mixture over the sore spot. Wrap the area loosely with gauze and keep it covered for about 20 minutes. You can buy arnica cream or the herb itself at health food stores.

to the brim. You can take 500 to 800 milligrams of each mineral daily while your muscles are on the mend, says Dr. Potthoff. Magnesium may cause diarrhea in some people. If this occurs, reduce the dose.

Ease it with E. Want to stop muscle pain before it starts? Take vitamin E before you exercise. This powerful antioxidant can offset muscle damage caused by exertion. About 400 IU will do the trick.

Go with the flow. When your body isn't well hydrated, muscle aches feel worse. Filling your water tanks helps your body get rid of toxins that contribute to muscle pain. When you're exercising or working hard, keep a bottle of water or sports drink nearby and take frequent sips.

Apply cream heat. Drugstores stock a number of creams and ointments designed to ease muscle soreness. Products such as Ben Gay and Icy Hot stimulate nerve endings on the surface of your skin, which makes it harder for "ouch" signals to reach your brain.

Warm up, then cool down. You're much less likely to get sore muscles if you ease them into exercise and bring them to a gradual stop when you're done. "If you're exercising for 30 minutes, you should spend at least 5 minutes warming up and 5 minutes cooling down," says Dr. Potthoff.

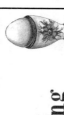

No Salt, No Swelling

Forget the chips, pretzels, and other salty foods when you're coping with muscle pain. Salt makes your body retain water, which can increase painful swelling inside your muscles. If you need a quick snack, fill up on grapes, orange slices, other fruits, or vegetables, which are naturally low in salt. They also contain a lot of water, which will help sore muscles stay hydrated and heal more quickly.

Post-Amputation Pain

Smoothing Out the Road Ahead

I asked Douglas G. Smith, M.D., associate professor of orthopedic surgery at the University of Washington in Seattle, how people usually cope with losing a limb. What's the secret that enables them to keep going after an experience that's so physically and mentally painful? He told me a story that really opened my eyes.

"One of my patients was a high school boy who had lost his leg in a farming accident," Dr. Smith said. On one occasion, the doctor had just left the room and was standing in the hall when one of the boy's friends arrived—a friend who had lost a leg the previous year. Dr. Smith overheard some of their conversation—things like "What do your buddies say?" and "Can you get a date?"

Dr. Smith laughed as he related their conversation. "He never would have asked me those questions, but they were the first things on his mind."

It makes sense. After all, what else would a teenage boy be

thinking about? That was when I realized that I'd been thinking the wrong way about amputation. It's not the lost limb that's so important; what really matters is the person who's still here.

PAIN AND LOSS

Pain is an inevitable consequence of any surgery, and amputation—whether it's the result of an accident or a disease like diabetes—is no exception. People who have lost a limb usually experience two kinds of pain in the weeks and months after the operation.

The first is phantom pain, in which the sensation of pain seems to come from the amputated limb. Doctors still don't know what causes it, but it affects nearly everyone who has undergone amputation. The pain is usually worst during the first year after surgery, then it gradually tapers off.

The second type is residual pain, which is simply pain in the remaining part of the limb. It's a normal part of the healing process, and it goes away when the healing is complete.

GETTING AHEAD OF PAIN

If you're recovering from amputation surgery, your doctor has probably already told you what to expect as you recuper-

---

Soothing Salves

HOT STUFF HELPS

The next time you experience residual pain, apply a little capsaicin cream, available in drugstores. It's made with the chemical compound that makes red pepper hot, so it heats and slightly irritates the area, blocking the transmission of pain signals.

Don't use capsaicin on the part of your limb that's covered by the prosthesis, however. You need air circulation to keep the cream from causing too much irritation. If you've never used capsaicin before, try a low strength; it comes in concentrations ranging from 0.025 to 0.075 percent.

ate. In addition, you may want to get in touch with the Amputee Coalition of America (www.amputee-coalition.org), a nonprofit organization that's a great resource for amputees and their families.

Amputation is a traumatic experience, physically as well as emotionally. While it's impossible to address in just a few pages all of the difficulties you're likely to experience, we've collected some very practical advice that will hopefully make things just a little easier.

Don't blame your head. People tend to blame their imaginations for phantom pain. Some even keep the pain a secret from family, friends, and even their doctors because they don't want to give the impression that they have psychological problems. Don't make that mistake, says Dr. Smith.

"Phantom pain is real," he says. "It's been described by patients for centuries, and today we think that it has something to do with the nerves that are left after the surgery and with the associated part of the brain."

Healing Hands

Massage is an important tool after an amputation, whether you're having phantom pain or residual limb pain, says Douglas G. Smith, M.D. Massaging the area improves circulation, reduces discomfort, and helps promote faster healing.

To add the healing properties of herbal oils, look for of St. John's wort oil (for soothing pain) or calendula oil (for healing damaged skin and preventing infection) wherever herbal products are sold. Add 6 to 12 drops of either herbal oil to an ounce of olive, almond, or sunflower oil, then use the mixture whenever you need a soothing rub.

His advice: Tell your doctor immediately if you're experiencing phantom pain. There are a number of treatments—including massage, biofeedback, and a variety of drugs—that will go a long way toward reducing the discomfort.

Use your prosthesis. Wearing an artificial limb is often the most effective way to cope with phantom pain. "Wearing a prosthesis can lessen the severity or frequency," Dr. Smith says.

Compress to fight distress. Most people who have had amputation surgery find that both phantom pain and pain in the remaining part of the limb are greatest in the first few months after surgery. That's when your body is healing and when you're making the biggest adjustments in your lifestyle.

One way to get through these difficult months is to wear a compressive wrap, or "shrinker sock," on the residual limb. Available from your doctor and some drugstores, compression wraps often reduce swelling and throbbing as well as pain.

Apply heat. When pain flares, apply a heating pad set on low to the affected area. Heat relaxes the muscles and makes the discomfort easier to bear.

Or ice it down. As with heat, applying cold is a quick way to take the edge off pain. When you're hurting, apply a cold pack or ice cubes wrapped in a small towel or a washcloth to the affected area. Keep the cold in place for 20 minutes

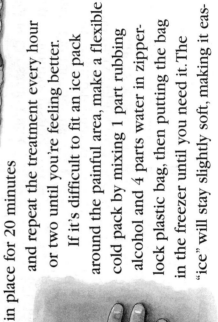

and repeat the treatment every hour or two until you're feeling better.

If it's difficult to fit an ice pack around the painful area, make a flexible cold pack by mixing 1 part rubbing alcohol and 4 parts water in zipperlock plastic bag, then putting the bag in the freezer until you need it. The "ice" will stay slightly soft, making it easier to mold around the area that hurts.

Use your imagination. A technique called visualization can be very effective for reducing phantom pain. At the simplest level, visualization may involve closing your eyes and mentally picturing the missing limb as still in place and moving. Doctors aren't sure why it helps, but people who practice this technique report that it can make a real difference.

Regular exercise is a must. It's a natural antidote for depression, it promotes healing by ensuring good blood flow to the residual limb, and it burns off any extra calories that you may be taking in.

Ask your doctor to help you set up an exercise program that will work for your particular situation, then do your best to stay active each and every day.

Make it a group effort. There are few experiences as devastating as amputation. "The response to losing part of your body is really tough," says Dr. Smith. Many people get so depressed that they withdraw from the world and even from the people closest to them.

Don't let this happen to you. Join a support group; it's one of the best ways to stay active and socially involved. "It's also a way to get questions answered, meet other folks who are working through the same problems, and talk about things that you're uncomfort-

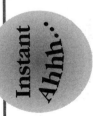

Instant Ahhh...

Keep the Muscles Moving

A fast way to stop pain in a residual limb is to exercise the area, says Douglas G. Smith, M.D. In fact, doing this regularly can help keep pain from getting started.

Suppose you're experiencing pain after a leg amputation. You might curl the toes of your remaining foot downward while imagining that you're doing the same thing on the side with the missing leg. "It gets the muscles that are still in the residual limb to contract and relax appropriately," Dr. Smith explains.

able discussing with family and friends," Dr. Smith says. The Amputee Coalition of America can put you in touch with a support group in your area.

Distract yourself. "Pain thrives on attention," says Dr. Smith. Whatever you can do to keep your mind busy—watching a video, working crossword puzzles, or phoning a friend, for example—will help make the pain a little less intense.

Keep it clean. Even after the surgical wound heals, the residual limb will be vulnerable to infection because it spends so much time cooped up inside the socket of a prosthesis. Be sure to wash the area daily with mild soap and water.

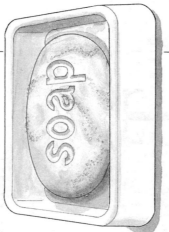

Watch for signs of infection, especially when the wound is still healing. Common signs include redness, swelling, pus, or an increase in pain. If you even suspect that an infection may be brewing, call your doctor right away.

Get a good fit. If your prosthesis doesn't fit the way it should, you may develop blisters, ulcers, or an infection. Don't put up with a prosthesis that's either too tight or too loose. Have it adjusted right away so that it's completely comfortable.

Postoperative Pain

After-Surgery Strategies

The other night, I asked two friends about their post-surgical experiences. Their situations were totally different. One is a competitive athlete who's always in great shape and had never been in a hospital until he had knee surgery in his thirties. The other had had several operations as a child and some follow-up procedures a few decades later.

Much to my surprise, they both agreed on two major points. First, one of the hardest things about recovering is wanting to be up and doing things before you're ready. Second, when you're stuck in a hospital room, it's people who make all the difference in the world.

As one friend said, "You want people to come and spend time with you. But you don't want them to be always asking about your operation or telling you what to do to get better. You want them to distract you, play a board game with you, or make you laugh."

Pain Anywhere (And Sometimes Everywhere!)

DOWN FOR REPAIRS

Most surgical procedures will leave you with some kind of pain during the recovery period. Different types of procedures produce different patterns of pain, and even two people who have had the same operation report different experiences.

Although pain after surgery is normal, most hospitals treat it aggressively. Controlling pain gets you back on your feet sooner and with fewer complications.

GOOD AS NEW

Don't hesitate to use the pain medications your health care team provides. Stopping pain quickly is the best way to ensure that it doesn't get any worse. Also, be sure to tell your doctor or nurse if the pain gets worse or the medicine doesn't seem to be working. They have a lot of different options in those little black bags, and there's no reason to suffer needlessly.

I spoke to a lot of experts about the things people could do themselves to keep their postoperative pain to a minimum. Obviously, each situation is different, and you'll want to check with your doctor before you try any of these approaches on your own. Nevertheless, there's a good chance that the following strategies will help you feel a lot more comfortable.

Soothing Salves

OIL AWAY SCARS

Once you've had your stitches removed, apply a thin layer of vitamin E oil to the area once or twice a day. "It can help reduce scarring," says Cristopher Bosted, N.D.

Cocoa butter and creams containing calendula, available at health food stores, also promote skin healing, he adds—or you can make a calendula poultice. Get some dried herb at a health food store, chop it, and add enough water to make a paste. Once or twice a day, apply it to the damaged skin for at least 20 minutes at a time.

Keep it up. As with any trauma to the body, surgery often results in swelling and inflammation. One simple inflammation-fighting strategy is to keep the affected body part elevated, which allows fluids to drain from the site of the surgery.

Whether this is possible, of course, depends on the type of surgery you've had. Ask your doctor if elevating that part of your body is likely to make a difference.

Ice is nice. You'll probably have medication to help control post-surgical pain, and that's a good thing. You'll get even more pain relief by using a cold pack, says Cristopher Bosted, N.D., a naturopathic physician and faculty member at Bastyr University near Seattle. "It generally helps to ice the post-surgical area during the first 24 to 72 hours," he says.

Keep the ice in place for no more than 20 minutes out of every hour. After three days or so, if there's no sign of swelling, you can use a heating pad set on low or a warm compress when pain is bothersome. Check with your doctor before using cold or heat treatments, though.

Take some bromelain. Your body will be quite busy

A Cup of Comfort

Chicken soup has a little bit of everything you need when you're on the mend after surgery, says Cristopher Bosted, N.D. "It has lots of vegetables in it, and some protein, and you can put in garlic and onions, which are helpful for healing and immunity," he says. If you're lucky enough to know someone who makes fresh chicken soup—or you can make it yourself—freeze several serving-size batches before your surgery, then thaw some every day to enjoy.

cleaning up the cellular debris and waste products created by the trauma of surgery. You can aid the cleanup by taking bromelain, an enzyme extracted from pineapple.

"It helps break up inflammation as well as any scar tissue that may be forming," Dr. Bosted says. Bromelain is available in drugstores and health food stores. Follow the directions on the label; a typical dose is three to nine capsules taken throughout the day. Don't take bromelain with food, though, as your digestive juices will make the enzyme ineffective.

Spice up your recovery. Did you know that turmeric is a healthful remedy as well as a tasty seasoning? Like bromelain, it helps your body clear away toxins that contribute to inflammation. Use it liberally in chicken and rice dishes.

Arnicate and recuperate. Anyone who knows about homeopathic remedies is quick to sing the praises of arnica. "It's a great remedy that's used specifically for trauma," says Dr. Bosted. "It can help people come out of anesthesia so they're not as groggy, and it decreases swelling and pain." He advises taking a 30C dose two or three times daily for a week or two after the surgery. It's available at health food stores.

Protein power. "You want to get enough protein in your diet for tissue healing and building," says Dr. Bosted. The exact amount you need depends on your weight and sex, so your doctor can advise you how much you should eat.

"Generally, 45 grams a day is a low to middle amount for a woman, and 60 grams a day is a low to middle amount for a man," Dr. Bosted says. Check food labels to see how much protein they provide. Typically, a few servings of protein-rich foods, such as fish, chicken, or peanut butter, will give you most of the protein you need.

Make a meal plan. Your doctor will probably recommend a specific diet that you should follow after the procedure. Get all the details in writing, then follow the diet to the letter.

"You might be on thin, clear liquids for a few days before moving on to thicker foods such as yogurt or Cream of Wheat," says Dr. Bosted.

Once you're ready for solid food, plan on eating plenty of fruit, vegetables, and whole grains. Not only are these healthful foods in general, but they're also recommended for preventing constipation, a common side effect of surgery.

Sink the sweets. If well-meaning visitors bring you candy while you're convalescing, thank them politely and offer them a piece. When they've left, hide the candy under your bed. Sugar shouldn't be on the menu when you're recovering from surgery.

You want to protect yourself from infections that may take hold while you're in a weakened state. Sugar, unfortunately, suppresses your immune system and could feed any bacteria that get past your defenses.

Invest in vitamins. Taking vitamin and mineral supplements will ensure that your body's repair systems are working at peak efficiency. A daily multivitamin is a good place to start—preferably before you even go to the operating room.

Restock your gut. A common side effect of surgery is the loss of beneficial types of bacteria that live in your digestive system. "Anesthesia kills them, and the antibiotics that people often take after surgery can also kill them," says Dr. Bosted.

Protect yourself by taking supplements that contain *Lactobacillus acidophilus* (avail-

MAXIMUM
Daily Pack

MULTIVITAMIN
& MINERAL SUPPLEMENT

able at health food stores), following the directions on the label. You can also get beneficial bacteria by eating a daily serving or two of live-culture yogurt.

Move it or lose it. You may not feel like being up and about, especially during your first days of recovery, and it's true that resting is a critical part of getting well. But it's also important to move around to the extent that you're able, says Dr. Bosted.

"The trend in hospitals these days is to get patients up and walking as soon as possible," he says. "Otherwise, your muscles atrophy, and you get weaker and weaker."

Your doctor can advise you on how much exercise, or simple movements, your situation will allow. A key point is to try to improve whatever capacity you already have.

"Just sitting up two or three times a day could be enough, if that's all you can do," says Dr. Bosted. "Then try to build on that, doing a little more every day."

Take a salty soak. Muscles that are tight and achy from spending so much time in bed will feel better after a bath with Epsom salts. Just add a cup of salts to your bath water and step in for a relaxing soak.

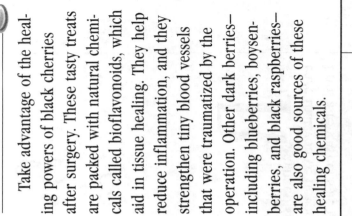

Cherry Power

Take advantage of the healing powers of black cherries after surgery. These tasty treats are packed with natural chemicals called bioflavonoids, which aid in tissue healing. They help reduce inflammation, and they strengthen tiny blood vessels that were traumatized by the operation. Other dark berries—including blueberries, boysenberries, and black raspberries—are also good sources of these healing chemicals.

Raynaud's Syndrome

Get the Blood Flowing

Raynaud's syndrome may be the most common disease that you've never heard of. I certainly hadn't heard of it until a few weeks ago, and I was surprised to learn that about 1 in 10 people have it to some degree. I was even more surprised to learn just how strange it really is.

People with Raynaud's have occasional attacks in which their hands or feet get cold, then begin changing colors—everything from white and blue to red. After a while, their hands get numb, then throb with pain.

Personally, I'd find these symptoms disturbing, if not downright frightening. But then I spoke to Magdalena Dziadzio, M.D., a faculty member in the department of internal medicine

Sweet Success

If you've got a sweet tooth, you're in luck. Two of the sweetest fruits, strawberries and papaya, are full of vein-strengthening vitamin C, which is helpful if you have Raynaud's. Once a day, slice up a cup of each and make a tasty fruit salad.

at the University of Ancona, Italy, and chair of the medical advisory committee for the International Scleroderma Network (scleroderma is a skin condition that sometimes causes Raynaud's). She told me that most people learn to anticipate the symptoms and take the necessary steps to relieve them.

"Most cases are mild," she says. "And there's much that can be done without the need for drugs."

THE COLD WAR

The most important parts of your body—namely, your brain, heart, lungs, liver, and other organs—are located in your head and chest. Your body is pretty efficient at protecting them. Part of this protection means keeping your core body temperature at the recommended 98.6°F.

Suppose that you step outside into a howling blizzard. Your body will detect the frigid temperatures, then take steps to ensure that your brain and trunk stay at the optimal temperature. It does this in part by narrowing blood vessels in your hands, arms, feet, and legs. Restricting blood flow to these areas ensures that more heat stays in your deeper tissues and organs.

In people with Raynaud's, however, this normal response is exaggerated, and so much circulation is rerouted to the trunk that very little blood reaches the hands or feet. This is what causes the numbness, color changes, and other symptoms.

Normal blood flow usually resumes within a few seconds or minutes, although some people may experience the effects for hours. When circulation resumes, there may be a tingling sensa-

Drink in Total Comfort

Cold beverage containers are a Raynaud's attack waiting to happen. To protect your hands, slip a cold can of soft drink into an insulating foam container, or sip your soda through a straw. That way, you can enjoy your drink without touching the cold can or bottle.

tion or perhaps throbbing pain. Attacks can be triggered by a cold day in February or even reaching into the freezer for ice cubes.

RESTORING WARMTH

You always need to see a doctor if you have Raynaud's symptoms. For one thing, the disease is sometimes triggered by other conditions, such as scleroderma, lupus, or other forms of arthritis. Even if your doctor can't pinpoint a cause—and in most cases, there isn't a known cause—you'll get plenty of good advice for preventing and stopping attacks.

In some cases, your doctor may prescribe medication to control the symptoms. More often, you'll learn about the many different ways to maintain normal circulation throughout your body, including your vulnerable hands and feet. Here are some of the best tips for keeping blood flowing.

Give your hands a hand. Avoiding extreme cold is the best way to prevent attacks. One useful strategy is to wear battery-heated gloves and socks, available in sporting goods stores, whenever you're going to be spending time in cold weather. "A belt-worn rechargeable battery pack can keep them powered for up to 3 hours," says Dr. Dziadzio. Those chemical hand

A Cup of Comfort

The herb ginkgo has traditionally been used for all sorts of circulatory problems, and there's some evidence that it may help if you have Raynaud's, says Magdalena Dziadzio, M.D. Add a teaspoon of dried ginkgo (available at health food stores) to a cup of freshly boiled water, steep for about 10 minutes, then strain and drink. If you take anticoagulant (blood-thinning) medications, talk to your doctor before using ginkgo.

warmers used by hunters, campers, and other outdoor enthusiasts are also good gadgets for people with Raynaud's. When you squeeze them, they release chemicals that fire up instant, hand-warming heat.

Use kitchen mittens. Keep a pair of warm mittens or insulated oven mitts hanging in a handy spot in your kitchen. You can use them to take cold items out of the refrigerator or freezer. Some people even use them when they handle frozen foods at the supermarket.

Avoid caffeine. The caffeine in coffee, tea, and some soft drinks causes blood vessels to constrict, which reduces crucial blood flow. You don't necessarily have to give up your favorite beverages, but you'll certainly want to limit yourself to one or two servings daily.

Save your soles. Don't neglect your feet when shopping for anti-cold clothing. "Shoes with padded soles will keep your feet warm and relieve pressure on your toes," says Dr. Dziadzio. "Pressure can also trigger the symptoms."

Wear easy-on, easy-off outerwear. Avoid coats, gloves, boots, and other kinds of outdoor clothing that have lots of snaps, zippers, or other fasteners. You'll find it almost impossible to get them off when your hands are cold. Try on outerwear in the store and be sure you can slip it over your head, or off your hands or feet, without having to fumble with hard-to-grip fasteners.

Bundle up all over. To prevent Raynaud's flare-ups, you have to keep your whole body warm, not just your hands and feet. Wear whatever you need to keep nice and toasty, from thermal underwear and tights to long coats, scarves, and earmuffs. The advantage of dressing in layers is that you'll find it easier to adjust your levels of insulation—and comfort—as the temperature changes.

Watch the weather. People with Raynaud's should always consider the local weather forecast when making daily plans. This is especially important in the early spring or fall, when temperatures can change dramatically. And don't take any chances on frigid days. If the weather is really cold, wet, or windy, stay inside in order to keep your hands and feet warm and symptom-free.

Be careful what you touch. When your hands are particularly cold or numb, you may have problems telling if a surface is hot or cold, or you may find it difficult to grip things securely. Think twice about what you're doing when symptoms strike, taking extra care to avoid accidents.

Oil your circulation. Evening primrose oil and fish oil, available

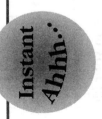

Instant Ahhh...

Wiggle and Warm

The quickest way to stop a Raynaud's attack is to warm up your hands and feet. Doctors recommend a five-step plan—and each of the steps starts with the letter W, which makes them easy to remember.

• Wiggle your toes or fingers to restore normal circulation.

• Windmills, in which you rotate your arms in large circles, will also boost circulation.

• Warm water is a great way to unchill your hands and feet instantly. Fill the sink or a basin with water, but don't make it too hot, because that can actually prolong an attack. Soak your hands or feet for about 5 minutes, or until they're feeling better.

• Warm pits (a way of referring to your armpits) are a handy source of heat. When your hands suddenly turn cold or numb, tuck them into your armpits and keep them there until circulation returns.

• Warmers, such as heated gloves or socks, will often stop a Raynaud's attack before it really gets under way.

in capsules at health food stores, appear to encourage vasodilation, the ability of blood vessels to expand and carry more blood, says Dr. Dziadzio. People with Raynaud's sometimes notice an improvement in their symptoms when they take the capsules daily, following the directions on the label.

Get extra nutrients. Vitamins C and E help reduce the harmful effects of free radicals, harmful oxygen molecules in the blood that may play a role in triggering Raynaud's, says Dr. Dziadzio. She recommends taking 100 to 400 IU of vitamin E and, if you don't have any stomach or kidney problems, 500 to 1,000 milligrams of vitamin C daily.

Beware of bad vibes. Sometimes, vibration can trigger an attack of Raynaud's. Causes of vibration may include using power tools, vigorous typing, or even working in the yard with a shovel or rake. Try to insulate yourself from vibration as much as possible by taking frequent breaks, for example, or using tools with thick foam handles.

Butts out. You shouldn't be smoking anyway, but here's one more reason to quit: Cigarettes impair circulation and can make Raynaud's much worse. "Stopping cigarette smoking can produce immediate benefits," says Dr. Dziadzio.

Review medications with your doctor. A number of medications, including a class of drugs called beta-blockers, sometimes aggravate Raynaud's symptoms. Make a list of all your medications and review it with your doctor. In some cases, just changing drugs will bring dramatic improvement in your symptoms.

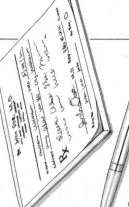

Index

Cluster headaches, 18–21
Coenzyme Q$_{10}$, 29, 45–46, 391
Cold air, trigeminal neuralgia and, 105–6
Cold compresses. *See* Ice packs and cold compresses
Cold sores, 22–25
Coleus, 54
Comfrey, for treating
  black eyes, 4
  burns, 365
  bursitis and tendinitis, 424
  dry skin, 376
  foot pain, 281, 283, 300
  muscle soreness, 457
  smashed fingers, 131
  splinters, 410
  sprains or strains, 278
  varicose veins, 337
Compression stockings, 278–79, 338
Compression wraps, 425, 463. *See also* RICE
Computer ergonomics, eye pain and, 41
Constipation
  as cause of hemorrhoids, 250–51
  as drug side effect, 192, 241
  effect on breast pain, 152–53
  treating, 188–92
Contrast hydrotherapy, for treating
  back pain, 172–73
  bruises, 358–59
  bursitis and tendinitis, 425–26
  carpal tunnel, 116
  eye injuries, 5, 58
  foot soreness, 299
  ingrown hairs, 391
  menstrual pain, 221
  penis and testicle pain, 261
  pressure ulcers, 397
  restless legs syndrome, 324
  shingles, 405
  sore throat, 79
  varicose veins, 340
Copper, 77
Coriander, 229–30
Corns, 294–96
Cornsilk tea, 215
Cornstarch, for chafing, 368

Cosmetics, reactions to, 17, 382, 401
Coughs, 154–58, 167–68
Cramp bark, 87, 255, 293
Cranberry juice, for UTIs, 267
Cumin, 229–30
Curcumin. *See* Turmeric
Cuts, 371–74

D

Dairy products, avoiding, 36, 168, 206, 230, 444
Dandelion greens, 152, 191, 201, 227
Dehydration. *See* Hydration
Dental visits, trigeminal neuralgia and, 105
Denture pain, 26–29
Detergents, as cause of folliculitis, 383
Diarrhea, 193–97
Diet and eating habits. *See also specific foods*
  as cause of
    anal itching, 241
    rashes, 400
  effect on
    breast pain, 151–53
    gallstones, 199–202
    gas, 204, 205
    Lyme disease, 450
    restless legs syndrome, 324–25
  for preventing
    chapped lips, 14
    diarrhea, 197
    headaches, 54–55, 77
    heartburn, 162–63
    menstrual pain, 219, 221
    muscle cramps, 455
    stomachaches, 228
    yeast infections, 271–72
  for treating
    anal pain, 239–40
    angina, 146–48
    back pain, 174
    cancer pain, 431, 433
    constipation, 190–91
    earaches, 36
    flu, 443–44
    hangover headaches, 48, 49–50

heartburn, 163
IBS, 210–11
intermittent claudication, 313–16
postoperative pain, 469–70
shingles, 404
sore throat, 81, 82
sunburn, 411
tooth and mouth pain, 11, 12, 25, 27–28, 71–72, 93
Digestion, 191, 205, 227
Disk pain, 170–74
Doulas, for childbirth, 246–47
Drugs, side effects of
  burning tongue syndrome, 8, 9
  constipation, 192, 241
  gallstones, 202
  gas, 207
  headaches, 21
  muscle cramps, 452
  Raynaud's syndrome, 477
  yeast infections, 271
Dry mouth, 98
Dry skin, 375–79

E

Earaches, 30–36
Ear piercing, pain following, 65–68
Eating habits. *See* Diet and eating habits
Echinacea, for treating
  folliculitis, 381
  headaches, 77
  pierced-ear pain, 67
  pneumonia, 167
  shingles, 404
  sore throat, 81
  splinters, 410
  UTIs, 265, 267
  yeast infections, 270
Elderberry, 77
Electrolyte balance, 50, 197, 454
Elevation. *See also* RICE
  for treating
    burns, 364
    bursitis and tendinitis, 425
    calf pain, 287–88
    foot pain, 302, 333
    frostbite, 386–87